Biomedical Imaging and Sensing: Clinical Applications

Biomedical Imaging and Sensing: Clinical Applications

Editor: Ricky Collier

AMERICAN
MEDICAL PUBLISHERS
www.americanmedicalpublishers.com

AMERICAN
MEDICAL PUBLISHERS
www.americanmedicalpublishers.com

Cataloging-in-Publication Data

Biomedical imaging and sensing : clinical applications / edited by Ricky Collier.
p. cm.
Includes bibliographical references and index.
ISBN 978-1-63927-602-8
1. Diagnostic imaging. 2. Biosensors. 3. Imaging systems in medicine. I. Collier, Ricky.
RC78.7.D53 B56 2023
616.075 4--dc23

American Medical Publishers,
41 Flatbush Avenue,
1st Floor, New York,
NY 11217, USA

ISBN 978-1-63927-602-8 (Hardback)

Contents

Preface

This book was inspired by the evolution of our times; to answer the curiosity of inquisitive minds. Many developments have occurred across the globe in the recent past which has transformed the progress in the field.

Biomedical sensing and imaging are technologies that are helpful in acquiring and processing biomedical information, significant for timely detection, quick diagnosis and accurate treatment of the diseases. Biomedical sensors are electronic devices, which transform the biomedical signals into electric signals that can be measured easily. They are a significant component in different medical diagnostic equipment and instruments. Generally used biomedical sensing technologies like invasive ultrasound, electrocardiogram and electroencephalogram have successful application in clinical medicine. Biomedical imaging presents a visual representation of internal structures, which are hidden beneath the skin and bones, and help in appropriate diagnosis and treatment of diseases. Generally utilized imaging technologies include radiology, radiography, ultrasound, magnetic resonance imaging, elastography and endoscopy. This book provides significant information to help develop a good understanding of the clinical applications of biomedical imaging and sensing techniques. It is a vital tool for all researching and studying this field.

This book was developed from a mere concept to drafts to chapters and finally compiled together as a complete text to benefit the readers across all nations. To ensure the quality of the content we instilled two significant steps in our procedure. The first was to appoint an editorial team that would verify the data and statistics provided in the book and also select the most appropriate and valuable contributions from the plentiful contributions we received from authors worldwide. The next step was to appoint an expert of the topic as the Editor-in-Chief, who would head the project and finally make the necessary amendments and modifications to make the text reader-friendly. I was then commissioned to examine all the material to present the topics in the most comprehensible and productive format.

I would like to take this opportunity to thank all the contributing authors who were supportive enough to contribute their time and knowledge to this project. I also wish to convey my regards to my family who have been extremely supportive during the entire project.

Editor

1

Colorimetric Diagnostic Capillary Enabled by Size Sieving in a Porous Hydrogel

John Mello Camille C. Guzman [1], Sheng-Min Hsu [2] and Han-Sheng Chuang [1,3,*]

[1] Department of Biomedical Engineering, National Cheng Kung University, Tainan 701, Taiwan; p86077038@ncku.edu.tw
[2] Department of Ophthalmology, National Cheng Kung University Hospital, Tainan 701, Taiwan; shengmin@mail.ncku.edu.tw
[3] Center for Micro/Nano Science and Technology, National Cheng Kung University, Tainan 701, Taiwan
* Correspondence: oswaldchuang@mail.ncku.edu.tw

Abstract: Handy and disposable point-of-care diagnostics facilitate the early screening of severe diseases in resource-limited areas. To address urgent needs in inconvenient sites, a simple colorimetric diagnostic device equipped with a capillary tube with porous hydrogel and immunocomplex particles was developed for the rapid detection of biomarkers (16 min). In this device, probe particles attach to capture particles (dp = 40 μm) and form sandwiched immunocomplexes in the presence of target biomarkers, and a red color progressively emerges when the sandwiched immunocomplex particles are blocked by the porous hydrogel embedded inside the glass capillary. Colorimetric aggregation was recorded using a smartphone and analyzed with imaging software. The limit of detection reached 1 ng/mL and showed a maximum of 79% accuracy compared with that obtained through a conventional spectrophotometric technique. The level of a diabetic retinopathy (DR) biomarker, lipocalin-1 (LCN-1), was measured in 1 μL of a human tear sample and used in testing the practicability of the proposed device. All healthy subjects showed lower intensity levels than the other diabetic counterparts (proliferative DR or nonproliferative DR patients), implying the potential of this device in clinical applications. Overall, the diagnostic device facilitates point-of-care-testing and provides a low-cost (~1 USD), compact, and reliable tool for early diagnosis in resource-limited areas.

Keywords: porous hydrogel; immunoassay; biomarker; lipocalin 1; colorimetry; gold nanoparticles

---

1. Introduction

Epidemics have been threatening public health for centuries. The battle has become increasingly fierce recently as the highly contagious disease, COVID-19, broke out in early 2020 and rapidly spread worldwide, raising an unprecedented crisis [1,2]. Although early diagnosis is an effective measure for containing mass transmission, heavy dependence on high-end instruments forms a barrier to facile realization [3]. The consequences impact healthcare systems, especially in resource-limited areas [4].

To deal with these challenges, microfluidic technology has evolved since its advent in the 1990s. It is a research frontier and a possible alternative for sophisticated instruments. This technology has demonstrated the feasibility of device miniaturization and the development of new art in the Lab-on-Chip (LoC) system for various chemical and biological applications [5]. LoC has emerged as a powerful tool in the field of biomedical engineering. In contrast to their macroscale counterparts, LoC devices have many advantages, including small volumes of sample/reagent (down to the nanoliter), fast throughput, low cost, operational simplicity, and good potential for disposability [6–8]. In the manufacture of an LoC device, one of the most important considerations is material selection. Different materials have been used in microfluidic platforms, such as silicon [9], glass [10,11], polymer like polydimethylsiloxane and poly(methyl methacrylate) [12–15] and paper [16–19]. Most of these materials are not well suited to point-of-care testing (POCT) applications for low-resource settings, such as developing nations. Nevertheless, paper has shown desirable results in analytical and clinical chemistry for a decade. Paper has been used as a substrate in analytical testing, but paper-based assays usually show only a positive or negative result in most cases. Thus, despite offering quantitative data, they cannot detect low-level concentration when samples with microlevel volumes are used, such as testing strips for pH, pregnancy, and diabetes [20]. Therefore, paper-based assays are still limited in terms of producing reliable tools for POCT diagnostics.

Currently, researchers are exploring novel approaches for addressing some of the limitations of paper-based assays in disease diagnosis at a POCT setting [21]. POCT can be implemented by untrained individuals at any location, allowing timely treatment [22]. The collection and analysis of samples, such as whole blood, urine, saliva, pathogens, and proteins, for diagnosis and disease management in hospitals, clinics, or even homes is therefore possible [23–27], based on the concept of POCT, Chin et al. [28] developed a new strategy that integrates an easy-to-use assay into a microfluidic device to replicate all ELISA steps in remote settings. Recently, Wang et al. [29] carried out POCT by developing microbeads conjugated with fluorescence-tagged probe antibodies on their microfluidic system for the early detection of diabetic retinopathy (DR). Existing techniques have issues about execution and assembly in large stationary laboratories [30]. For simplicity, researchers have recently shifted their focus to developing various smart phone-based detection systems for handy POCT applications. Smartphone cameras can be used in identifying color variations in colorimetric assays. With this capability, smartphone photography and image analysis are adopted to read the value of solution color for the quantitative analysis of urinary glucose [31]. In another study, Oncescu et al. [32] successfully demonstrated the applicability of smartphones to sweat and saliva biomarker detection.

Given the popularity of POCT and smartphones in modern times, we proposed an integrated diagnostic platform equipped with a modified capillary-based device, a sandwiched immunocomplex, and a portable detection system for the rapid detection (16 min) of biomarkers in early disease diagnosis or low-abundance analytes (1 pg/mL) (Figure 1). A porous hydrogel was fabricated inside the microchannel through sol−gel chemistry. For the preparation of immunoassay, capture particles (d_p = 40 μm) and gold nanoparticles (AuNPs) as probe particles were bound using sandwiched immunocomplexes. For a proof of concept, LCN-1 was selected as a biomarker in the preparation of the sandwiched immunocomplexes. Liquid samples containing LCN-1 were firstly mixed with the capture and probe particles, and then injected into a modified capillary that filled with a porous hydrogel for color development. Subsequently, a smartphone was used to record the images for quantitative analysis. The limit of detection (LOD) reached 1 ng/mL. Only a small drop of a sample, as low as 1 μL, was required for effective measurement. The practicability of the proposed device was demonstrated by measuring LCN-1 in tear samples collected from seven volunteers. All healthy subjects showed considerably lower intensities, implying that their LCN-1 concentrations were markedly lower than those of the other clinically confirmed proliferative DR (PDR) and nonproliferative DR (PDR) patients. To a large extent, the proposed diagnostic platform shows great potential in the advancement of reliable diagnostic tools. The integration of this platform into smartphones and their applications for lens-less imaging will enable rapid disease diagnosis in resource-constrained areas.

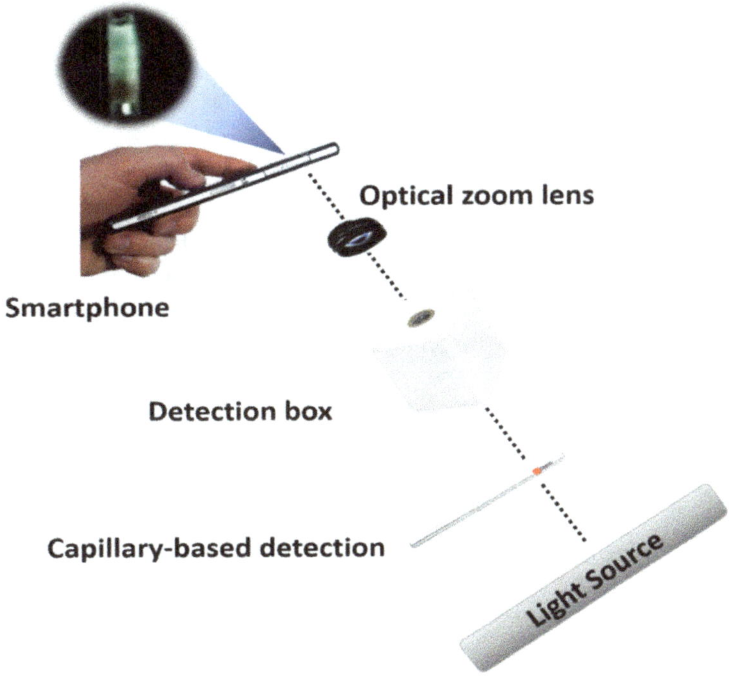

Figure 1. Illustration of an integrated platform consisting of a modified capillary device, a sandwiched immunocomplex and a portable detection system.

2. Materials and Methods

2.1. Reagents

All solvents and chemicals were of reagent quality. Poly(ethylene glycol) diacrylate (PEGDA) Mn 250, 2-hydroxy-2-methylpropiophenone 97%, 2-(N-morpholino) ethanesulfonic acid (M3671), and N-hydroxysuccinimide (6066-82-6) were purchased from Sigma–Aldrich, St. Louis, MO, USA. Monoclonal Anti-LCN1 IgG (a7611) and a gold conjugation kit (ab154873) were purchased from Abcam, Cambridge, UK. Polyclonal anti-LCN1 IgG (17900-1-AP) was purchased from Proteintech. 1-(3-dimethylaminopropyl)-3-ethylcarbodiimide hydrochloride 98+% (A10807) was purchased from Alfa Aesar, Ward Hill, MA, USA. AuNPs (40 nm, 20 OD, C12-25-980-TA-50) were purchased from Nanopartz Inc., Loveland, CO, USA. Amine-modified polystyrene (PS) particles (40 μm, 01-01-404) were purchased from Micromod Partikeltechnologie GmbH, Germany and used in capturing AuNPs. Plain PS particles (45 μm) were purchased from Polysciences Asia Pacific, Inc., Taiwan for the fabrication of porous hydrogels.

2.2. Assembly of the Diagnostic Capillary with a Porous Hydrogel

For the fabrication of a porous hydrogel (Figure 2), a plain PS particle suspension was injected into a capillary tube and dried in a ventilated hood at 30 °C for 4 h. Surface tension gradually drove the particles to form a hexagonal close-packed structure during evaporation. Subsequently, 2 μL of 99 wt% PEGDA Mn 250 and 1 wt% 2-hydroxy-2-methylpropiophenone mixture was injected into the same capillary tube to fill the interstitial spaces within the self-assembled PS particle scaffold. After positioning the capillary vertically for 5 min, the hydrogel was photo-polymerized with a 312 nm UV lamp (EBF-280C, ALT) for 10 min. Excess capillary was cut for subsequent particle dissolution by the solvent. The capillary with the self-assembled structure was soaked in toluene and agitated in a shaker for 4 h for the removal of the PS particles. The treated hydrogel was later soaked in 0.1 M acetone for 1 h and then rinsed with deionized water three times for the removal of residual PS particles in the hydrogel. The porous hydrogel was relocated into another sterilized capillary tube (Supplementary Material Section S1 and Figures S1 and S2). In addition, a sponge plug was inserted into the new capillary tube and positioned next to the porous hydrogel to induce self-driving background flow. Given that colorimetric intensity may be influenced by sample volume, a mark was set on the capillary tube to define the appropriate sample volume to intake.

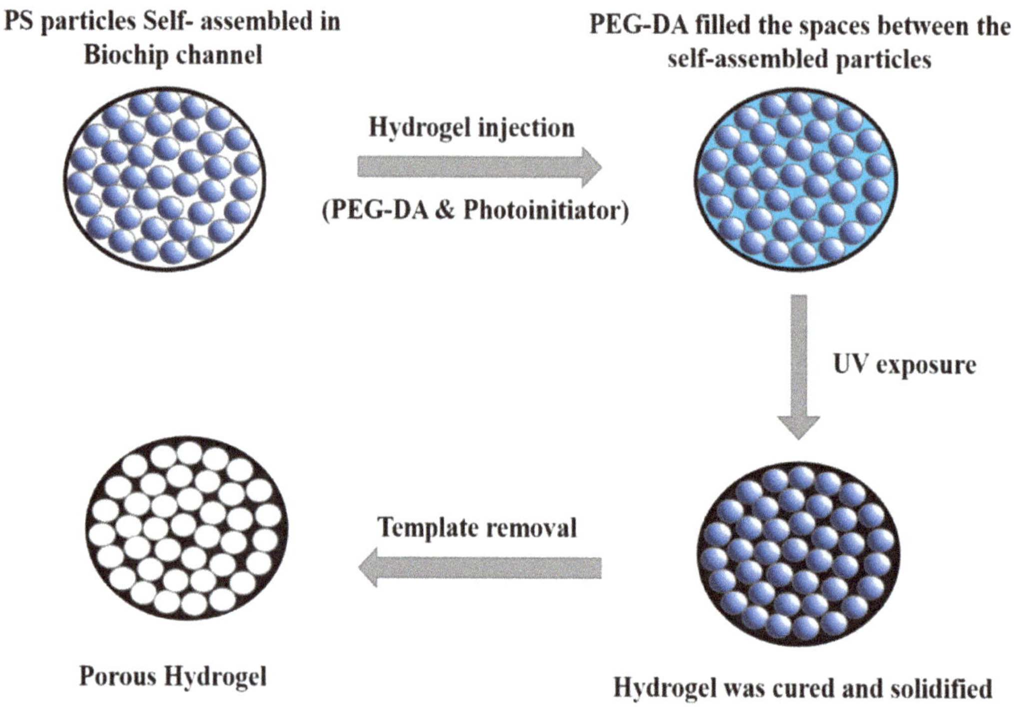

Figure 2. Schematic representation of the step-by-step formation of porous hydrogel.

2.3. Preparation of Sandwiched Immunocomplex

2.3.1. Functionalization of Capture Particles

In this study, 40 µm amine-modified PS particles were used in preparing the capture particles. Successful sieving by the porous hydrogel was ensured by setting capture particle diameter close to the pore size. For particle surface treatment, 2-(N-morpholino) ethanesulfonic acid (M3671, Sigma, St. Louis, MO, USA) was used in centrifugally washing 20 µL of the selected particle twice. Unexpected aggregation was prevented by vortexing and sonicating the particle suspension in a sonicator for 30 min. Meanwhile, 2 µL of 10 mg/mL 1-ethyl-3-(3-dimethylaminopropyl)-carbodiimide (A10807, Alfa Aesar, Ward Hill, MA, USA), 4 µL of 10 mg/mL N-hydroxysuccinimide (6066-82-6, Sigma, St. Louis, MO, USA), and 10 µL of 50 mM (pH = 5.5) 2-(N-morpholino) ethanesulfonic acid (M3671, Sigma, St. Louis, MO, USA) buffer were added to 4.5 µL of 0.5 µg/µL mouse monoclonal anti-LCN-1 immunoglobulin G (IgG) (a76611, Abcam, Cambridge, UK) to activate the carboxyl groups on the capture antibody. Lastly, the antibody solution and the particle suspension were mixed and incubated in a thermal shaker at 800 rpm and 4 °C for 4 h for the conjugation of the antibodies and PS particles (Figure 3). Free-suspending antibodies were eventually washed away through centrifugation three times, and 1% bovine serum albumin (A2153, Sigma, St. Louis, MO, USA) was added to the particle suspension at 25 °C in a shaker for 1 h to block nonspecific binding.

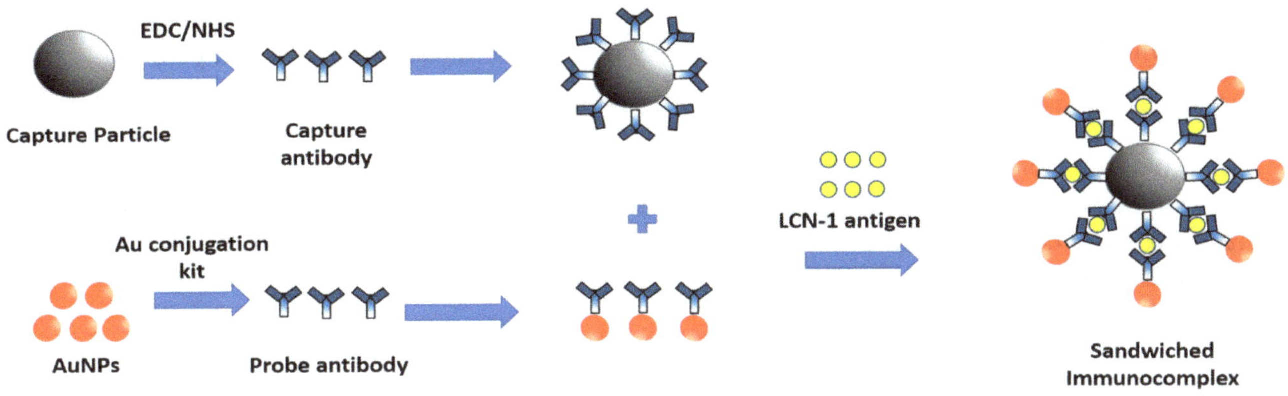

Figure 3. Illustrations for preparing sandwiched immunocomplex and detection process.

2.3.2. Functionalization of Probe Particles

Probe particles were obtained by covalently conjugating the probe antibody, rabbit polyclonal anti-LCN-1 IgG (17900-1-AP, Proteintech, Rosemont, IL, USA), to AuNPs according to the protocol of the gold conjugation kit (ab154873, Abcam, Cambridge, UK). To this end, the probe antibody solution was diluted to 0.1 mg/mL with the gold antibody diluent provided in the kit. Afterward, 12 μL of diluted antibody solution was thoroughly mixed with 42 μL of gold reaction buffer. The mixed solution was then added to the AuNP suspension to enable conjugation in a shaker at 400 rpm for 20 min. Finally, 5 μL of gold quencher was added to the mixture for the complete conjugation of the antibodies and AuNPs. The antibody-conjugated AuNPs were stored at 4 °C for subsequent use.

2.3.3. Formation of Sandwiched Immunocomplex

The sandwiched immunocomplex was synthesized by mixing 20 μL of antibody-conjugated capture particles with 10 μL of the desired concentration of LCN-1 (a76611, Abcam, Cambridge, UK), incubating at 25 °C in a shaker for 15 min, and mixing with 15 μL of antibody-conjugated AuNPs. The formation of sandwiched immunocomplex eventually resulted in the colorimetric aggregation of probe particles because they were blocked along with large capture particles by the porous hydrogel.

2.4. Measurement Platform

For visual observation, the capillary-based detection device (i.e., a capillary filled with a porous hydrogel and a sponge plug) was sufficient to provide qualitative information. However, for quantitative analysis, additional components, including a backlight source, a detection box, and a smartphone, were required. The backlight was generated from the LCD screen of a laptop (Pavilion 15-au109TX, HP). A capillary tube holder and a reference capillary tube were placed inside the detection box, and an optical zoom lens (0.67×) having a working distance of 3.9 cm, was clamped on the camera of a smartphone to facilitate closeup imaging. In the LCN-1 detection process, a modified capillary was dipped into a vial containing the immunocomplexed particle solution until it reached the mark on the capillary. Subsequently, the capillary was flipped to stand vertically and allow the sandwiched immunocomplex solution to flow freely downward until the solution passed through the hydrogel. The capillary was then inserted into the capillary tube holder in the detection box, and the backlight was adjusted to 20% of full grayscale intensity (standard for reference) for the best and optimal image in detection (Supplementary Material Section S2 and Figures S3 and S4). Colorimetric aggregation inside the capillary was captured using a smartphone. The region of interest (ROI) was the particle aggregate in front of the porous hydrogel. The captured images were then quantitatively analyzed using ImageJ (https://imagej.net/Fiji). Finally, the concentration of the biomarkers was determined by analyzing the grayscale intensity of the aggregated particles in the image. Notably, the reference capillary tube in the study served as a standard when a different backlight source or smartphone was used. For instance, an intensity of the ROI in the reference capillary tube higher or lower than the standard would need to be readjusted to the same value before measurement could proceed.

2.5. Statistical Analysis

All data were obtained from independent tests and presented as mean ± standard deviation (SD). Comparison between the values was performed using student's *t*-test. The significance level was set at 95% ($p < 0.05$) and the GraphPad Prism 5.0 software package (GraphPad Software Inc., San Diego, CA, USA) was used for data analysis.

3. Results and Discussion

3.1. Formation of Porous Hydrogel

A porous PEGDA hydrogel was obtained after completely dissolving the 45 μm PS particles with toluene. The fabrication process and the appearance of the porous hydrogel were observed with a microscope (Olympus, IX71, Tokyo, Japan). First, the self-assembled PS particles formed a hexagonal close-packed structure after evaporation (Figure 4a). Notably, evaporation is commonly used in promoting self-assembly for colloidal suspensions due to its simplicity and high reliability [33]. However, rapid evaporation may impair the order of self-assembly [34]. To avoid this unexpected disorder, the capillary tube was used for the self-assembly of particles. For 5 μL of colloidal suspension, the evaporation took 4 h to complete in a ventilated hood. A PEGDA solution was prepared and poured into the capillary tube to fill the interstitial space within the self-assembled structure. After the PS particles were removed with toluene, a raw porous PEGDA hydrogel was obtained (Figure 4b). The cross-sectional image of the porous hydrogel showed that the pore size remained close to the original template. The useful porous hydrogel section was obtained by cutting the capillary tube and transferring the remaining hydrogel to a new capillary tube. The front and side images of the transferred hydrogel inside the capillary tube were examined. The capillary tube was completely filled with the porous hydrogel (Figure 4c,d), indicating the successful fabrication of the diagnostic capillary.

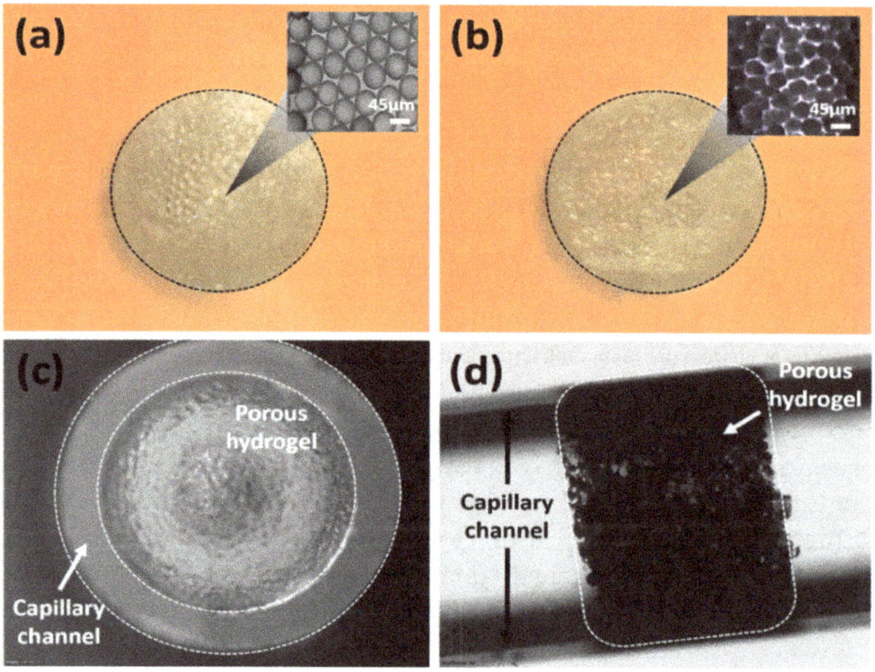

Figure 4. Microscope image of porous hydrogel (image scale 500 μm): (**a**) hydrogel filled the spaces of the self-assembled particles and closely-packed colloidal structure; (**b**) porous hydrogel after the removal of the template and the microstructure of the porous hydrogel; (**c**) frontal view of the porous hydrogel inside the capillary channel; (**d**) side view of the porous hydrogel inside the capillary channel.

3.2. *Sandwiched Immunocomplex Detection*

In our design, the capture and probe particles formed a sandwiched immunocomplex in the presence of LCN-1, resulting in colorimetric aggregation. By dipping the diagnostic capillary into the immunocomplexed solution and reaching a depth defined by a mark, a certain volume of immunocomplexed solution was dragged into the capillary tube through capillary force. When an appropriate amount of the solution was held in the tube, the capillary was then flipped over such that the sample would fall through the porous hydrogel through gravitational force (Figure 5a). When the sample reached the sponge plug at the other end of the porous hydrogel, powerful suction forced the remaining immunocomplexed solution to move forward until it dried out. The porous hydrogel served as a semipermeable barrier, and the sensing mechanism was realized by blocking the sandwiched immunocomplex to form colorimetric aggregation (Figure 5b). In the absence of target antigens, only plain capture particles stacked up, but free-suspending probe particles (AuNPs) passed through the porous hydrogel, leaving no noticeable emergence of color. Conversely, the presence of target antigens in the sample induced a sandwich formation on the immunocomplex. When this sandwiched immunocomplex was run through the capillary, they were blocked by the porous hydrogel because of size sieving. The aggregation of the sandwiched immunocomplex then produced a dark red color band because of stacked AuNPs, indicating a positive response (Supplementary Material Section S3 and Figure S5). Surface plasmon resonance on the stacked AuNPs induced the red color. However, the red color turned dark as more AuNPs stacked up to deplete light intensity in the presence of more LCN-1.

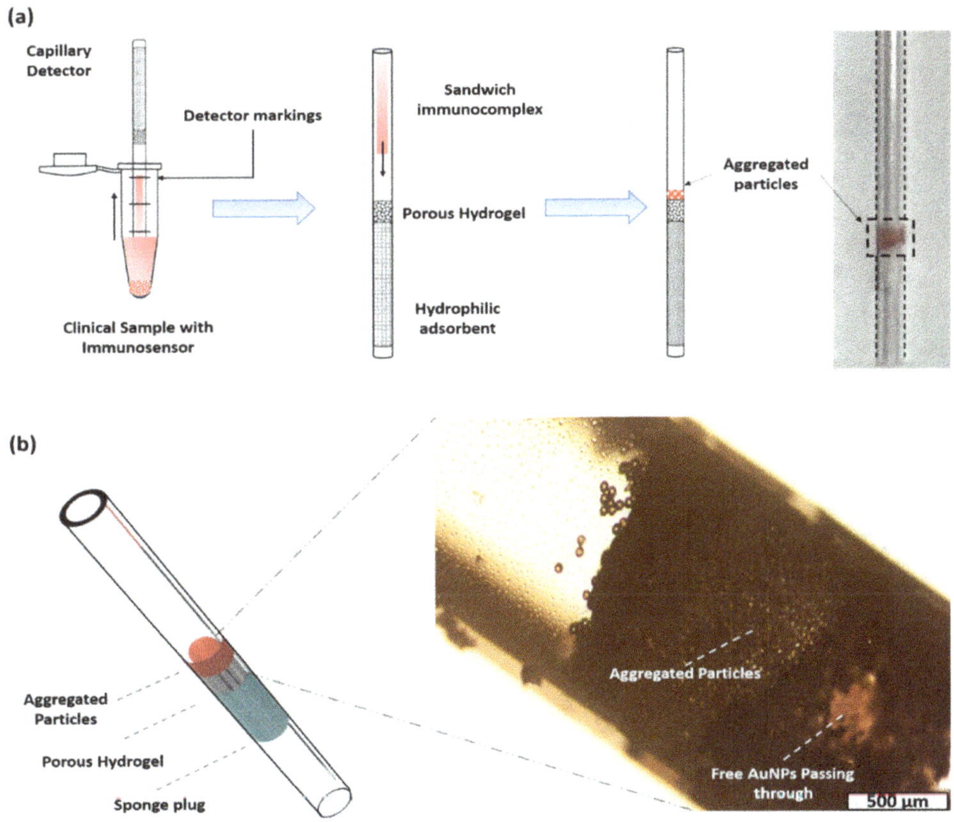

Figure 5. (**a**) Sandwiched immunocomplex detection process; (**b**) 3D model of capillary detector and aggregation of immunocomplex.

3.3. *Colorimetric Assessment for Direct Visualization*

The images of the colorimetric aggregation were further recorded for the investigation of the relationship between color change and LCN-1 concentration. A ROI that covered the particle aggregate in the image was firstly selected. The ROI was then split into three output images according to RGB value (Figure 6a). These values were converted into (x, y) coordinates defining the color profile of the aggregated particles in the CIE 1931 chromaticity space. Through this process, the actual color of the aggregated sandwiched immunocomplex within the capillary device was determined. The RGB levels and color profiles of the sandwiched immunocomplex with six different concentrations of LCN-1 were plotted (Figure 6b). For the RGB variations in the immunocomplex at different antigen concentrations, the red value dramatically increased with antigen concentration. Notably, this color enhancement simply resulted from stacked AuNPs rather from the red shifting effect due to changes in the sizes of the aggregated AuNPs [35]. Furthermore, the CIE 1931 chromaticity space was used in quantitatively illustrating the color change resulting from the different concentrations of antigens (Figure 6c). Increase in antigen concentration led to increase in red intensity, which was the basis for macroscopic concentration reading.

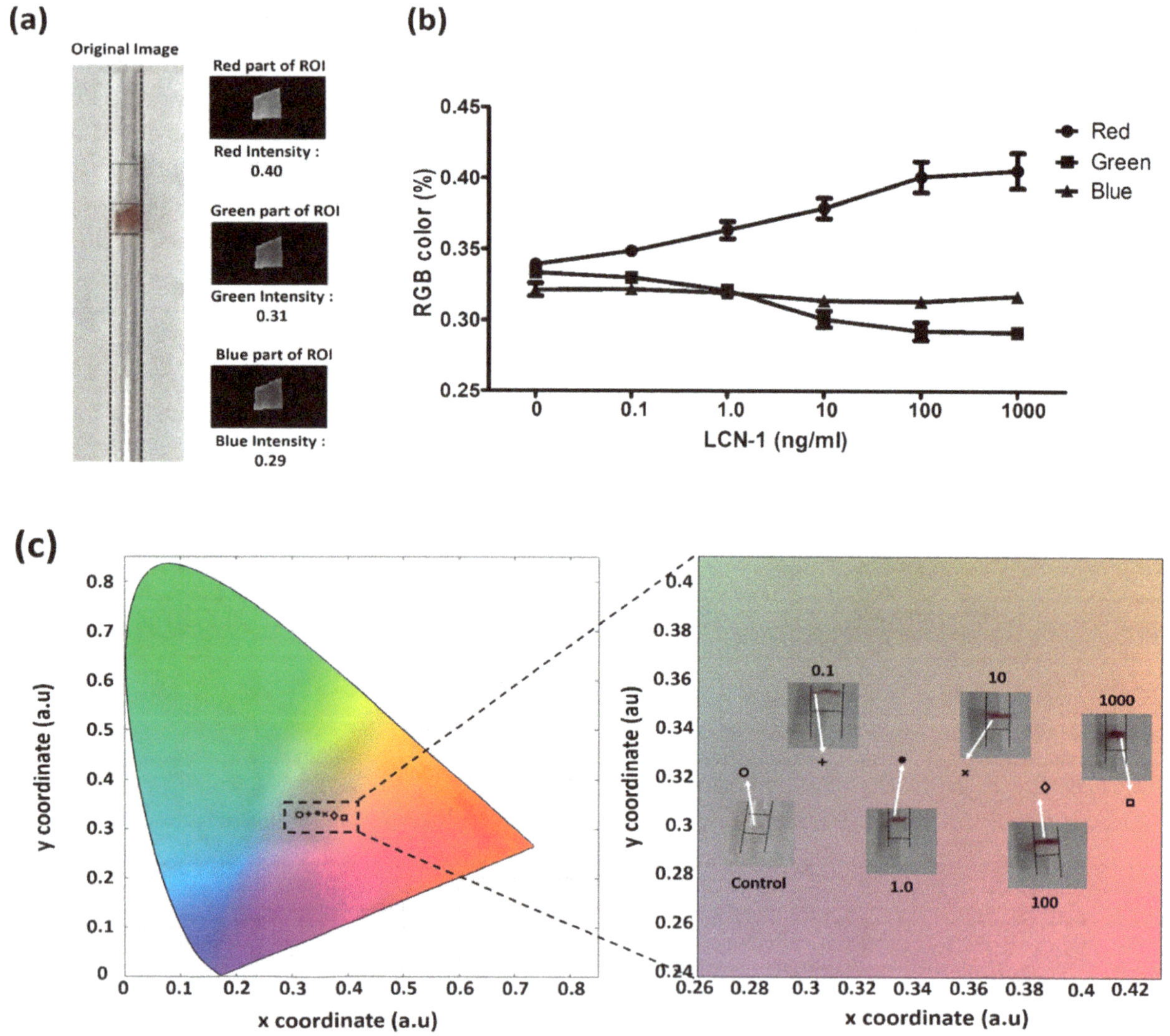

Figure 6. (**a**) MATLAB interface for image processing for color profile; (**b**) percentage of RGB of the sandwiched immunocomplex at different antigen concentrations; (**c**) CIE 1931 color profile of aggregated sandwiched immunocomplex for visualization with the naked eye. The unit of the numbers in the insets is ng/mL.

3.4. Quantitative Assessment with the Measurement Platform

In addition to direct visualization, the capillary device was also evaluated through quantitative analysis. Unlike the previous color mode that showed potential for quick screening by direct visualization, a grayscale mode exhibited a linear relationship between the light intensity and protein concentration. Given the background noise resulting from different measurement conditions, the capillary device was measured in a customized detection box. The detection box provided a dark environment with a controllable light source supplied from the laptop screen. For quantitative imaging, a smartphone was connected to an optical lens holder and attached to the detection box. Images recorded by the smartphone were converted into grayscale, and their average ROI intensity was calculated (Figure 7a). Grayscale intensity was obtained over a concentration ranging from 100 pg/mL to 1 μg/mL, covering three orders of magnitude. The results indicated that a high antigen concentration increased the quantity of the sandwiched immunocomplex aggregates and grayscale intensity. Based on the intersection of the threefold error bars of the control and linear trend line, the estimated LOD level for the target biomarker was 1 ng/mL. (Figure 7b).

For the investigation of binding specificity, two irrelevant antigens, VEGF and TNF-α, were used in the study. All of the three antigens, including LCN-1, were prepared (10 ng/mL) and separately mixed with the capture and probe particles. According to their grayscale intensities (Figure 7c), although VEGF and TNF-α seemed to induce some nonspecific bindings, they both showed lower immune responses than LCN-1. The higher grayscale intensity of LCN-1 as compared with the intensities of the other two antigens showed that the current capture and probe particles were specifically responsive to LCN-1.

Another experiment was performed to investigate the stability of the sandwiched immunocomplex. The grayscale intensities of the five different concentrations of the LCN-1 control samples were continuously monitored for over 720 min (Figure 7d). Notably, the grayscale intensities of all the samples appeared to have maintained their levels in the first 300 min and then gradually decreased over time afterward. This trend was likely due to the degradation of the antibody in a moderate environment, specifically at room temperature, which led to disintegration of capture and probe particles. Accordingly, it was recommended to complete the color reading within 5 h after the samples were injected into the capillary tube.

Lastly, LCN-1 was also measured using a UV–VIS spectrophotometer (NanoDrop One, Thermo Scientific) for validation. The protein concentration was determined by the absorbance peak at 280 nm according to the instrument standard protocol. A calibration curve (i.e., absorbance vs. protein concentration) from 30 pg/mL to 3 mg/mL using bovine serum albumin was established. Subsequently, four control samples with LCN-1 concentration ranging from 100 pg/mL to 100 ng/mL were prepared and then separately measured with the spectrophotometer and our diagnostic capillary (Figure 7e). When spectrophotometric results were used herein as reference values, the accuracy of the proposed diagnostic device (Equation (1)) varied between 44.28% (0.1 ng/mL of antigen) and 79% (100 ng/mL of antigen), implying that the current diagnostic device remained incapable of low concentrations below 1 ng/mL. For diseases with rich biomarkers, such as LCN-1 in DR, however, this device is suitable as a rapid screening tool and can provide valuable information about the presence of biomarkers in samples.

$$\text{Accuracy (\%)} = \left(1 - \left|\frac{\text{diagnostic device} - \text{macroscale method}}{\text{macroscale method}}\right|\right) \times 100 \quad (1)$$

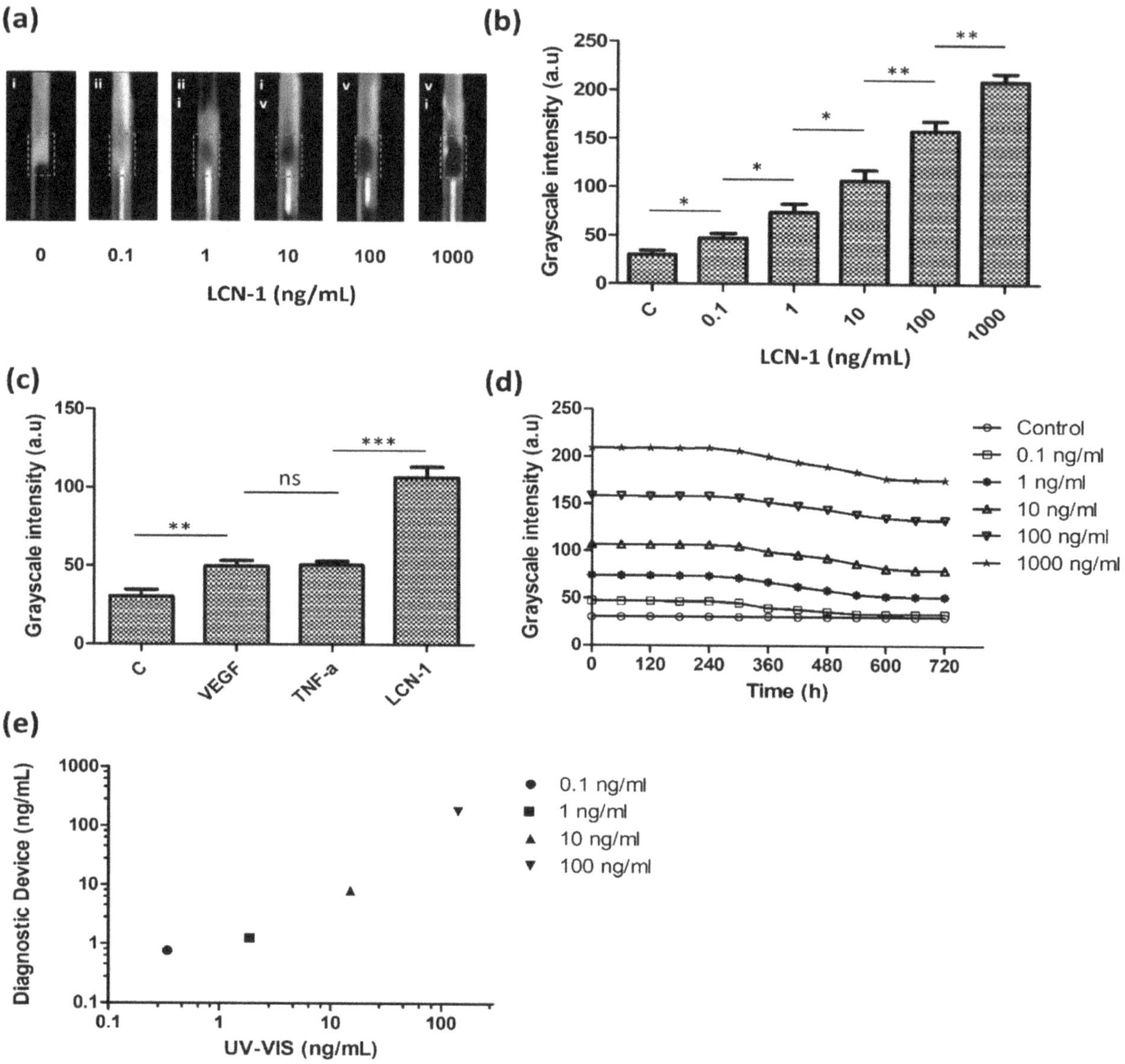

Figure 7. Quantitative assessment of the detection platform: (**a**) grayscale images of diagnostic tool inside the detection box; (**b**) calibration of the grayscale intensity of sandwiched immunocomplex with respect to different lipocalin-1 (LCN-1) concentrations ranging from 100 pg/mL to 1 µg/mL; (**c**) binding specificity of the capture and probe particles in the presence of different antigens; (**d**) binding stability of sandwiched immunocomplex with respect to different times; (**e**) reliability of the detection platform. Comparison of LCN-1 concentration detection results between the proposed diagnostic tool and spectrophotometer. The symbols "*", "**", "***", "ns" denote $p < 0.05$, $p < 0.01$, $p < 0.001$, and $p > 0.05$, respectively, under student's t test ($n = 5$). The error bars represent standard deviation.

3.5. Detection of Biomarker LCN 1 in Clinical Tear Samples

The practicability of the diagnostic capillary device was evaluated according to the measured concentration of the DR biomarker LCN-1 in tear samples collected from seven clinical volunteers. The volunteers included four healthy subjects and three DR patients. Tear sample collection was conducted by a medical specialist at the Department of Ophthalmology, National Cheng Kung University Hospital (NCKUH) in compliance with the IRB agreement # A-ER-105-113. The patients were initially preselected by the ophthalmologist. The exclusion criteria included dry eye syndrome, macular degeneration, and under drug treatments. Approximately 10 µL of tear fluid was extracted from the lower eyelid of each volunteer through a sterilized glass tube. To this end, the lower eyelid was firstly pulled downward, revealing the conjunctival sac into which the glass tube was held horizontally. Owing to the capillary effect, the tear fluid then automatically flowed into the glass tube. When sufficient tear fluid was collected, the tear sample was pipetted out of the glass tube and injected into a microcentrifuge tube. The tube was stored in a refrigerator at −70 °C for subsequent use. Notably, unlike in the previous calibration steps, the clinical samples were diluted with 1× PBS + 0.1% Tween 20 (PBST) 100-fold. This step ensured that LCN-1 level was within the dynamic range of measurement (1 pg/mL–1 μg/mL). Afterward, the final LCN-1 concentration was obtained by multiplying the measured data 100-fold. Among these volunteers, four healthy subjects (S1–S4) were diagnosed with no clinical history of diabetes or any other reported eye-related diseases, two (S5, S6) were clinically confirmed as PDR patients, and one (S7) was a NPDR patient. The LCN-1 concentrations of the seven clinical samples were obtained using the proposed capillary device (Figure 8). As expected, the healthy subjects appeared to show lower concentrations than the other PDR and NPDR patients. However, the measured LCN-1 concentrations in all the samples were lower than the previously reported threshold of LCN-1 (1–2 mg/mL) [36] in healthy tear fluids. The dramatic deviations were likely due to the multiple dilutions performed during sample preparation. The original concentration was not linearly proportional to the dilution ratio. Nevertheless, the significant LCN-1 level differences between the healthy subjects and the patients with PDR or NPDR implied that potential patients with PDR or NPDR may be diagnosed accurately with the proposed diagnostic tool. This diagnostic device provides a rapid screening tool for performing preventive DR treatments in the early stage.

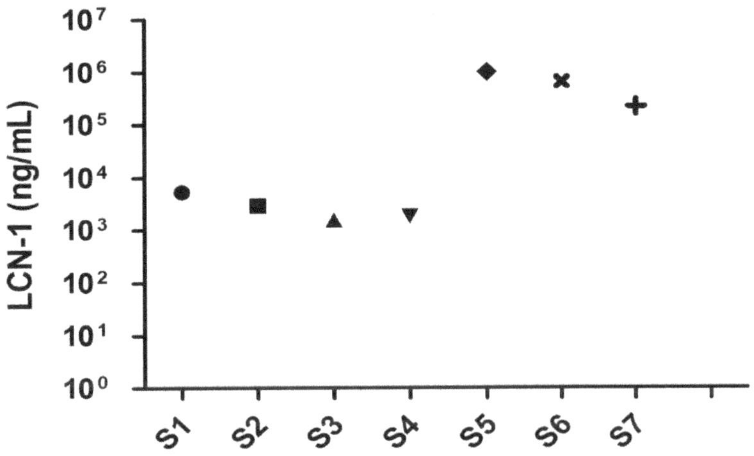

Figure 8. Preclinical test with four healthy subjects (**S1–S4**), two (**S5, S6**) clinically diagnosed proliferative diabetic retinopathy (PDR) patients, and one (**S7**) diagnosed nonproliferative diabetic retinopathy (NPDR) patient.

4. Conclusions

This study presents a simple method for detecting small molecules or low-abundance biomarkers with a modified capillary tube and a portable detection platform for color profiling. In the proposed detection method, the capillary tube was modified by embedding a porous hydrogel, which served as a filter and sponge plug to drag liquid samples to accelerate detection. In addition, capture and probes particles were conjugated with selected antibodies. In the presence of antigen, the two particles would be linked together forming a sandwiched immunocomplex. In the detection process, the capillary tube was submerged into the vial containing the sandwiched immunocomplex up to the markings. Through capillary force, the immunocomplex was dragged into the capillary tube, and upon sucking enough sample, the detector was flipped over for additional gravitational force. When the sample reached the sponge plug on the other end of the porous hydrogel, powerful suction kept dragging the remaining immunocomplex solution to move forward until it dried out. The porous hydrogel served as a semipermeable barrier and its sensing mechanism was dependent on blocking sandwiched immunocomplex particles to form color. In the absence of target antigens, only plain capture particles stacked up, and free-suspending probe particles passed through the porous hydrogel, and thus no noticeable color was observed. The aggregated immunocomplex was observed and quantified by the grayscale intensity of an image. The LOD of the technique reached as low as 1 ng/mL. The evaluation results revealed that accuracy was as high as 79% and high binding specificity to the target biomarker LCN-1. The suitability of the proposed detection system for real-world detection applications was investigated by measuring LCN-1 in tear samples collected from volunteers. Significant differences in the LCN-1 level between the healthy subjects and patients with PDR or NPDR implied that potential patients with PDR or NPDR may be accurately diagnosed with the proposed diagnostic tool. Finally, this diagnostic device provides a low-cost (~1 USD) and rapid screening tool (1 min of colorimetry) for preventive DR treatments in the early stages.

Author Contributions: J.M.C.C.G. conducted the experiments, wrote, and revised the manuscript; S.-M.H. provided the clinical tear samples and clinical diagnosis; H.-S.C. wrote, reviewed and revised the manuscript, and formulated and supervised this study. All authors have read and agreed to the published version of the manuscript.

Acknowledgments: We would like to thank the clinical samples obtained from the volunteers authorized by the IRB project # A-ER-105-113 and all the technical assistance provided by the staff at National Cheng Kung University Hospital.

References

1. Mirzaie, A.; Halaji, M.; Dehkordi, F.S.; Ranjbar, R.; Noorbazargan, H. A narrative literature review on traditional medicine options for treatment of corona virus disease 2019 (COVID-19). *Complement. Ther. Clin. Pract.* **2020**, *40*, 101214. [CrossRef] [PubMed]
2. Zhou, M.; Zhang, X.; Qu, J. Coronavirus disease 2019 (COVID-19): A clinical update. *Front. Med.* **2020**, *14*, 126–135. [CrossRef] [PubMed]
3. Zhu, X.; Wang, X.; Han, L.; Chen, T.; Wang, L.; Li, H.; Li, S.; He, L.; Fu, X.; Chen, S.; et al. Multiplex reverse transcription loop-mediated isothermal amplification combined with nanoparticle-based lateral flow biosensor for the diagnosis of COVID-19. *Biosens. Bioelectron.* **2020**, *166*, 112437. [CrossRef]
4. Chuang, H.-S.; Chen, Y.-J.; Cheng, H.-P. Enhanced diffusometric immunosensing with grafted gold nanoparticles for detection of diabetic retinopathy biomarker tumor necrosis factor-α. *Biosens. Bioelectron.* **2018**, *101*, 75–83. [CrossRef]
5. Yang, R.-J.; Hou, H.-H.; Wang, Y.-N.; Fu, L.-M. Micro-magnetofluidics in microfluidic systems: A review. *Sens. Actuators B Chem.* **2016**, *224*, 1–15. [CrossRef]
6. Guzman, J.M.C.C.; Tayo, L.L.; Liu, C.-C.; Wang, Y.-N.; Fu, L.-M. Rapid microfluidic paper-based platform for low concentration formaldehyde detection. *Sens. Actuators B Chem.* **2018**, *255*, 3623–3629. [CrossRef]
7. Zhong, Q.; Ding, H.; Gao, B.; He, Z.; Gu, Z. Advances of Microfluidics in Biomedical Engineering. *Adv. Mater. Technol.* **2019**, *4*, 1800663. [CrossRef]
8. Luka, G.; Ahmadi, A.; Najjaran, H.; Alocilja, E.C.; DeRosa, M.C.; Wolthers, K.R.; Malki, A.; Aziz, H.A.; Althani, A.A.; Hoorfar, M. Microfluidics Integrated Biosensors: A Leading Technology towards Lab-on-a-Chip and Sensing Applications. *Sensors* **2015**, *15*, 30011–30031. [CrossRef] [PubMed]
9. Caputo, D.; De Angelis, A.; Lovecchio, N.; Nascetti, A.; Scipinotti, R.; De Cesare, G. Amorphous silicon photosensors integrated in microfluidic structures as a technological demonstrator of a "true" Lab-on-Chip system. *Sens. Bio-Sens. Res.* **2015**, *3*, 98–104. [CrossRef]
10. Fu, L.-M.; Ju, W.-J.; Yang, R.-J.; Wang, Y.-N. Rapid prototyping of glass-based microfluidic chips utilizing two-pass defocused CO2 laser beam method. *Microfluid. Nanofluidics* **2012**, *14*, 479–487. [CrossRef]

11. Smejkal, P.; Breadmore, M.C.; Guijt, R.M.; Grym, J.; Foret, F.; Bek, F.; Macka, M. Separation of carboxylic acids in human serum by isotachophoresis using a commercial field-deployable analytical platform combined with in-house glass microfluidic chips. *Anal. Chim. Acta* **2012**, *755*, 115–120. [CrossRef]
12. Fan, X.; Jia, C.; Yang, J.; Li, G.; Mao, H.; Jin, Q.; Zhao, J. A microfluidic chip integrated with a high-density PDMS-based microfiltration membrane for rapid isolation and detection of circulating tumor cells. *Biosens. Bioelectron.* **2015**, *71*, 380–386. [CrossRef]
13. Kunstmann-Olsen, C.; Hanczyc, M.M.; Hoyland, J.; Rasmussen, S.; Rubahn, H.-G. Uniform droplet splitting and detection using Lab-on-Chip flow cytometry on a microfluidic PDMS device. *Sens. Actuators B Chem.* **2016**, *229*, 7–13. [CrossRef]
14. Masrie, M.; Majlis, B.Y.; Yunas, J. Fabrication of multilayer-PDMS based microfluidic device for bio-particles concentration detection. *Bio-Med. Mater. Eng.* **2014**, *24*, 1951–1958. [CrossRef] [PubMed]
15. Yavuz, C.; Oliaei, S.; Çetin, B.; Yesil-Celiktas, O. Sterilization of PMMA microfluidic chips by various techniques and investigation of material characteristics. *J. Supercrit. Fluids* **2016**, *107*, 114–121. [CrossRef]
16. Ahmed, S.; Bui, M.-P.N.; Abbas, A. Paper-based chemical and biological sensors: Engineering aspects. *Biosens. Bioelectron.* **2016**, *77*, 249–263. [CrossRef] [PubMed]
17. Dou, M.; Sanjay, S.T.; Benhabib, M.; Xu, F.; Li, X. Low-cost bioanalysis on paper-based and its hybrid microfluidic platforms. *Talanta* **2015**, *145*, 43–54. [CrossRef]
18. Pena-Pereira, F.; Lavilla, I.; Bendicho, C. Paper-based analytical device for instrumental-free detection of thiocyanate in saliva as a biomarker of tobacco smoke exposure. *Talanta* **2016**, *147*, 390–396. [CrossRef] [PubMed]
19. Xia, Y.; Si, J.; Li, Z. Fabrication techniques for microfluidic paper-based analytical devices and their applications for biological testing: A review. *Biosens. Bioelectron.* **2016**, *77*, 774–789. [CrossRef]
20. Martinez, A.W.; Phillips, S.T.; Whitesides, G.M.; Carrilho, E. Diagnostics for the Developing World: Microfluidic Paper-Based Analytical Devices. *Anal. Chem.* **2010**, *82*, 3–10. [CrossRef]
21. Singh, A.T.; Lantigua, D.; Meka, A.; Taing, S.; Pandher, M.; Camci-Unal, G. Paper-Based Sensors: Emerging Themes and Applications. *Sensors* **2018**, *18*, 2838. [CrossRef] [PubMed]
22. Luppa, P.B.; Müller, C.; Schlichtiger, A.; Schlebusch, H. Point-of-care testing (POCT): Current techniques and future perspectives. *TrAC Trends Anal. Chem.* **2011**, *30*, 887–898. [CrossRef] [PubMed]
23. Song, Y.; Huang, Y.-Y.; Liu, X.; Zhang, X.; Ferrari, M.; Qin, L. Point-of-care technologies for molecular diagnostics using a drop of blood. *Trends Biotechnol.* **2014**, *32*, 132–139. [CrossRef] [PubMed]
24. Gubala, V.; Harris, L.F.; Ricco, A.; Tan, M.X.; Williams, D.E. Point of Care Diagnostics: Status and Future. *Anal. Chem.* **2012**, *84*, 487–515. [CrossRef] [PubMed]
25. Vashist, S.K.; Luppa, P.B.; Yeo, L.Y.; Ozcan, A.; Luong, J.H.T. Emerging Technologies for Next-Generation Point-of-Care Testing. *Trends Biotechnol.* **2015**, *33*, 692–705. [CrossRef] [PubMed]
26. Chen, H.; Liu, K.; Li, Z.; Wang, P. Point of care testing for infectious diseases. *Clin. Chim. Acta* **2019**, *493*, 138–147. [CrossRef]
27. Yang, J.; Wang, K.; Xu, H.; Yan, W.; Jin, Q.; Cui, D. Detection platforms for point-of-care testing based on colorimetric, luminescent and magnetic assays: A review. *Talanta* **2019**, *202*, 96–110. [CrossRef]
28. Chin, C.D.; Laksanasopin, T.; Cheung, Y.K.; Steinmiller, D.; Linder, V.; Parsa, H.; Wang, J.; Moore, H.; Rouse, R.; Umviligihozo, G.; et al. Microfluidics-based diagnostics of infectious diseases in the developing world. *Nat. Med.* **2011**, *17*, 1015–1019. [CrossRef]
29. Wang, J.-Y.; Kwon, J.-S.; Hsu, S.-M.; Chuang, H.-S. Sensitive tear screening of diabetic retinopathy with dual biomarkers enabled using a rapid electrokinetic patterning platform. *Lab Chip* **2020**, *20*, 356–362. [CrossRef]
30. Wang, S.; Inci, F.; De Libero, G.; Singhal, A.; Demirci, U. Point-of-care assays for tuberculosis: Role of nanotechnology/microfluidics. *Biotechnol. Adv.* **2013**, *31*, 438–449. [CrossRef]
31. Wang, T.-T.; Lio, C.K.; Huang, H.; Wang, R.-Y.; Zhou, H.; Luo, P.; Qing, L.-S. A feasible image-based colorimetric assay using a smartphone RGB camera for point-of-care monitoring of diabetes. *Talanta* **2020**, *206*, 120211. [CrossRef] [PubMed]
32. Oncescu, V.; O'Dell, D.; Erickson, D. Smartphone based health accessory for colorimetric detection of biomarkers in sweat and saliva. *Lab Chip* **2013**, *13*, 3232–3238. [CrossRef]
33. Van Dommelen, R.; Fanzio, P.; Sasso, L. Surface self-assembly of colloidal crystals for micro- and nano-patterning. *Adv. Colloid Interface Sci.* **2018**, *251*, 97–114. [CrossRef] [PubMed]

34. Maki, K.L.; Kumar, S. Fast Evaporation of Spreading Droplets of Colloidal Suspensions. *Langmuir* **2011**, *27*, 11347–11363. [CrossRef]
35. Pluchery, O.; Remita, H.; Schaming, D. Demonstrative experiments about gold nanoparticles and nanofilms: An introduction to nanoscience. *Gold Bull.* **2013**, *46*, 319–327. [CrossRef]
36. Csosz, E.; Boross, P.; Csutak, A.; Berta, A.; Toth, F.; Poliska, S.; Török, Z.; Tőzsér, J. Quantitative analysis of proteins in the tear fluid of patients with diabetic retinopathy. *J. Proteom.* **2012**, *75*, 2196–2204. [CrossRef] [PubMed]

2

Urinalysis Using a Diaper-Based Testing Device

Wei-Hsuan Sung [1,2], Ching-Yi Liu [3], Chung-Yao Yang [2,3], Cheng-Han Chen [4,5,6], Yu-Ting Tsao [6], Ching-Fen Shen [7,*] and Chao-Min Cheng [6,*]

1 College of Medicine, Chang Gung University, Taoyuan 33302, Taiwan; w.h.sung0109@gmail.com
2 Chang Gung Memorial Hospital Linkou Medical Center, Taoyuan 33305, Taiwan; cyyang@hygeiatouch.com
3 Hygeia Touch Inc., Taipei 10441, Taiwan; itis3636@gmail.com
4 Department of Emergency Medicine, Taipei Veterans General Hospital, Taipei 11217, Taiwan; gdc123.tw@gmail.com
5 School of Medicine, National Yang-Ming University, Taipei 11221, Taiwan
6 Institute of Biomedical Engineering, National Tsing Hua University, Hsinchu 30013, Taiwan; sherry450047@gmail.com
7 Department of Pediatrics, National Cheng Kung University Hospital, College of Medicine, National Cheng Kung University, Tainan 70403, Taiwan
* Correspondence: drshen1112@gmail.com (C.-F.S.); chaomin@mx.nthu.edu.tw (C.-M.C.)

Abstract: Urinary tract infections (UTI), one of the most common bacterial infections, annually affect 150 million people worldwide. Infants and the elderly are likely to have missed or delayed diagnosis of UTI due to difficulty clearly describing their symptoms. A rapid screening method for UTI is a critical and urgent need for these populations. The aim of our study is to develop a diaper-based testing device to assay urine biomarkers including pH, leukocyte, and nitrite level. This all-in-one device assists in urine collection and testing using a colorimetric approach to provide easily read visual results on the outside surface of a test strip-integrated diaper. In this study, we tested samples from 46 patients using testing strips and examined the results from 7 patients recruited to validate the strip-integrated diaper. In conclusion, this new diaper-based testing device is easy to use, rapid, and inexpensive, all of which imbue it with tremendous potential for development into a commercially viable UTI screening system.

Keywords: urinary tract infection; UTI; urinalysis; diaper-based testing device; pH; leukocyte; nitrite

1. Introduction

Diagnosis of a urinary tract infection (UTI) indicates the presence of infection anywhere in the urinary tract. Common manifestations include bacterial infections in the kidney (pyelonephritis), urethra (urethritis), and bladder (cystitis), of both genders and at a variety of ages [1]. Fever, pain in the back, burning sensation or pain when urinating, and frequent urination are common UTI symptoms [2]. UTI is one of the most common bacterial infections, annually affecting 150 million people worldwide [3]. In 2010, the direct and indirect costs of UTI in the United States amounted to approximately $2.3 billion [4]. The diagnosis of UTI depends on the execution of a urinary culture for the identification of bacterial species in the presence of clinical symptoms [5]. Consequently, UTI diagnosis, and subsequent treatment, are often missed or delayed due to the 24 to 72 h required to complete a urinary culture process. Rapid screening for urinary tract infection can reduce the costs and effort for medical treatment before it becomes more serious, especially when patients exhibit minor symptoms.

The professional urinary testing process is complicated for most people to accomplish. On the other hand, for those who may not have specific symptoms or who may have trouble describing their symptoms clearly, like infants, children, and the elderly, a rapid and easily operated urinary screening method is an urgent need [6]. The introduction of point-of-care testing (POCT) allows for more timely diagnosis and rapid clinical decisions toward targeted treatment [7]. Urine dipsticks are a prominently used example of a commercially produced POCT tool for rapid urinary infection testing [8]. There is, however, still room to consider and develop a urine-sampling POCT device that is less costly and more user-friendly. Several groups have developed the concept of a cotton-based smart diaper. Cotton, a natural material, provides excellent flexibility and biocompatibility for detection devices. Lin et al. have underscored the particular advantages of a cotton-based testing device by accurately obtaining semi-quantitative information in a buffer system [9]. Seo et al. presented a diaper-embedded and self-powered UTI monitoring sensor module [10]. Couto et al. described an eight-layer microfluidic paper-based device for screening and analysis of multiple biomarkers from urine samples on diapers [11,12].

Above all, there has been an urgent need to integrate urine sampling, testing, and analysis to build a convenient UTI screening solution that would benefit specific, at-risk populations, especially those who are have difficulty clearly describing their symptoms. We felt that novel advances could be made to improve the efficiency of UTI screening by using point-of-care testing (POCT) techniques that simultaneously integrated urine collection, screening, and analysis. In this study, we aimed to develop an accurate, inexpensive, rapid, and easy to use in-vitro diagnostic device (IVD) to detect UTIs in infants and the elderly. Leveraging the characteristics of cotton and using specific biological indicators for bacterial infection, i.e., pH value, leukocyte, and nitrite concentrations in urine, we have developed a diaper-based testing device that integrates sampling and UTI detection in a single, convenient package.

2. Materials and Methods

2.1. Screening Reagents for Urinary Tract Infections (UTI) Detection

For UTI biomarker selection and for screening reagent formulation, we used Hygeia Touch Urinary Tract Infection Test Strips (US FDA listing, Hygeia Touch Inc., Hsinchu, Taiwan). It has been suggested that the use of POCT urine analyzers would increase the quality of urinalysis. With the introduction of commercially available POCT urine analyzers, it may be possible to improve the quality of urinalysis in general practice, but such analyzers must demonstrate good analytical performance and agreement with laboratory standards, and data to support these qualities is still lacking. The Hygeia brand test strips can be used as a quick self-screening aid to detect UTI, for people with symptoms such as fever, back pain, uncomfortable burning or pain upon urinating, and frequent urination. The test strips simultaneously identify three UTI indicators: urinary pH value, leukocyte level, and nitrite level. The screening reagents for each indicator are coated on independent test pads, and act as the reaction zone of each strip.

The screening reagents were formulated for a colorimetric assay to provide unique UTI-associated gradient color changes associated with UTI infection. When the urine being tested contains bacteria, these reagents change in color from light orange to dark green to indicate a high pH value, from light yellow to pink or purple to indicate the abnormal presence of leukocytes, and from light yellow to pink to indicate a high nitrite level. The colorimetric reaction of each reagent is based on chemical reactions with specific components in urine. The leukocyte testing reagent, i.e., 0.5% *w/w* pyrrole amino acid ester (CAS No. 100750-39-8, Santa Cruz Biotechnology, Dallas, TX, USA) + 0.4% *w/w* diazonium salt (CAS No. 101-89-3, MilliporeSigma, St. Louis, MO, USA) detects leukocyte esterase hydrolysis of ester derivatives, the nitrite testing reagent detects the formation of diazonium compounds based on the reaction of nitrite and 4.5% *w/w* p-arsanilic acid (CAS No. 98-50-0, MilliporeSigma, St. Louis, MO, USA), and the pH testing reagent uses dual indicators, i.e., 0.5% *w/w* methyl red sodium salt (CAS No. 845-10-3, MilliporeSigma, St. Louis, MO, USA) + 5% *w/w* bromthymol blue (CAS No. 76-59-5, Tokyo Chemical Industry, Tokyo, Japan). We immersed the test strip into reagents for 5 min and then allowed it to dry for 24 h.

2.2. *Clinical Evaluation for UTI Test Strip*

A comparison test was performed to evaluate screening reagent capability. A clinical evaluation (N = 49) of Hygeia Touch Urinary Tract Infection Test Strips was used to evaluate the accuracy of the testing reagents, which were then integrated into our diaper-based testing device. The urine test strip detection results were compared to the laboratory analysis from Artemis Hospital (Kaohsiung, Taiwan) as our laboratory reference standard. UTI diagnosis is based on the detection of pathogens in the presence of clinical symptoms. However, laboratory urinalysis, not clinical diagnosis, was selected as the reference standard in this study because clinical diagnosis of UTI is not necessarily related to the presence of nitrite, leukocyte, or high alkalinity level in urine. The standard was calibrated prior to executing the study. All urine testing and results reading procedures were performed at Artemis Hospital (Kaohsiung, Taiwan). The study flowchart is presented in Figure 1. Forty-nine urine samples were collected from patients who delivered a urine sample for a routine investigation. Women above 18 years old were included, and those with severe comorbidities were excluded. Each subject was enrolled only once. Three subjects without complete urine analysis data were excluded from analysis.

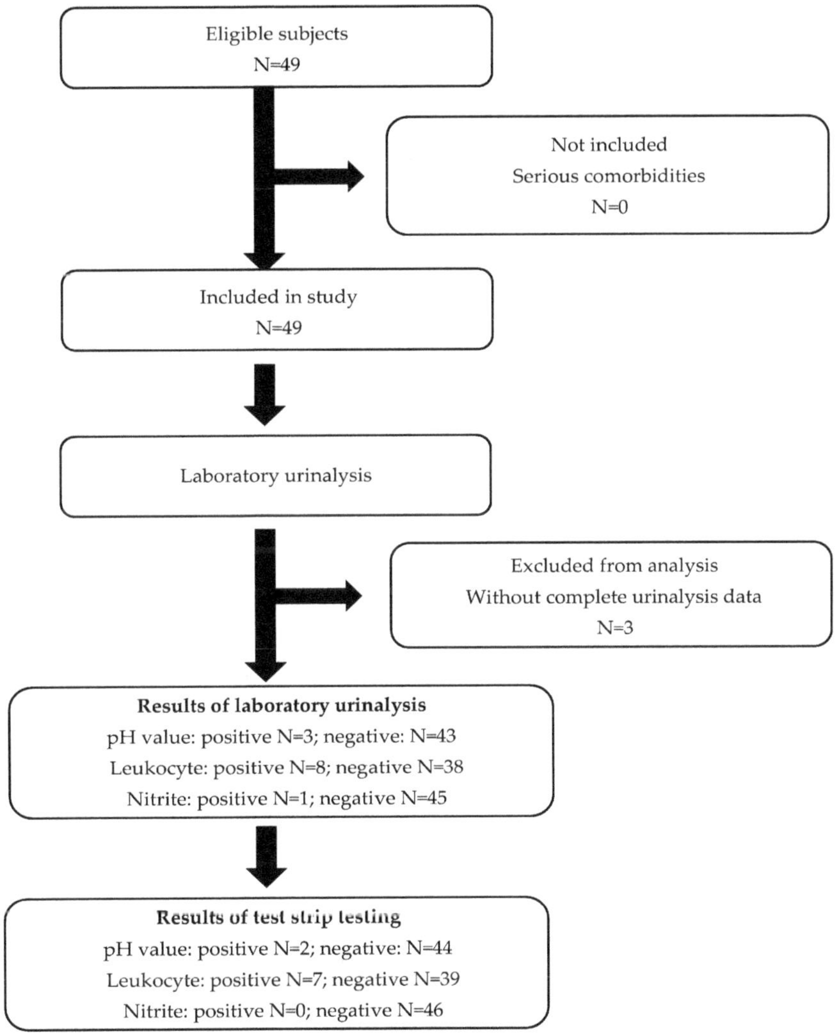

Figure 1. An overview of the clinical evaluation and process flow. Urine samples were provided by all subjects for comparative analysis. Samples were evaluated using typical laboratory urinalysis and test strips, and results from both methods were compared.

2.3. Diaper-Based Testing Device Fabrication

The diaper-based testing device was designed to provide multiple biomarker detection values with a focus on accuracy, ease-of-use, and cost-effectiveness. A schematic of the fabrication process is provided in Figure 2A. The diaper-based testing device comprised two primary parts: (1) a test strip (Hygeia Touch Inc., Hsinchu, Taiwan); and, (2) a multi-layered cotton diaper with an outer layer of plastic substrate [9]. As shown in Figure 2B, urine was deposited onto the first layer of cotton. The function of the first layer was to pass the liquid to the subsequent absorbent layer. The reverse side of this layer was hydrophobic and prevented urine backflow toward the skin. The function of the second layer was to absorb the liquid sample and deliver it to the third layer. The third layer was constructed of the same type of cotton as the first layer—it absorbed urine, passed urine to the outer hydrophobic side, and prevented backflow toward the second layer. The biomarker-impregnated test strips were implanted between this layer and the final plastic back layer, which was designed to keep liquid inside without leaving the diaper. We leveraged these material characteristics to create effective, one-directional flow for urine sample delivery, allowing fluid to pass to the target test strips while removing impurities. As samples reached the test strips, a colorimetric reaction ensued. The entire procedure, from sample to test, was completed in a single step. This facilitated urine sampling and testing in real time.

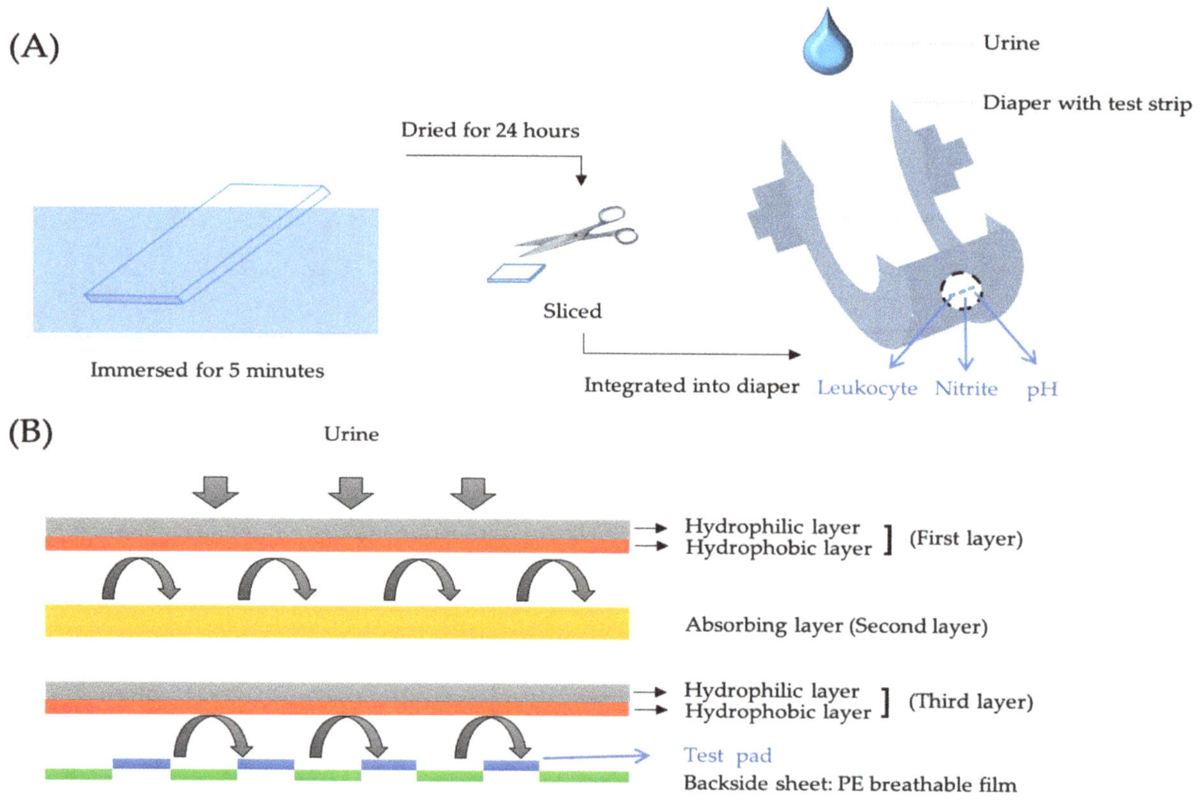

Figure 2. (**A**) The fabrication process for our diaper-based testing device. The test strip was immersed into various diagnostic reagents for 5 min and dried for 24 h at room temperature. The test strip was integrated into a diaper, attached to the breathable plastic backside sheet, allowed the results to be visible from the outside. (**B**) Schematic of the structure of our diaper-based testing device. The test strip was integrated between the third layer and backside sheet, which allowed the colorimetric result to be visible from the outside.

2.4. Statistics Analysis

We analyzed, evaluated, and compared data collected from test strips and regular laboratory urinalysis method from Artemis Hospital. To compare UTI test strip performance regarding pH value, leukocyte level, and nitrite level with the laboratory reference standard, we used contingency (2×2) tables to calculate sensitivity, specificity, agreement, positive predictive value (PPV), negative predictive value (NPV). Sensitivity referred to how often the test was positive when the result of the laboratory reference standard was positive, while specificity indicated how often the test was negative when the result of the laboratory reference standard was negative. The overall agreement was defined as the consistent probability between the test strip results and the laboratory reference standard results. The positive predictive value (PPV) was defined as the probability that a positive result truly indicated the presence of infection. The negative predictive value (NPV) was the probability that a normal result indicated the patient did not have an infection. Statistical analyses were performed using SPSS computer software (SPSS Inc., Chicago, IL, USA).

3. Results

To evaluate the accuracy of the three UTI detection reagents used in this study, we collaborated with Artemis Hospital to employ Hygeia Touch Urinary Tract Infection Test Strips for preliminary screening. We enrolled patients for eligibility over a two-month period from March 1st, 2018 to April 30th, 2018. During this time, 49 participates agreed to join our study. An overview of subject inclusion and exclusion details is provided in Figure 1. The age of subjects ranged from 22 to 40 years (30.3 ± 4.9 years), and all of them were female. Forty-nine anonymous urine samples from subjects were collected and analyzed. Samples were first analyzed using laboratory-standard methods in Artemis Hospital and then analyzed with urine test strips. Both processes were performed by a well-trained, registered nurse, who was responsible for test strip operation, colorimetric result reading, and data recording. All testing was anonymized.

There were no subjects with severe comorbidities. Therefore, all 49 subjects were enrolled in this study. From the results of laboratory urinalysis, three samples did not have complete nitrite test results, and were excluded from data analysis. The laboratory results indicated that four samples were alkaline ($pH > 8$, indicating bacterial infection), nine samples were leukocyte positive (>5 leukocytes per high power field), and one sample was nitrite positive. From the test strip results, two samples had positive pH values, seven samples were leukocyte positive, and none were nitrite-positive samples. All of the included data were analyzed and are statistically summarized in Table 1. Data includes sensitivity, specificity, PPVs, and NPVs, as well as the agreement for pH, leukocyte, and nitrite values for both the test strip and the reference-standard laboratory urinalysis. By plotting the pairs of sensitivity and corresponding specificity, we obtained a receiver operating characteristic (ROC) curve (Figure 3). Clinical validation of the test strip showed that, for pH value, the specificity, agreement, PPV, and NPV were high (100%, 97.83%, 100%, 97.73%), despite the sensitivity (66.67%). Leukocyte detection showed a similar status, with the specificity, agreement, PPV, NPV of 94.74%, 89.13%, 71.43%, 92.31%, but lower sensitivity (62.5%). For the nitrite test, the specificity, agreement, and NPV showed positive results for the nitrite detection reagent (100%, 97.83%, 97.83%). We were unable to calculate sensitivity and PPV because the sample number for nitrite-positive urine was less for both the laboratory standard and the test strip. As a result, sensitivity and PPV were not applicable for the nitrite test. Since our inclusion criteria did not specifically include patients with UTI, values for pH, leukocyte-, or nitrite-positive urine sample size was too small to reflect sensitivity in both the laboratory urinalysis and the UTI test strip testing. This is because the sensitivity and PPV decrease as prevalence decreases. For a mathematical explanation of this phenomenon, we can use PPV as an example. PPV is defined as (sensitivity $\times$ prevalence)/[(sensitivity $\times$ prevalence) + ((1 $-$ specificity) $\times$ (1 $-$ prevalence))]. Therefore, as prevalence decreases toward zero, the value of (sensitivity $\times$ prevalence) goes towards zero, driving the whole denominator to smaller and smaller values as prevalence decreases. That is to say, if our series had a higher prevalence of UTI, there would be an increase in PPV along with a decrease of NPV. However, our current study demonstrates that when the test strips generated positive results for high pH or leukocytes, urinalysis results showed similar results. These results indicate the applicable potential for clinical adoption of these UTI detection reagents as a tool for UTI screening.

This confirms that the currently tested POCT urine analyzer performed sufficiently well for use in primary care practices.

Table 1. The clinical evaluation summary of urinary tract infections (UTI) detection reagents. Comparisons of pH value, nitrite, and leukocyte concentration between the test strip and clinical laboratory urinalysis are shown. Sensitivity, specificity, agreement, positive predictive value (PPV), and negative predictive value (NPV) were analyzed in this study. (PPV, positive predicted value. NPV, negative predictive value. N, the sample number in each condition.).

		pH Value		
			Laboratory urinalysis (N)	
		Positive	Negative	Total
Test strip (N)	Positive	2	0	2
	Negative	1	43	44
	Total	3	43	46
Validity	**Specificity**	**Agreement**	**PPV**	**NPV**
66.67%	100.00%	97.83%	100.00%	97.73%
		Leukocyte Level		
			Laboratory urinalysis (N)	
		Positive	Negative	Total
Test strip (N)	Positive	5	2	7
	Negative	3	36	39
	Total	8	38	46
Validity	**Specificity**	**Agreement**	**PPV**	**NPV**
62.50%	94.74%	89.13%	71.43%	92.31%
		Nitrite Level		
			Laboratory urinalysis (N)	
		Positive	Negative	Total
Test strip (N)	Positive	0	0	0
	Negative	1	45	46
	Total	1	45	46
Validity	**Specificity**	**Agreement**	**PPV**	**NPV**
N/A	100.00%	97.83%	N/A	97.83%

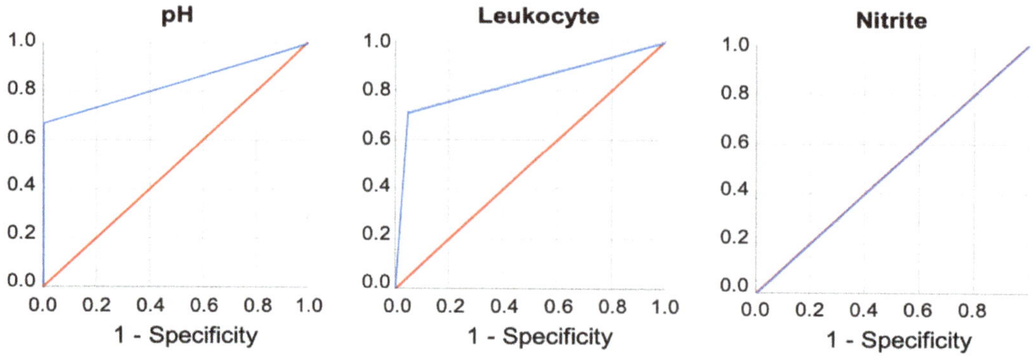

Figure 3. Receiver operating characteristic (ROC) curves of pH, leukocyte, and nitrite. The realization of the receiver operating characteristic (ROC) curve found the area under the curve (AUC) of 0.833 in pH, 0.832 in leukocyte and 0.5 in nitrite.

After evaluating the results from using the UTI detection reagents coated on the UTI test strip, we further developed the diaper-based testing device. The sample volume used was 10 mL. This protocol has been approved by Institutional Review Board of Taipei Veterans General Hospital (IRB 2019-10-001B approved 25 October 2019). The test strips were coated with detection reagents separately and then integrated into the diaper, as shown in Figure 2A. To prevent the reagent from coming into direct contact with human skin, and to provide a better result reading process, the test pad (of the test strip) was embedded into a diaper. The outer surface of the test pad was visible on the outer surface of the diaper. This design allowed for efficient and safe sample collection and readily observable colorimetric results.

Figure 2B is a schematic of the diaper-based testing device construction. In this device, urine contacts the first, initial layer of the diaper and is absorbed so that it flows from one side of that layer to the other side and then to the second layer. The side of the first layer that is away from the body has hydrophobic properties that inhibit urine flow back toward the body. Urine is absorbed into the second absorption layer and then passed to the third layer. The test strip is embedded on the other side of this third layer, so that it absorbs the urine sample. The diaper-based testing device prototype is shown in Figure 4. We fabricated the diaper-based testing device prototype as shown in Figure 4A. The left picture shows the device post-production and demonstrates how the test strip was adhered to the back of the diaper under a transparent layer of plastic, which allows the test pad (of the test strip) to be visible from the outside. Test strips were coated with indicated reagents to detect urinary leukocyte, nitrite, and pH levels (from left to right). Test strips were integrated into the back of the diaper and under a transparent plastic film so that results were visible on the outside of the device. The colorimetric results from case 2 showed no color changes; the device did not detect leukocytes, nitrite, or a pH value of 6 or greater. The colorimetric results from case 4 showed color changes from light yellow to light pink (indicating leukocyte detection), from light yellow to pink (indicating nitrite detection), and from light orange to dark green (indicating the detection of a pH value of 7). The colorimetric results from case 6 showed color changes from light yellow to purple (indicating leukocyte detection), and no other color changes that would indicate the presence of nitrite or a pH value of 6 or greater. After waiting for an hour, we also observed the inside surface of the diaper, to evaluate whether there was any backflow; in Figure 4B, images from inside the diaper show the clean surface, which indicates that the diaper displayed great absorption and prevented backflow. In Table 2, we provide patient demographics to include gender, age symptoms, underlying diseases, results of urinalysis and diaper-based testing device. These results indicate that our test-strip-integrated diaper is suitable for detecting the presence of urine constituents such as nitrite and leukocytes. The embedded test strip design facilitated outside visibility, a user-friendly feature, and did not affect colorimetric reaction efficiency.

Table 2. The demographics of patients enrolled in the diaper-based testing device including gender, age symptoms, underlying diseases, results of urinalysis, and diaper-based testing device results.

	Gender	Age	Symptoms				Underlying Diseases			Urinalysis			Diaper-Based Testing Device		
			Shaking Chills	Dysuria	Increased Urinary Frequency	Flank Pain	DM	Uremia	CKD	pH	Leukocyte	Nitrite	pH	Leukocyte	Nitrite
Case 1	F	84	N	N	N	N	P	P	P	6	N	N	5	N	N
Case 2	F	72	N	N	N	N	N	P	P	6	N	N	6	N	N
Case 3	M	88	N	N	N	N	N	N	N	7	N	N	5	N	N
Case 4	M	67	N	N	N	N	P	N	N	6.5	P	P	7	P	P
Case 5	M	66	N	N	N	N	N	N	N	5.5	N	N	6	N	N
Case 6	F	57	P	P	P	P	N	N	N	6	P	N	6	P	N
Case 7	F	69	N	N	N	N	N	N	N	5	N	N	5	N	N

F: female; M: male; N: negative; P: positive; DM: Diabetes Mellitus; CKD: Chronic Kidney Disease.

The visually recognizable colorimetric results provided by our testing device support its potential for laboratory-based studies, clinical use, and personal use at home. By embedding UTI detection reagents into test strips that were then integrated into a diaper, we created a diaper-based testing device prototype. The colorimetric method provides clear results for caregivers to observe possible UTI, which is especially helpful for individuals who face difficulties expressing symptoms, i.e., infants, children, and the elderly.

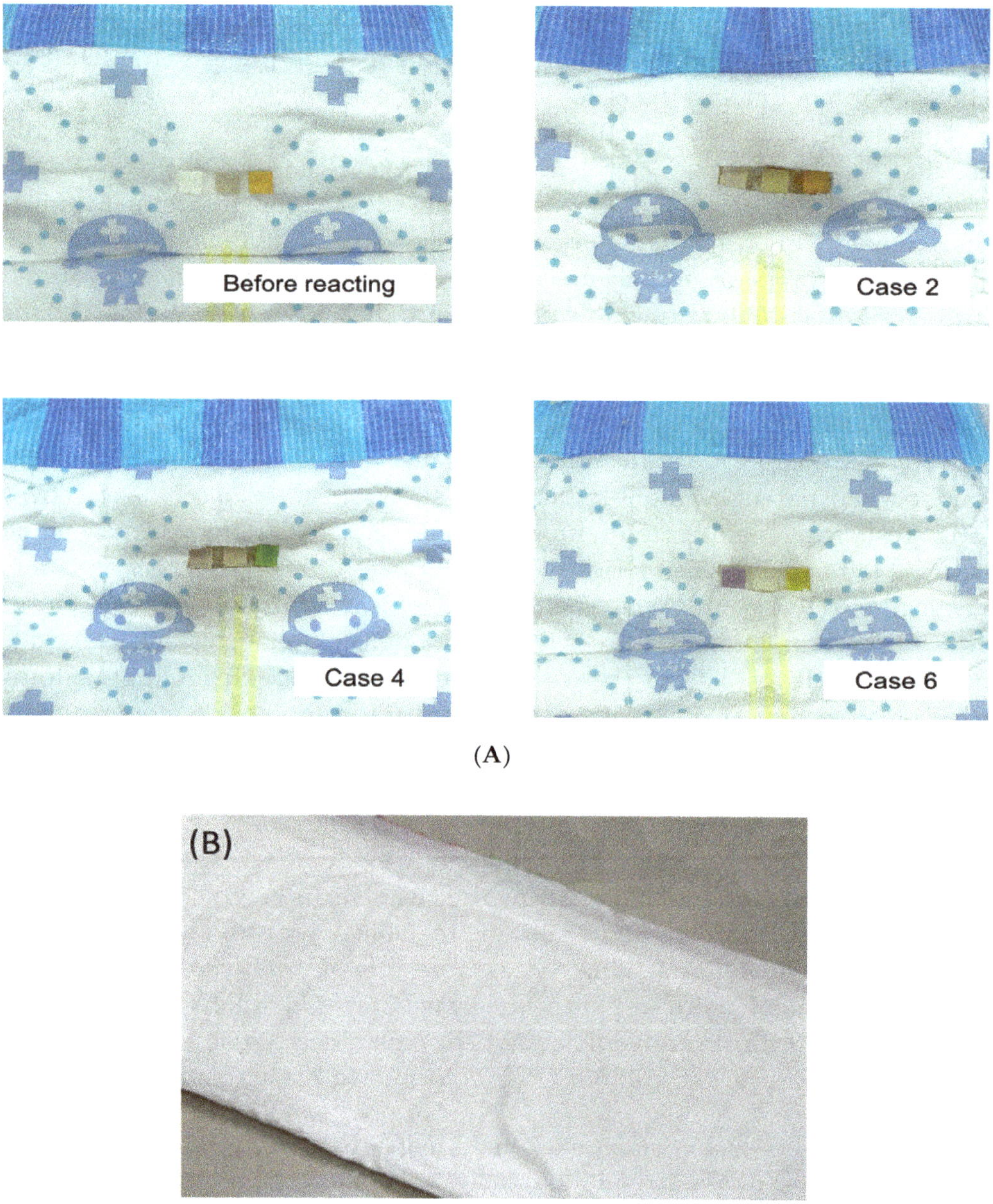

Figure 4. The representative images of the diaper-based testing device prototype. (**A**) Test strips were coated with indicated reagents to detect urinary leukocyte, nitrite, and pH levels (from left to right). The colorimetric results from case 2 showed no color changes. The colorimetric results from case 4 showed positive results for the detection of leukocytes and nitrite. The colorimetric results from case 6 showed positive results for the detection of leukocytes, and no other color changes. (**B**) After reacting for 1 h, no backflow appeared on the inside of the used diaper.

4. Discussion

In this study, it was shown that the UTI screening reagents could be applied in an interesting way to screen for UTI in a variety of populations and across age groups, especially in infants, children, and the elderly. These populations are at high risk of UTI due to consistent diaper wearing, and they may face difficulties expressing symptoms of infection. UTI diagnosis is often missed during physical examinations due to the non-specific symptoms and signs, such as fever, dysuria, frequency, urgency, suprapubic pain, or hematuria in these age groups [13]. It would be particularly useful for them to have a rapid, early-stage, user-friendly approach for UTI screening. For this reason, we created a device that integrated urine collection, biomarker-based screening, and results reading.

Screening and early diagnosis of UTI during infancy is highly recommend, since Infantile UTI possibly is associated with urinary tract malformations and therefore contributes to renal scarring and consecutive chronic kidney disease (CKD) [14]. Notably, integrating the screening reagents into a diaper will help obtain and process urine samples quickly and easily, reduce the risk of using invasive sampling methods, such as transurethral bladder catheterization or suprapubic aspiration. The highest prevalence of UTI is actually in the overall elderly population.

UTI strongly influences not only community-dwelling elderly but also highly functionally impaired long-term care facility residents [15]. The diagnosis of symptomatic UTI in older adults with associated disorders such as Alzheimer's disease, Parkinson's disease, and stroke are extremely challenging [16]. Elderly patients suffering from functional or cognitive impairments have great difficulty communicating localized genitourinary symptoms [2]. Our testing devices may help urine sample collection and bacteriuria screening in these populations [17]. The design of the testing device promoted urine flow to our test strips and facilitated results observation from the outside, which provided considerable convenience for users and caregivers.

Normal urine pH is slightly acidic, ranging from 4.5 to 8.0. A urine pH of 8.5 or 9.0 is indicative of urea-splitting organisms [18]. In a previous study, a portable electronic pH meter was found to provide more accurate results than commonly used dipsticks or test strips [19]. In comparison, our UTI testing reagents were based on colorimetric analysis and demonstrated considerable specificity, agreement, PPV, and NPV, without electrically powered or complicated machine readers. This screening method might be more convenient for general users to read results and perform urinary screening.

For the detection of leukocytes, we compared the analytical performance of our test strip with reagents to other commercially available POCT urine analyzers (see Table 3) [20]. Our test strip demonstrated comparable specificity, NPV, and agreement. The sensitivity and PPV of our test strip were lower than those for other POCT urine analyzers, but this may be due to the fact that few UTI-positive subjects enrolled in our study.

Table 3. Comparisons of leukocyte detection capability of test strips. Comparison of the sensitivity, specificity, PPV, NPV, and agreement for the leukocyte reagent used in this study, and other point-of-care testing (POCT) urine analyzers in the detection of leukocytes.

	Sensitivity (Validity)	Specificity	PPV	NPV	Agreement
Hygeia Touch Test Strip	62.50%	94.74%	71.43%	92.31%	89.13%
Clinitek Status (Siemens)	56%	100%	100%	76%	60.04%
Uryxxon Relax (Macherey Nagel)	94%	98%	97%	96%	91.94%
Urisys 1100 (Roche)	78%	100%	100%	87%	80.67%
Aution micro (Menarini)	94%	98%	97%	96%	91.94%
Aution 11 (Menarini)	93%	96%	94%	96%	89.31%
Urilyzer (Analyticon)	66%	100%	100%	80%	69.05%

For nitrite, our test strip has comparable specificity, agreement, and NPV compared to the reference method [20]. However, the sensitivity and PPV were not applicable for our nitrite tests due to the limited number of nitrite-positive urine samples. The sensitivity of the nitrite-detecting reagent requires more data for better analysis—we believe that increasing the number of study subjects would provide a more convincing result.

There are some limitations to our study. First, we included only a small number of patients, i.e., 46 patients for testing strips (note that only 3, 8, and 1 patients displayed positive results for the detection of pH, leukocyte, and nitrite, respectively, using laboratory urinalysis), and 7 patients for the strip-integrated diaper, which makes it difficult to draw strong conclusions. Second, our approach itself is the difficulty isolating and capturing midstream samples, which would be more ideal for urine test accuracy. Third, although our diaper-based testing device was sterilized following production and both sampling and biomarker detection were executed in a single step, there is still a chance of contamination due to collection under non-sterile conditions. The test strip test area remains stable for two years. The test strips on our diaper-based testing device prototype are stable for at least one month, a timespan that will be improved to two years following additional engineering efforts. Fourth, just like most of other urinary POCT device, our testing device detects a possible UTI, but does not identify the precise casual pathogenic microorganism. Although we have evaluated the UTI detecting reagents, clinical validation of our diaper-integrated test strip requires more clinical evidence to improve the sensitivity and specificity.

Overall, in comparison to conventional detection methods, our diaper-based testing device prototype features many advantages: (1) it detects multiple clinical targets in a single step using one device, which provides better user-friendliness; and, (2) it is inexpensive and can be used as a POCT device with little training or equipment. The novelty of the design is primarily derived from the capacity for simultaneous detection of urine pH, nitrite, and leukocyte levels combined with the complexity for collecting and testing using a single, diaper-based POCT device. Further, we expect this particular diaper-based testing device technology to translate well into the development of a commercial POCT device correlated due to the high degree of technical capability. Notably, this device may offer significant advantages for screening in a variety of areas, including rural/remote areas and long-term healthcare centers.

5. Conclusions

In this study, we demonstrated a diaper-based testing device that is inexpensive, portable, and easy to use. UTI-screening diapers integrated with biomarker-impregnated test strips would offer great potential for use with infants, children, and the elderly. This methodology may be used at home and in short- and long-term healthcare settings and offers promise for convenient UTI screening of individuals in remote and resource-poor areas.

Author Contributions: Conceptualization, C.-F.S. and C.-M.C.; methodology, W.-H.S., C.-Y.L. and C.-Y.Y.; validation, W.-H.S., C.-Y.L., C.-Y.Y., C.-H.C. and Y.-T.T.; formal analysis, W.-H.S., C.-Y.L., C.-Y.Y., C.-H.C. and Y.-T.T.; investigation, W.-H.S., C.-Y.L., C.-Y.Y., C.-H.C., Y.-T.T.; resources, C.-F.S. and C.-M.C.; data curation, all authors; writing—original draft preparation, W.-H.S., C.-F.S. and C.-M.C.; writing—review and editing, all authors; visualization, W.-H.S. and C.-Y.Y.; supervision, C.-F.S. and C.-M.C.; project administration, C.-F.S. and C.-M.C.; funding acquisition, C.-M.C. All authors have read and agreed to the published version of the manuscript.

References

1. Heilberg, I.P.; Schor, N. Diagnosis and clinical management of urinary tract infection. *Rev. Assoc. Med. Bras.* **2003**, *49*, 109–116. [CrossRef] [PubMed]
2. Geerlings, S.E. Clinical Presentations and Epidemiology of Urinary Tract Infections. *Microbiol. Spectr.* **2017**, 27–40. [CrossRef]
3. Flores-Mireles, A.L.; Walker, J.N.; Caparon, M.; Hultgren, S.J. Urinary tract infections: Epidemiology, mechanisms of infection and treatment options. *Nat. Rev. Microbiol.* **2015**, *13*, 269–284. [CrossRef] [PubMed]
4. Foxman, B. The epidemiology of urinary tract infection. *Nat. Rev. Urol.* **2010**, *7*, 653–660. [CrossRef] [PubMed]
5. Schmiemann, G.; Kniehl, E.; Gebhardt, K.; Matejczyk, M.M.; Hummers-Pradier, E. The diagnosis of urinary tract infection: A systematic review. *Dtsch. Arztebl. Int.* **2010**, *107*, 361–367. [CrossRef] [PubMed]
6. Holm, A.; Aabenhus, R. Urine sampling techniques in symptomatic primary-care patients: A diagnostic accuracy review. *BMC Fam. Pract.* **2016**, *17*, 72. [CrossRef] [PubMed]

7. Weir, N.M.; Pattison, S.H.; Kearney, P.; Stafford, B.; Gormley, G.J.; Crockard, M.A.; Gilpin, D.F.; Tunney, M.M.; Hughes, C.M. Criteria required for an acceptable point-of-care test for UTI detection: Obtaining consensus using the Delphi technique. *PLoS ONE* **2018**, *13*, e0198595. [CrossRef] [PubMed]
8. Mambatta, A.K.; Jayarajan, J.; Rashme, V.L.; Harini, S.; Menon, S.; Kuppusamy, J. Reliability of dipstick assay in predicting urinary tract infection. *J. Fam. Med. Prim. Care* **2015**, *4*, 265–268. [CrossRef] [PubMed]
9. Lin, S.C.; Hsu, M.Y.; Kuan, C.M.; Wang, H.K.; Chang, C.L.; Tseng, F.G.; Cheng, C.M. Cotton-based diagnostic devices. *Sci. Rep.* **2014**, *4*, 6976. [CrossRef] [PubMed]
10. Seo, W.; Yu, W.; Tan, T.; Ziaie, B.; Jung, B. Diaper-Embedded Urinary Tract Infection Monitoring Sensor Module Powered by Urine-Activated Batteries. *IEEE Trans Biomed. Circuits Syst.* **2017**, *11*, 681–691. [CrossRef] [PubMed]
11. Couto, A.; Dong, T. Design of a microfluidic paper-based device for analysis of biomarkers from urine samples on diapers. *Conf. Proc. IEEE Eng. Med. Biol. Soc.* **2017**, 181–184.
12. Chen, C.; Dong, T. Microfluidic paper-based analytical devices for colorimetric detection of urinary tract infection biomarkers on adult diapers. *Conf. Proc. IEEE Eng. Med. Biol. Soc.* **2015**, 5892–5895.
13. Zorc, J.J.; Kiddoo, D.A.; Shaw, K.N. Diagnosis and management of pediatric urinary tract infections. *Clin. Microbiol. Rev.* **2005**, *18*, 417–422. [CrossRef]
14. Okarska-Napierala, M.; Wasilewska, A.; Kuchar, E. Urinary tract infection in children: Diagnosis, treatment, imaging—Comparison of current guidelines. *J. Pediatr. Urol.* **2017**, *13*, 567–573. [CrossRef]
15. Nicolle, L.E. Urinary Tract Infections in the Older Adult. *Clin. Geriatr. Med.* **2016**, *32*, 523–538. [CrossRef] [PubMed]
16. Rowe, T.A.; Juthani-Mehta, M. Diagnosis and management of urinary tract infection in older adults. *Infect. Dis. Clin. N. Am.* **2014**, *28*, 75–89. [CrossRef] [PubMed]
17. Detweiler, K.; Mayers, D.; Fletcher, S.G. Bacteruria and Urinary Tract Infections in the Elderly. *Urol. Clin. N. Am* **2015**, *42*, 561–568. [CrossRef] [PubMed]
18. Bono, M.J.; Reygaert, W.C. Urinary Tract Infection. In *StatPearls*; StatPearls Publishing LLC.: Treasure Island, FL, USA, 2020.
19. De Coninck, V.; Keller, E.X.; Rodríguez-Monsalve, M.; Doizi, S.; Audouin, M.; Haymann, J.-P.; Traxer, O. Evaluation of a Portable Urinary pH Meter and Reagent Strips. *J. Endourol.* **2018**, *32*, 647–652. [CrossRef] [PubMed]
20. Schot, M.J.C.; van Delft, S.; Kooijman-Buiting, A.M.J.; de Wit, N.J.; Hopstaken, R.M. Analytical performance, agreement and user-friendliness of six point-of-care testing urine analysers for urinary tract infection in general practice. *BMJ Open* **2015**, *5*, e006857. [CrossRef] [PubMed]

3

CO_2 Laser Photoacoustic Spectrometer for Measuring Acetone in the Breath of Lung Cancer Patients

Mitrayana [1,*], Donni Kis Apriyanto [2] and Mirza Satriawan [1]

1 Department of Physics, Universitas Gadjah Mada, Yogyakarta 55281, Indonesia; mirza@ugm.ac.id
2 Department of Physics, University of Lampung, Bandar Lampung 35141, Indonesia; donni.kis@fmipa.unila.ac.id
* Correspondence: mitrayana@ugm.ac.id

Abstract: A CO_2 laser has the advantages of being high in power and having many laser lines in the 9–11 μm infrared region. Thus, a CO_2 laser photoacoustic spectrometer (PAS) can have a multi-component measurement capability for many gas compounds that have non-zero absorption coefficients at the laser lines, and therefore can be applied for measuring several volatile organic compounds (VOCs) in the human breath. We have developed a CO_2 laser PAS system for detecting acetone in the human breath. Although acetone has small absorption coefficients at the CO_2 laser lines, our PAS system was able to obtain strong photoacoustic (PA) signals at several CO_2 laser lines, with the strongest one being at the 10P20 line. Since at the 10P20 line, ethylene and ammonia also have significant absorption coefficients, these two gases have to be included in a multi-component measurement with acetone. We obtained the lowest detection limit of our system for the ethylene, acetone, and ammonia are 6 ppbv, 11 ppbv, and 31 ppbv, respectively. We applied our PAS system to measure these three VOCs in the breath of three groups of subjects, i.e., patients with lung cancer disease, patients with other lung diseases, and healthy volunteers.

Keywords: lung cancer; acetone; volatile organic compounds; CO_2 laser photoacoustic

---

1. Introduction

In the last several decades, the gas chromatography - mass spectrometry (GC-MS) method has become the common method used for the study of the volatile organic compound (VOC) in the human breath [1,2]. Unfortunately, the GC-MS method is considered not practical, needs thorough sample preparation and experts for operation [3]. It method is also unreliable for detecting gas concentration less than ppbv. Moreover, the detection of these VOC gases needs to be performed in a one-time setup for several gases, which is difficult to be realized in the GC-MS method. These reasons motivate many scientists to develop more practical and highly sensitive tools for detecting VOCs in human breath. Some of those tools are enhancement and perfection of the mass spectroscopy methods, like the Selected Ion Flow Tube (SIFT)-MS [4,5], and the Proton Transfer Reaction (PTR)—MS [6]. Other use different approach, like the laser spectroscopy method, that uses the electromagnetic radiation absorption of the targeted gas compound. The sensitivity of the detection in the laser spectroscopy method can be increased using some methods, like Multi-pass Cell Spectroscopy [3], Cavity Ring-Down Spectroscopy (CRDS) [7], and Photo Acoustic Spectroscopy [8].

Photoacoustic spectroscopy (PAS) method is considered to be reliable in detecting trace gases directly with simple sample preparation [9]. PAS is based on the concept of generating acoustic pressure waves from certain targeted gas molecules [9]. The molecules absorbed electromagnetic radiation and released the energy in the form of collisions to other surrounding molecules, and this will then heat the surrounding gas. Modulating the electromagnetic radiation at acoustic frequency will modulate the heat at the same frequency and thus creating acoustic pressure waves, which can be detected using microphones. In order to increase the sensitivity of the microphone detection, the whole process of acoustic pressure waves generation should take place inside an acoustic resonance cell, i.e., the photoacoustic cell. If the modulated acoustic waves have the same frequency as the resonance frequency of the PA cell, the acoustic signal detected by the microphone will increase. The targeted gas may have large absorption coefficients at certain characteristic wavelengths, thus by using radiation source whose wavelength is match with the characteristic wavelength of the targeted gas, one can selectively detect the targeted gas compound. For the infrared spectrum region, these characteristic wavelengths correspond to the vibrational frequencies of the gas compound. The produced PA signal is proportional to the targeted gas concentration, the gas absorption coefficient, and the power of the radiation source. Even though usually one uses the characteristic wavelength of the targeted gas, it is actually possible to use other wavelength to produce the PA signal, as long as the gas has non-zero absorption coefficient at that wavelength. But in this case, the selectivity capability is loss.

In the last two decades, there have been many studies on the PAS method with various radiation sources for detecting several VOCs in human breath. Among the radiation sources for the PAS system, the CO_2 laser has many advantages of being high in power with many easily tunable laser lines in the infrared region. There are several reports on the measurement of VOCs in the human breath using a CO_2 laser PAS system, especially for measuring ethylene and ammonia [10–17]. Those are because the ethylene and ammonia have strong absorption coefficients at several CO_2 laser lines. Ammonia is one of the major compound in the human breath, with a typical concentration in human breath around 422–2389 ppbv [18]. An increased concentration of ammonia in the human breath is thought to be related to several diseases like a renal failure [19], liver dysfunction [20], and Alzheimer's disease. Dumitras, et. al. have measured the absorption coefficient of ammonia at several CO_2 laser lines, with the largest is $\alpha = 57.12$ cm^{-1} atm^{-1} at 9R30 line [12]. Unlike ammonia, ethylene occurs in smaller amounts in the human breath, but its concentration in a healthy human can reach several tens ppbv [21]. The trace of ethylene has been measured using the CO_2 laser PAS system for many applications because one of the strongest absorption coefficients of ethylene coincides with the CO_2 laser line, i.e., the 10P14 where $\alpha = 30.4$ cm^{-1} atm^{-1}. An increase in ethylene breath concentration is linked to oxidative stress in a person, like in patients on hemodialysis [16], inflammatory disorder [22], and ultraviolet damage of the skin [23]. This ethylene production has been attributed to the lipid peroxidation [22].

A multicomponent detection of breath VOCs using the CO_2 laser PAS system was first done by Popa et al., who have measured ammonia and ethylene from patient breath with renal failure [15]. Recently, Popa et al. have used a CO_2 laser PAS system for multi-component detection of carbon dioxide, ammonia, ethanol, methanol, and ethylene in the mouth breathing vs nasal breathing study [24]. Ammonia, ethanol, methanol, and ethylene are among major VOCs in human breath with a typical concentration of up to 100 ppbv. Besides these four gases, other major breath VOCs with typical concentration up to 100 ppbv are methane, hydrogen sulfide, carbon monoxide, acetone, and isoprene. Base on IR spectrum data from NIST [25], among these other VOCs, acetone has significant, although small absorption coefficient at the CO_2 laser lines. Acetone has a characteristic absorption coefficient $\alpha = 0.27$ cm^{-1} atm^{-1} (calculated from acetone infrared absorbance spectrum in [25]) at the wavelength of 9.166 μm, corresponds to a weak 9R42 line of the CO_2 laser. In the 10–11 μm region, acetone has a small but non-zero absorption coefficient around $\alpha = 0.1$ cm^{-1} atm^{-1} [25]. Together with its large typical concentration in the breath, acetone should be detectable using the CO_2 laser PAS system.

There have been many studies regarding acetone concentration in the human breath. Turner, et al., using the SIFT-MS method, measured the breath acetone concentrations in the healthy human, the breath acetone concentration in healthy person falls in the range 148 to 2744 ppbv [26]. Schwarz et al. have studied the variations of breath acetone concentrations with age, gender and body-mass index (acetone concentration range: 281 ppbv to 1246 ppbv for subjects with no dietary control) [27]. Spanel et al. have shown that breath acetone has a wide variation of concentration due to diurnal increase and varying diet [28]. With this wide variation of concentration in human breath, it is debatable whether acetone can be used as a biomarker of some disease.

Nevertheless, breath acetone has been considered as a potential biomarker of some diseases. For example, it is known that there is a significant increase of acetone concentration in the breath of a patient with diabetes [29,30], There have been many studies using many methods for detecting acetone in human breath. Among those many methods, only Tyas et al. that has reported the use of CO_2 laser PAS for measuring breath acetone concentration, where they measured the acetone concentration in the breath of a patient with type II diabetes mellitus, and obtained increased acetone concentration on the breath of type II diabetes mellitus patients with acetone concentration in the range of 1.01–1.62 ppmv compared to 0.15–0.85 ppmv in the healthy group [31]. Another interesting case is the acetone concentration in the breath of a patient with a lung cancer disease. There are various conflicting reports in the literature about the concentration of acetone in the breath of lung cancer patients. Bajtarevic et al. reported that the acetone concentration in the breath of lung cancer patients is somewhat less than in healthy patients [32]. Oppositely, Ulanowska et al. reported that the acetone concentration is relatively high in the breath of lung cancer patients compared to healthy patients [33]. Kischkel et al., on the other hand, reported a significantly larger acetone concentration in the breath of lung cancer patients compared to the smokers, but not significantly larger compared to the healthy patient [34].

In this paper, we present our study of using CO_2 laser PAS system to detect acetone, and its application for detecting breath acetone in the lung cancer patients. Even though acetone has some large absorption coefficient at the 9R42 CO_2 lines, we did not use this line for detecting acetone, since at that line the ethanol and methanol have strong absorption coefficients also ($\alpha = 2.0$ cm^{-1} atm^{-1} and 0.1 cm^{-1} atm^{-1}, respectively [25]), moreover, the 9R42 CO_2 laser line had relatively low power. Instead, we used the strongest line of the CO2 laser, i.e., the 10P20 lines for detecting acetone. Since at 10P20 ammonia and ethylene also had strong absorption coefficients ($\alpha = 0.2$ cm^{-1} atm^{-1} and 1.84 cm^{-1} atm^{-1}, respectively [12,35]), we included these two gases in a multicomponent measurement together with the acetone. We chose the 10R14 and 10P14, where the ammonia and ethylene had strong absorption coefficients [12,35], while other major breath compounds had relatively small ones [25]. In the measurement of a sample that has many compounds like in the breath sample, one has to include all compounds that have non zero absorption coefficients at the laser lines that being used. The PA signal recorded at a line comes from the PA signal contribution from several gas compounds. For N gas compounds with a non zero absorption coefficient, one needs at least N laser lines where the N gas should have different absorption coefficients on those laser lines.

This study aims to show the possibility of detecting acetone, using the CO_2 laser PAS system, together with ethylene and ammonia in a multi-component measurement setup, with its real-life application in the detection of breath acetone from lung cancer patients. Ethylene and ammonia in the breath are not directly related to lung cancer disease. Their inclusion in the measurement was required by the multicomponent PAS method, as described above.

As a comparison we also took breath samples from patients who have other lung diseases and from healthy patients (confirmed by their medical record). We only used a limited number of patients for this study: eleven patients who have lung cancer disease, nine patients who have other lung diseases, and ten healthy volunteers. The lung cancer patients were selected from the lung cancer patients of the Sardjito Hospital that did not have other lung disease. They did not have diabetes, renal disease, or inflammatory disorder. The patients who had other lung disease had bronchitis, pneumonia, or asthma, with no known additional chronic diseases. All non-healthy subjects were patients of Dr. Sardjito Hospital in Yogyakarta, Indonesia, and the ethical committee of Dr. Sardjito Hospital approved this study. Due to a limited number of patients and volunteers involved, this study was not aimed to show acetone as a potential biomarker for lung cancer.

2. Materials and Methods

The schematic of our lab-built CO_2 laser PAS system is shown in Figure 1. The three main components of the system include the CO_2 laser system, the photoacoustic (PA) cell system, and the electronics system (lock-in amplifier and the data acquisition interface).

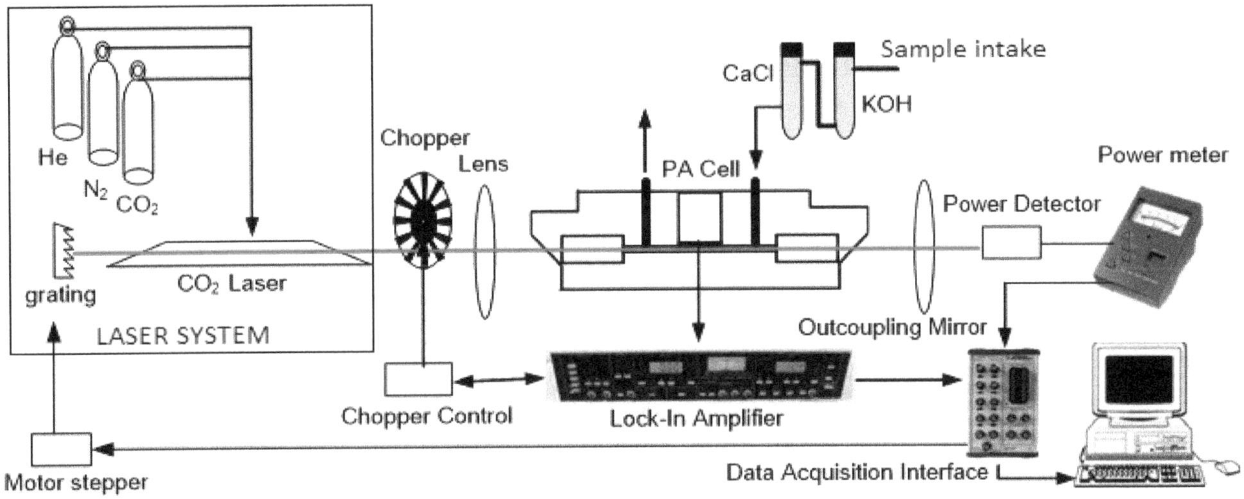

Figure 1. Schematic of the CO_2 laser photoacoustic spectrometer.

Our CO_2 laser was an axial flowing type gas laser, operating on a continuous wave mode at a tunable frequency using a grating, emitting radiation from many CO_2 lines in the 9–11 μm regions. The CO_2 laser used He, N_2, and CO_2 gases as active laser components, that were kept at a pressure of 30 mbar, 50 mbar, and 50 mbar, respectively. A power supply (HCN 350-20.000) was used to create an electrical discharge to excite the active laser gases. To optimize the laser power, there were several factors to be considered, namely setting the laser tube position alignment with the PA cell, controlling the composition ratio of the active ingredient of the CO_2 laser, i.e., He, N_2, and CO_2, and the voltage and current regulation of the CO_2 laser operation. For the laser operation, the current is set at 14.79 mA and the voltage at 9.61 kV with a negative polarity.

We used a PA cell with an intra-cavity setup where the cell was put inside the laser resonator. In this way, the laser light passed the PA cell several times, increasing the chance of laser light absorption by the gases inside the cell. The PA cell geometry was an H-type cylinder with a buffer at both ends that had windows positioned at a Brewster angle. The cylinder length was 100 mm, with its diameter was 6 mm. The buffer length was 50 mm, and its diameter 20 mm. Three microphones (Knowles EK 3033) were positioned in the middle of the cylinder symmetrically flushed on the cylinder wall. A chopper was placed in front of the CO_2 laser tube to modulate the laser radiation. The chopping frequency of the chopper should be set to match the acoustic resonance frequency of the PA cell. The three microphones in the PA cell were connected to the lock-in amplifier (EQ & G model 5210) to amplify the signal with the same frequency of the chopper. A Zn Se lens was positioned in between the chopper and the PA cell, for focusing the laser beam into the PA cell. At the far end of the PA cell, after an outcoupling mirror, we positioned a power meter (OPHIR model AN2), for measuring the laser power.

Before applying the PAS system for measuring the VOCs concentration in the human breath, we conducted the calibration and characterization of the PAS system. These included: Scanning the CO_2 laser lines to find the suitable line for acetone, ethylene, and ammonia; plotting the resonance curve to find the resonance frequency and the quality factor, i.e., the Q value of the PA cell; measuring the noise and the background signal; plotting the linearity curves of the PA signal versus the acetone, ethylene, and ammonia concentrations; and determining the lowest detection limit. As a reference standard, the various concentration of acetone, ethylene, and ammonia gases were obtained from the standard dilution process. The ethylene gas was provided by a certified local gas supplier, supplying a standardized concentration with a 99.95% purity. The acetone and ammonia gases were obtained from the standard solutions being vaporized. We performed a standard dilution procedure for those three gases to obtain different concentrations of the gases.

The volunteer's breath was taken by asking them to exhale using their mouth into a container bag (Tedlar bag). Prior to the breath sample taking, the patients were required to not be taking any medication or drug on that day and to not eat anything for at least one hour before the samples were taken. All samples were then taken to the lab where measurements of acetone, ethylene, and ammonia concentrations were taken using the PAS system. Each breath sample was passed through the KOH and $CaCl_2$ scrubber to remove the CO_2 and the water vapor from the sample. The breath gas was then flown into the PA cell for the PA signal measurement after passing through the scrubber.

3. Results and Discussion

The scanning result of the CO_2 laser wavelength with the acetone gases flowing inside the PA cell tube is shown in Figure 2. From Figure 2, it seems that there were several large PA signals at almost all the 10 μm region of the CO_2 laser lines. The largest PA signal in Figure 2 corresponds to the CO_2 laser line 10P20, i.e., at the wavelength of 10.59 μm.

The PA signal would be strong if the generated acoustic signal matched the resonance frequency of the PA cell. Therefore, the frequency modulation or the chopper frequency should be set at the acoustic resonance frequency of the PA cell, which can be found from the PA resonance curve. To produce the PA resonance curve, we filled the PA cell with one of the standard gases to be detected and set the laser grating to the respective line correspond to the strongest PA signal of the gas. The chopper frequency was then varied, and the PA signal was detected and measured by the microphone. The measured PA signal was normalized concerning laser power.

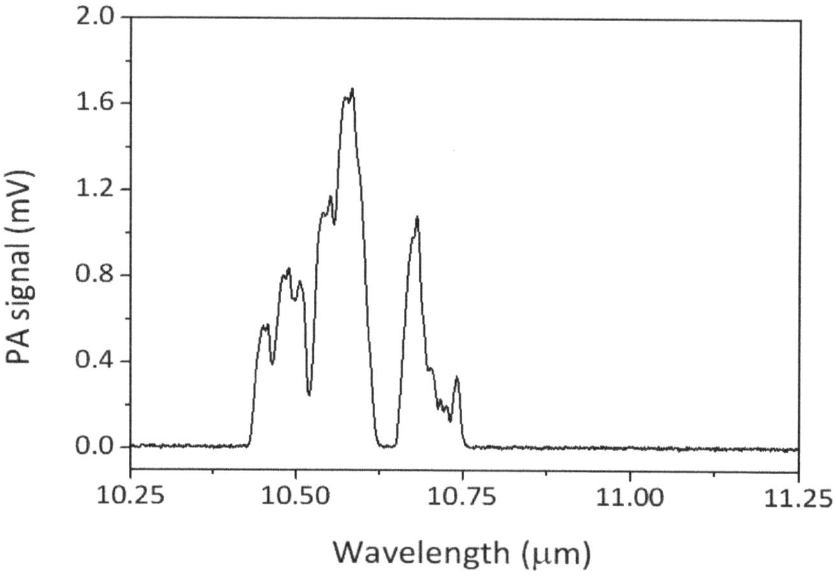

Figure 2. The scanning result of the photoacoustic (PA) signal of the acetone.

Figure 3 shows the resonance curve of the PA cell using acetone as the standard gas, which has a resonance frequency at (1650 ± 5) Hz. The same resonance frequency is also found in the case of ethylene and ammonia. The *Q* value can be obtained from the resonance curve. The greater the *Q* value, the better the photoacoustic cell [36]. The quality factor can be used as a measure of the power loss during the production of the standing waveform from the acoustic waves of every wave cycle [37]. The loss occurs typically as the result of heat conduction and viscosity. In some experiments, loss factor may also result from small leaks on the microphone's installation joint or other sources, diminishing the value of *Q* factor [37]. From Figure 3, we found the quality factor for the acetone gas at line 10P20 is (27 ± 4). For the other two gases, the ethylene at line 10P14, and the ammonia at line 10R14, we found the Q values are (31 ± 6), and (45 ± 10) respectively.

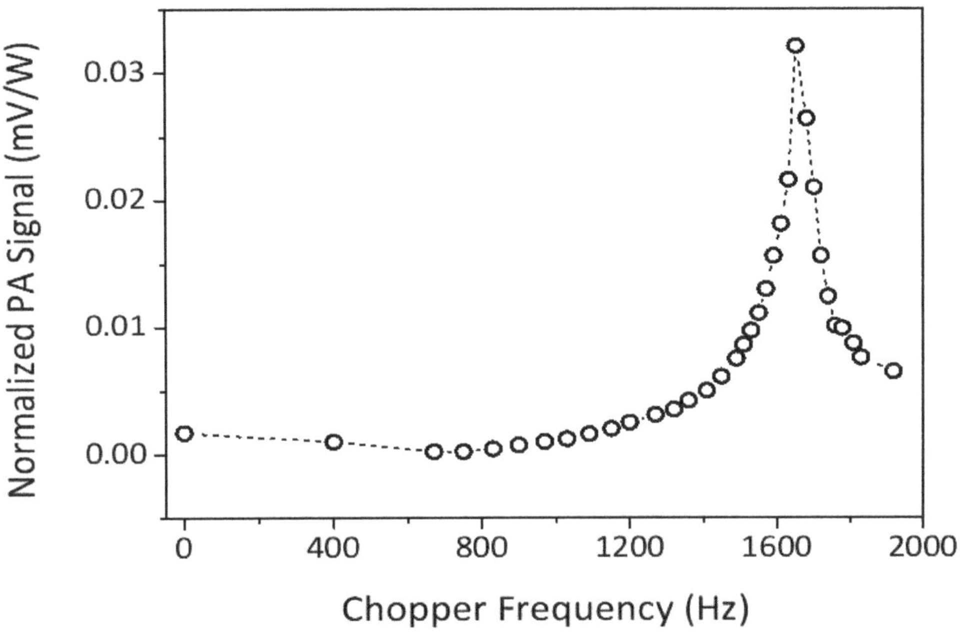

Figure 3. Acetone gas PA signal resonance curve at line 10P20.

The noise in the instrument comes mainly from the electronics, i.e., from the microphones and the lock-in amplifier. To measure the noise, we ran the instrument with the CO2 laser is off, and no gases in the PA cell. We measured the noise by measuring the signal from the microphone picked up by the lock-in amplifier, with only electronics running. The noise measured at the resonance frequency was 0.31 $\mu V/\sqrt{Hz}$. This noise determined the lowest detection limit of gas once we got the linear calibration factor and converted the normalized noise voltage into the gas concentration.

To measure the background signal, the PA cavity was filled with inert gas concerning the CO_2 laser (i.e., the N_2). With the CO_2 laser running, and the chopper set at the resonance frequency of the PA cell, we measured the background acoustic signal detected in the microphone. This background signal came primarily from the laser power absorption in the PA cell windows. We obtained the background signal normalized to the laser power for the line 10P14, 10P20, and 10R14 were 3.79 μV/W, 4.31 μV/W, and 4.52 μV/W, respectively. These background signals were subtracted from any PA-signal measurement in those laser lines.

Our PAS system is capable of doing a multi-component measurement, where there is a mixture of several gases inside the PA cell. In this multi-component setup, for each laser line, the generated PA signal is the linear sum of the PA signal from several trace gas components. Thus, the normalized PA signal (the PA signal divided with the laser power for that line) can be written as [38]

$$(V/P)_i = \sum_{j=1}^{N} K_{ij} C_j, \tag{1}$$

where $(V/P)_i$ is the normalized PA signal for the i-th laser line, C_j is the concentration of the j-th trace gas, and K_{ij} is the linear calibration factor, which is proportional to the PA absorption coefficient of the j-th trace gas at the i-th laser line times the PA cell responsivity.

To obtain the multi-component matrix calibration, we plotted the linear response of the PA signal concerning the gas concentration. The CO_2 laser was set at the main absorption line for one of the gas, and the PA signal was then measured for the various concentration of the three gases. The linearity curve of ethylene, acetone, and ammonia gas for the PA signal at 10P14, 10P20, and 10R14, respectively, are given in Figure 4 (there are other linearity curves for each laser line concerning the other two gases that we do not show in the figures). The slopes of the linearity curves were then used to construct the multi-component matrix calibration.

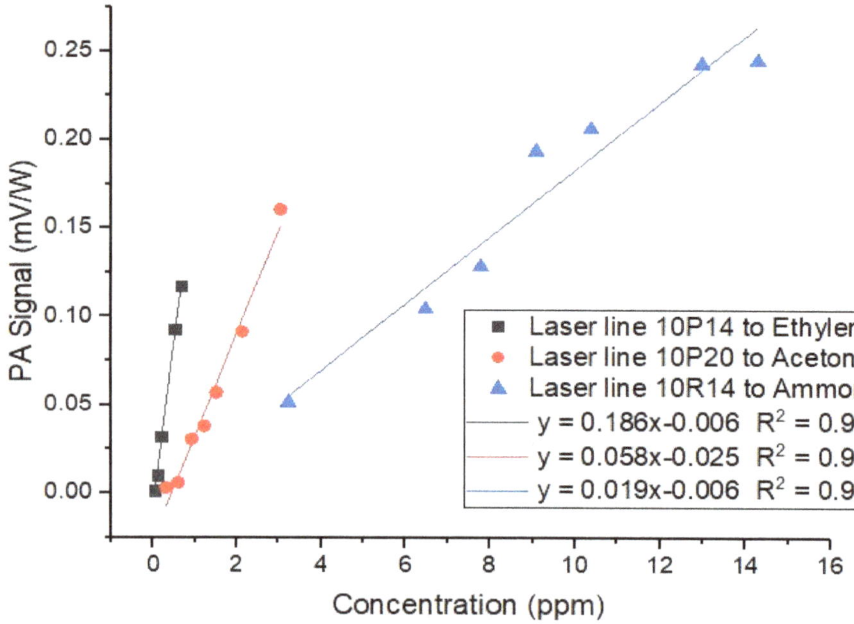

Figure 4. Linearity curves for the normalized PA signal versus ethylene, acetone, and ammonia concentration at 10P14, 10P20, and 10R14 lines, respectively.

The gradients of the linear relation between the normalized PA signal and the gas concentration were used to obtain the calibration factor K_{ij} in Equation 1. We obtained the following relation

$$\begin{pmatrix} (S/P)_1 \\ (S/P)_2 \\ (S/P)_3 \end{pmatrix} = \begin{bmatrix} 0.186 & 0.007 & 0.0011 \\ 0.011 & 0.058 & 0.004 \\ 0.003 & 0.0007 & 0.019 \end{bmatrix} \begin{pmatrix} C_1 \\ C_2 \\ C_3 \end{pmatrix}, \tag{2}$$

where $(S/P)_1$, $(S/P)_2$, and $(S/P)_3$ are the normalized PAS signal for the 10P14, 10P20, and 10R14 lines, respectively (in mV/W). While C_1, C_2, and C_3 are the concentration of the ethylene, acetone, and ammonia gases, respectively (in ppbv). Inverting the matrix in Equation (2) above, we have the relation for the gas concentration as a function of the measured normalized PA signal, as follows

$$\begin{pmatrix} C_1 \\ C_2 \\ C_3 \end{pmatrix} = \begin{bmatrix} 5.416 & -0.614 & -0.171 \\ -1.011 & 17.40 & -3.972 \\ -0.704 & -0.557 & 52.80 \end{bmatrix} \begin{pmatrix} (S/P)_1 \\ (S/P)_2 \\ (S/P)_3 \end{pmatrix}. \tag{3}$$

Equation (3) can be used to determine the concentration of ethylene (C_1), acetone (C_2), and ammonia (C_3) in each breath sample, based on the measured normalized PA signals. The CO_2 laser is then tuned into line 10R14, 10P14, and 10P20 for the measurement of each sample to get the corresponding PA signal. For each line, the measured PA signal (after amplified by the lock-in amplifier) and the laser power will give us the normalized PA signal (*S/P* = PA signal over laser power). The normalized PA signal is then used to obtain the acetone, ethylene, and ammonia concentration of the breath gas samples. Using the matrix in Equation (3) and the noise level obtained above, we found the lowest detection limit for ethylene is 6 ppbv, for acetone is 11 ppbv, and for ammonia gas is 31 ppbv.

The means and the standard deviations of the ethylene, acetone, and ammonia concentrations for all subjects in the three groups are presented in the form of graphics in Figure 5. We performed the Student's t-test for the two means of any two groups for acetone, ethylene, and ammonia concentrations. The results are given in Table 1. From Table 1, we can conclude that there was no significant difference among the three groups for the case of the ethylene and ammonia concentration in their breath. Oppositely, there was a significant difference in the concentration of acetone for patients who have lung cancer, compared to the other two groups.

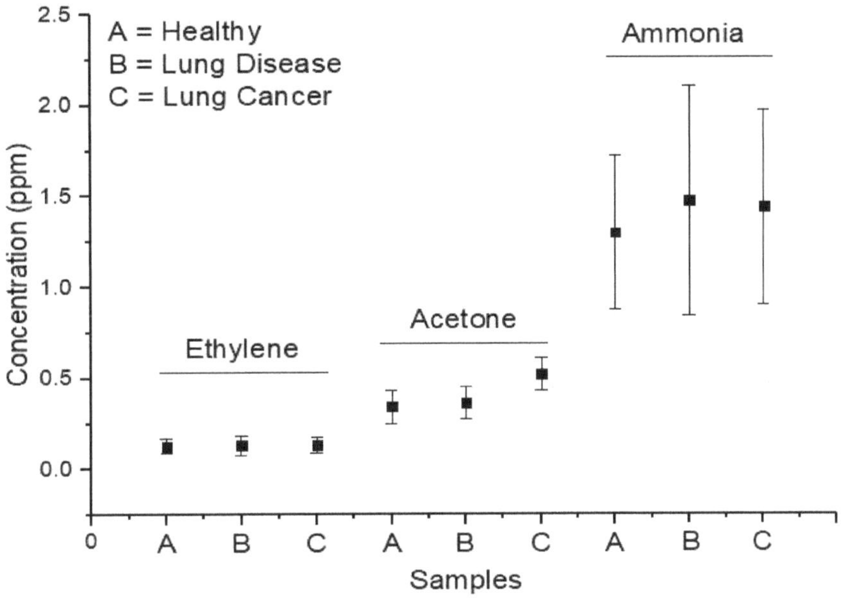

Figure 5. The means and the standard deviations of the ethylene, acetone, and ammonia concentrations for all patients in the three groups.

Table 1. The Student's t-test result for any two groups for the concentration of acetone, ethylene, and ammonia.

Groups Compared for Each Gas	T-Test	P-Value	Note
Acetone			
Lung Cancer vs. Healthy	4.47714	0.000258	Significant at $p < 0.01$
Lung Cancer vs. Other Lung Disease	3.92928	0.000983	Significant at $p < 0.01$
Healthy vs. Other Lung Disease	0.53065	0.602526	Not significant at $p = 0.05$
Ethylene			
Lung Cancer vs. Healthy	0.27623	0.785351	Not significant at $p = 0.05$
Lung Cancer vs. Other Lung Disease	0.03193	0.974876	Not significant at $p = 0.05$
Healthy vs. Other Lung Disease	0.19831	0.845155	Not significant at $p = 0.05$
Ammonia			
Lung Cancer vs. Healthy	0.66217	0.515817	Not significant at $p = 0.05$
Lung Cancer vs. Other Lung Disease	0.13711	0.892466	Not significant at $p = 0.05$
Healthy vs. Other Lung Disease	0.72381	0.479025	Not significant at $p = 0.05$

The use of a CO_2 laser PAS system for detecting trace acetone in human breath is a novelty that worth to be studied further. Base on the available IR absorption data of acetone, there is no significant absorption line of acetone in the 9–11 μm region of the CO_2 laser. From our study, however, it turns out that acetone did produce significant PA signals in almost all the CO_2 laser lines, with the strongest being at 10P20, as shown in Figure 2. Since the strength of the PA signal in Figure 2 seems to be proportional to the CO_2 laser power, there may be hidden broadband IR absorption lines for the acetone in the 10 μm region. Nevertheless, the fact that we got the linearity curve for the acetone (as in Figure 4) shows the validity of our result: that trace acetone concentration can be measured using a CO_2 laser PAS system.

Moreover, the validity of the ability of our CO_2 laser PAS system to measure trace acetone can also be seen from the successful application of our system for measuring the acetone in human breath.

Our measurement results for the acetone concentration in the healthy peoples fall in the range 200–450 ppbv. This result is somewhat smaller than the measurement range obtained by Wang and Sahay in [7], in which they reported that the acetone concentration in the breath of the healthy people varies from 0.39 ppmv to 0.85 ppmv. For the acetone concentration in the breath of patients with lung cancer, our result falls in the range 400–720 ppbv, while for the patients with other lung diseases, the range is 222–487 ppbv. These three ranges are still inside the typical acetone concentration range in normal human breath [26]. Thus, although the above statistical test showed that there is a significant difference between the acetone concentration in the lung cancer group and the other two groups, but to claim acetone as a potential biomarker for lung cancer disease still needs further studies.

For the ethylene and ammonia concentrations, our results for the three groups of subjects do not show any significant difference. The ethylene concentrations from the three groups fall in the range 39–201 ppbv, while the ammonia concentrations from the three groups fall in the range 685–2364 ppbv. The ethylene concentrations range that we obtained is somewhat larger than the typical concentrations in the healthy human. Meanwhile, the ammonia concentrations fall in the same typical range of concentrations in the healthy human.

4. Conclusions

Using a high-power CO_2 laser PAS system, we were able to measure the acetone concentration in the human breath together with measuring the ethylene and ammonia concentrations. Although acetone only has small absorption coefficients in the 10P and 10R CO_2 laser lines, we found a strong PA signal in almost all lines of CO_2 laser around the 10 μm region. We applied our system for measuring acetone, ethylene, and ammonia in three groups of people: Lung cancer patients, patients with other lung diseases, and healthy peoples. This multi-component capability is another advantage feature of our PAS system. For those three gases, the CO_2 laser PAS can measure the three VOCs concentration up to the ppbv level, with the lowest detection limit are 6 ppbv, 11 ppbv, and 31 ppbv for ethylene, acetone, and ammonia, respectively. There is no significant difference in the concentration of ethylene and ammonia among those three groups (with p-value > 0.1). While for acetone, we found a significant difference in its concentration between the lung cancer group and the other two groups (with p-value < 0.01), i.e., the patient with lung cancer has a larger concentration of acetone in their breath compared to the other two groups.

Author Contributions: Conceptualization, M.; Data curation, D.K.A.; Formal analysis, M. and M.S.; Funding acquisition, M.; Investigation, D.K.A.; Methodology, M.; Project administration, M.; Resources, M.; Supervision, M., and M.S.; Validation, M.S.; Visualization, M., and D.K.A.; Writing—original draft, M.; Writing—review and editing, M.S. All authors have read and agreed to the published version of the manuscript.

Acknowledgments: We would like to thank Kuwat Triyana for his valuable suggestions and discussion.

References

1. Ulanowska, A.; Trawiańska, E.; Sawrycki, P.; Buszewski, B. Chemotherapy control by breath profile with application of SPME-GC/MS method. *J. Sep. Sci.* **2012**, *35*, 2908–2913. [CrossRef] [PubMed]
2. Mazzone, P.J. Exhaled breath volatile organic compound biomarkers in lung cancer. *J. Breath Res.* **2012**, *6*, 02716. [CrossRef] [PubMed]
3. Buszewski, B.; Grzywinski, D.; Ligor, T.; Stacewicz, T.; Bielecki, Z.; Wojtas, J. Detection of volatile organic compounds as biomarkers in breath analysis by different analytical techniques. *Bioanalysis* **2013**, *5*, 2287–2306. [CrossRef] [PubMed]
4. Smith, D.; Španěl, P. Selected ion flow tube mass spectrometry (SIFT-MS) for on-line trace gas analysis. *Mass Spectrom. Reviews* **2005**, *24*, 661–700. [CrossRef] [PubMed]

5. Boshier, P.R.; Cushnir, J.R.; Mistry, V.; Knaggs, A.; Španěl, P.; Smith, D.; Hanna, G.B. On-line, real time monitoring of exhaled trace gases by SIFT-MS in the perioperative setting: A feasibility study. *Analyst* **2011**, *136*, 3233–3237. [CrossRef] [PubMed]
6. Cikach, F.S.; Dweik, R.A. Cardiovascular Biomarkers in Exhaled Breath. *Prog. Cardiovasc. Dis.* **2012**, *55*, 34–43. [CrossRef]
7. Wang, C.; Sahay, P. Breath analysis using laser spectroscopic techniques: Breath biomarkers, spectral fingerprints, and detection limits. *Sensors* **2009**, *9*, 8230–8262. [CrossRef]
8. Popa, C.; Petrus, M.; Bratu, A.M. Ammonia and ethylene biomarkers in the respiration of the people with schizophrenia using photoacoustic spectroscopy. *J. Biomed. Opt.* **2015**, *20*, 057006. [CrossRef]
9. Harren, F.J.M.; Mandon, J.; Cristescu, S.M. Photoacoustic Spectroscopy in Trace Gas Monitoring. *Encycl. Anal. Chem.* **2012**, *3*, 1–24.
10. Dumitras, D.C.; Giubileo, G.; Puiu, A. Investigation of human biomarkers in exhaled breath by laser photoacoustic spectroscopy. *Adv. Laser Technol.* **2004**, *5850*, 111–121.
11. Giubileo, G.; Puiu, A.P.; Dumitras, D.C. Detection of ethylene in smokers breath by laser photoacoustic spectroscopy. *Proc. SPIE* **2004**, *5486*, 23–34.
12. Dumitras, D.C.; Dutu, D.C.; Matei, C.; Cernat, R.; Banita, S.; Pathachia, M.; Bratu, A.M.; Petrus, M.; Popa, C. Evaluation of ammonia absorption coefficients by photoacoustic spectroscopy for detection of ammonia levels in human breath. *Laser Phys.* **2011**, *21*, 796–800. [CrossRef]
13. Wang, J.; Zhang, W.; Li, L.; Yu, Q. Breath ammonia detection based on tunable fiber laser photoacoustic spectroscopy. *Appl. Phys. B Lasers Opt.* **2011**, *103*, 263–269. [CrossRef]
14. Puiu, A.; Giubileo, G.; Bangrazi, C. Laser sensors for trace gases in human breath. *Int. J. Environ. Anal. Chem.* **2005**, *85*, 1001–1012. [CrossRef]
15. Popa, C.; Cernat, R.; Dutu, D.C.A.; Matei, C. Ethylene and ammonia traces measurements from the patients' breath with renal failure via LPAS method. *Appl. Phys. B Lasers Optics.* **2011**, *105*, 669–674. [CrossRef]
16. Popa, C.; Bratu, A.M.; Matei, C.; Cernat, R.; Popescu, A.; Dumitras, D.C. Qualitative and quantitative determination of human biomarkers by laser photoacoustic spectroscopy methods. *Laser Phys.* **2011**, *21*, 1336–1342. [CrossRef]
17. Cernat, R.; Matei, C.; Bratu, A.; Popa, C.; Dutu, D.C.A.; Patachia, M.; Petrus, M.; Banita, S.; Dumitras, D.C. Laser photoacoustic spectroscopy method for measurements of trace gas concentration from human breath. *Rom. Report Phyics.* **2010**, *62*, 610–616.
18. Diskin, A.M.; Španěl, P.; Smith, D. Time variation of ammonia, acetone, isoprene and ethanol in breath: A quantitative SIFT-MS study over 30 days. *Physiol. Meas.* **2003**, *24*, 107–119. [CrossRef] [PubMed]
19. Davies, S.; Spanel, P.; Smith, D. Quantitative analysis of ammonia on the breath of patients in end-stage renal failure. *Kidney Int.* **1997**, *52*, 223–228. [CrossRef] [PubMed]
20. Essiet, I. Diagnosis of kidney failure by analysis of the concentration of ammonia in exhaled human breath. *J. Emerg. Trends Eng. Appl. Sci.* **2013**, *4*, 859–862.
21. Petrus, M.; Bratu, A.M.; Popa, C. Spectroscopic analysis of breath ethylene and oxidative stress relation with glycaemic status in type 2 diabetes. *Opt. Quantum Electron.* **2017**, *49*, 1–12. [CrossRef]
22. Paardekooper, L.M.; Bogaart, G.V.D.; Kox, M.; Dingjan, I.; Neerincx, A.H.; Bendix, M.B.; Beest, M.T.; Harren, F.J.M.; Risby, T.; Pickkers, P.; et al. Ethylene, an early marker of systemic inflammation in humans. *Sci. Rep.* **2017**, *7*, 1–10. [CrossRef] [PubMed]
23. Harren, F.J.M.; Berkelmas, R.; Kuiper, K.; Hekkert, S.T.L.; Scheepers, P.; Dekhuijzen, R.; Hollander, P.; Parker, D.H. On-line laser photoacoustic detection of ethene in exhaled air as biomarker of ultraviolet radiation damage of the human skin. *Appl. Phys. Lett.* **1999**, *74*, 1761–1763. [CrossRef]
24. Popa, C.; Bratu, A.M.; Petrus, M. A comparative photoacoustic study of multi gases from human respiration: Mouth breathing vs. nasal breathing. *Microchem. J.* **2018**, *139*, 1700552. [CrossRef]
25. NIST Standard Reference Database Number 69. Available online: https://webbook.nist.gov/chemistry/ (accessed on 24 May 2020).
26. Turner, C.; Španěl, P.; Smith, D. A longitudinal study of ammonia, acetone and propanol in the exhaled breath of 30 subjects using selected ion flow tube mass spectrometry, SIFT-MS. *Physiol. Meas.* **2006**, *27*, 321–337. [CrossRef]

27. Schwarz, K.; Pizzini, A.; Arendacka, B.; Zerlauth, K.; Filipiak, W.; Schmid, A.; Dzien, A.; Neuner, S.; Lechleitner, M.; Burgi, S.S.; et al. Breath acetone - Aspects of normal physiology related to age and gender as determined in a PTR-MS study. *J. Breath Res.* **2009**, *3*, 027003. [CrossRef]
28. Španěl, P.; Dryahina, K.; Rejšková, A.; Chippendale, T.W.E.; Smith, D. Breath acetone concentration; Biological variability and the influence of diet. *Physiol. Meas.* **2011**, *32*, N23–N31. [CrossRef]
29. Wang, C.; Mbi, A.; Shepherd, M. A study on breath acetone in diabetic patients using a cavity ringdown breath analyzer: Exploring correlations of breath acetone with blood glucose and glycohemoglobin A1C. *IEEE Sens. J.* **2010**, *10*, 54–63. [CrossRef]
30. Wang, Z.; Wang, C. Is breath acetone a biomarker of diabetes? A historical review on breath acetone measurements. *J. Breath Res.* **2013**, *7*, 037109. [CrossRef] [PubMed]
31. Tyas, F.H.; Nikita, J.G.; Apriyanto, D.K.; Mitrayana, M.N. The Performance of CO2 Laser Photoacoustic Spectrometer in Concentration Acetone Detection as Biomarker for Diabetes Mellitus Type 2. *J. Phys. Conf. Ser.* **2018**, *1011*, 012056. [CrossRef]
32. Bajtarevic, A.; Ager, C.; Pienz, M.; Klieber, M.; Schwarz, K.; Ligor, M.; Ligor, T.; Filipiak, W.; Denz, H.; Fiegl, M.; et al. Noninvasive detection of lung cancer by analysis of exhaled breath. *BMC Cancer* **2009**, *9*, 348. [CrossRef]
33. Ulanowska, A.; Kowalkowski, T.; Trawińska, E.; Buszewski, B. The application of statistical methods using VOCs to identify patients with lung cancer. *J. Breath Res.* **2011**, *5*, 12–19. [CrossRef] [PubMed]
34. Kischkel, S.; Miekisch, W.; Sawacki, A.; Straker, E.M.; Trefz, P.; Amann, A.; Schubert, J.K. Breath biomarkers for lung cancer detection and assessment of smoking related effects—confounding variables, influence of normalization and statistical algorithms. *Clin. Chim. Acta.* **2010**, *411*, 1637–1644. [CrossRef] [PubMed]
35. Brewer, R.J.; Bruce, C.W.; Mater, J.L. Optoacoustic spectroscopy of C_2H_4 at the 9- and 10-μm $C^{12}O_2{}^{16}$ laser wavelengths. *Appl. Opt.* **1982**, *21*, 4092–4100. [CrossRef] [PubMed]
36. Chang, T.Y. Accurate frequencies and wavelengths of CO2 laser lines. *Opt. Commun.* **1970**, *2*, 77–80. [CrossRef]
37. Rosencwaig, A. Photoacoustic spectroscopy. *Annu. Rev. Biophys. Bioeng.* **1980**, *9*, 31–54. [CrossRef]
38. Dumitras, D.C.; Dutu, D.C.; Matei, C.; Magureanu, A.M.; Petrus, M.; Popa, C. Laser photoacoustic spectroscopy: Principles, instrumentation, and characterization. *J. Optoelectron. Adv. Mater.* **2007**, *21*, 3655–3701.

4

Advances in Sensing Technologies for Monitoring of Bone Health

Seema Rani [1], Sanchita Bandyopadhyay-Ghosh [1,*], Subrata Bandhu Ghosh [1] and Guozhen Liu [2]

1 Engineered Biomedical Materials Research and Innovation Centre (EnBioMatRIC), School of Automobile, Mechanical and Mechatronics Engineering (SAMM), Manipal University Jaipur, Rajasthan 303007, India
2 Graduate School of Biomedical Engineering, Faculty of Engineering, The University of New South Wales, Sydney NSW 2052, Australia
* Correspondence: sanchitab.ghosh@jaipur.manipal.edu

Abstract: Changing lifestyle and food habits are responsible for health problems, especially those related to bone in an aging population. Poor bone health has now become a serious matter of concern for many of us. In order to avoid serious consequences, the early prediction of symptoms and diagnosis of bone diseases have become the need of the hour. From this inspiration, the evolution of different bone health monitoring techniques and measurement methods practiced by researchers and healthcare companies has been discussed. This paper focuses on various types of bone diseases along with the modeling and remodeling phenomena of bones. The evolution of various diagnosis tests for bone health monitoring has been also discussed. Various types of bone turnover markers, their assessment techniques, and recent developments for the monitoring of biochemical markers to diagnose the bone conditions are highlighted. Then, the paper focuses on the potential assessment of the recent sensing techniques (physical sensors and biosensors) that are currently available for bone health monitoring. Considering the importance of electrochemical biosensors in terms of high sensitivity and reliability, specific attention has been given to the recent development of electrochemical biosensors and significance in real-time monitoring of bone health.

Keywords: bone; bone remodeling; bone biomarkers; bone diseases; osteoporosis; biosensors

---

1. Introduction

Growing and living bone tissue forms part of the vertebrate skeleton. Bone is basically a combination of organic matrix, inorganic minerals (calcium phosphate), and vitamins that makes the structural framework. Type I collagen forms approximately 94% of the organic bone matrix. During development of skeleton, modeling and remodeling of bone occur simultaneously [1]. Bone modeling is a slow and continuous formation of bones by connective tissues until the age of adolescence, as bones are not fully developed at the time of birth. Bone remodeling is also a continuous process by which mature bone tissues are removed and replaced with newly synthesized bone. This process is also known as bone turnover. Osteogenic cells, osteoblasts, osteoclasts, and osteocytes are four different type of bone cells involved in progression of bone modeling and remodeling [2]. Osteoblasts are responsible for bone formation; osteoclasts enable the bone resorption. Bone lining cells cover bone surfaces that take minerals directly and release them in bone and osteocytes behave as natural mechanosensors [3]. During osteoblastic bone formation, procollagen I aminioterminal propeptide (PINP) and osteocalcin (non-collagenous protein) are either found in the cavities of bone matrix or in the blood circulation [4,5]. In osteoclastic resorption, collagen is degraded, and small peptide fragments are released in the blood. In addition, bone resorption markers such as cross-linked N-terminal and C-terminal telopeptides of type I collagen are released in urine. The degraded collagen and peptides behave as biochemical markers [6]. The identification of bone biomarkers is important in the timely diagnosis of diseases such as osteoporosis, bone cancer, and infections, with their underlying processes involved. Biomarkers for bone health can be specific cells, enzymes or hormones, and gene products. The accurate recognition and appearance of specific bone biomarkers can be supportive in staging the diagnosis and effective treatment of bone diseases [7]. An electronic device is needed to process this biological information into readable output. However, it is quite challenging to connect such a device to a biological environment due to the complexity of attaching the device and processing the electronic signals. Besides, such devices are costly, require expertise, and can detect bone health only after large amounts of degradation of bone.

In this regard, several studies have reported that more sensitive and real-time assessment tools are required. Research has been continuously going on in the field of biosensors for the assessment of bone health by using biochemical markers present in biological samples such as blood or urine [8]. Biosensors collect information from biofluid and convert it into an electronic signal. In recent years, literature regarding biosensor technology has shown its potential as a tool for the prognostic monitoring of abnormal changes in bone mineral density. The development of bone biosensors is one of the rapidly emerging fields of biosensors. Researchers started exploring this area in the mid-1980s and only after 2005 did work on bone biosensors started gearing up. Later on, a significant rise in publication can be observed (Figure 1), demonstrating the increasing need and importance of working on bone biosensors.

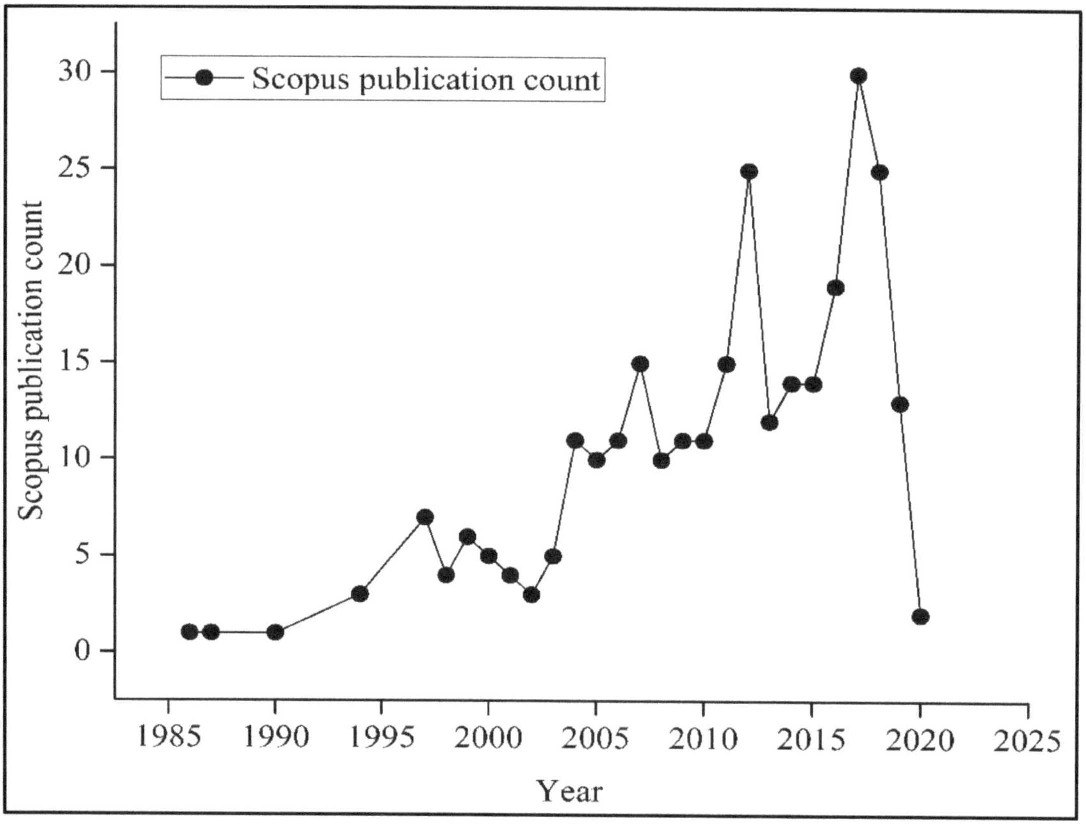

Figure 1. Research documents published on bone biosensors by year (Scopus data up to 15 January 2020).

Against the above background, this paper reviews and provides a potential assessment of recent bone biosensing techniques based on biochemical marker-based sensors. Biosensors for the detection of biomarkers to indicate bone health are increasingly becoming popular, since biomarkers are readily available in serum or urine carrying bone health information. In the following section, various methods for diagnosis based on biochemical changes associated with bone formation and resorption along with the analytical techniques for their measurements have also been reported. Finally, reports of traditional and emerging technologies on the development of biosensors for the assessment of bone health have been discussed.

2. Bone Remodeling

Bone remodeling is a lifelong process of new bone formation and the resorption of old bones. Osteoblasts synthesize and release a range of proteins such as extracellular matrix proteins, collagen, cytokines, and growth factors responsible for bone formation and changes in the extracellular matrix into bone through mineralization [9]. The components available prior to the formation of the organic matrix are called osteoids, and their mineralization is dependent on Ca^{2+} available in plasma [10]. Simultaneously, osteoclast cells accountable for resorption of bone are also found on the small depressions of bone surface. A variety of enzymes produced by osteoclasts dissolve the calcium of bone and the bone matrix. Mineralized bone is broken down, and collagen threads are absorbed by osteoclasts. Bone remodeling is controlled through the interplay between osteoblast differentiation and osteoclast activation and varies with age, as shown in Figure 2 [11]. Bone turnover markers (BTM) give real-time information about the bone remodeling process. It is useful for the monitoring of bone health [12].

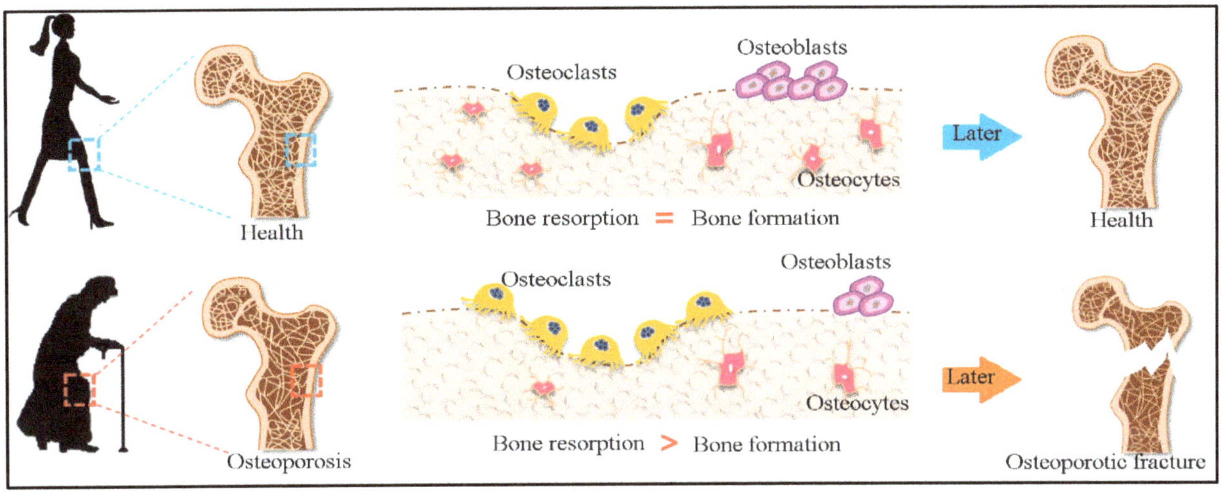

Figure 2. The process of bone remodeling, resulting from continuous bone resorption and bone formation with increasing age, and the balance shifts to more bone resorption than bone formation, causing osteoporosis (reproduced with permission from reference [9]).

3. Bone Diseases

The skeleton stores calcium and minerals for its proper operation. These calcium and minerals are not synthesized by body but taken from food. If enough calcium is not taken in the diet, the stored calcium of bone is utilized for the proper functioning of the body, making bones weaker [13–16]. Metals and minerals such as phosphorus, calcium, magnesium, sodium, potassium, sulfur, iodine, iron, molybdenum, manganese, and zinc are very important for human health. However, little deficiency or an excess of them can upset a delicate health balance of body. In addition, they are considered infamous for encouraging many chronic situations, including carcinogenesis [17,18]. Calcium is the most important mineral for bone strength and health, as a deficiency of calcium may cause various diseases. The body absorbs calcium from food with the help of vitamin D to build bones and teeth; a poor lifelong intake of calcium and vitamin D causes weaker bone growth and leads to disorders [19].

There are various types of bone problems such as osteoporosis, low bone density, osteogenesis imperfecta, and Paget's disease. These diseases of bone make them weak [20]. The World Health Organization (WHO) has reported various bone densities associated with normal and diseased bone [21] and categorized them on the basis of T-score range where the standard deviation (SD) of bone mineral density (BMD) of young adult reference mean indicates bone health. Adding to the above, increasing the metal intoxication and contaminated environment due to human activities has brought significantly adverse effects on health. Toxic metals such as lead can enter into the body, get deposited in different organs including bone, and cause serious damages [22]. Similarly, low concentrations of aluminium, zinc, chromium, arsenic, copper, nickel, and mercury are also found to be toxic for bone cells and may get accumulated in the bone matrix, causing various diseases [23].

The following section covers different type of bone diseases, their underlying mechanisms, and associated problems:

3.1. Osteoporosis

In this silent disease, bone becomes fragile and porous, and it may easily break (Figure 3). During growing age, bone formation is faster than resorption, which makes bone heavier, denser, and stronger. Balance in this process enables proper bone growth, failing which may cause a lowering of bone mass and structural weakening of bone tissues, which leads to osteoporosis and makes them prone to fracture at the wrist, spine, and hip. There are various habits of poor lifestyle such as less physical work, smoking, drinking alcohol, habits of junk food, and less intake of vitamin D that can result in osteoporosis [24,25]. Low bone density or osteopenia is a state of reaching the threshold value of BMD for osteoporosis. Osteopenia is not considered under any disease category. Similar to how prehypertension and prediabetes are early signs of hypertension and diabetes, osteopenia gives early indications of osteoporosis.

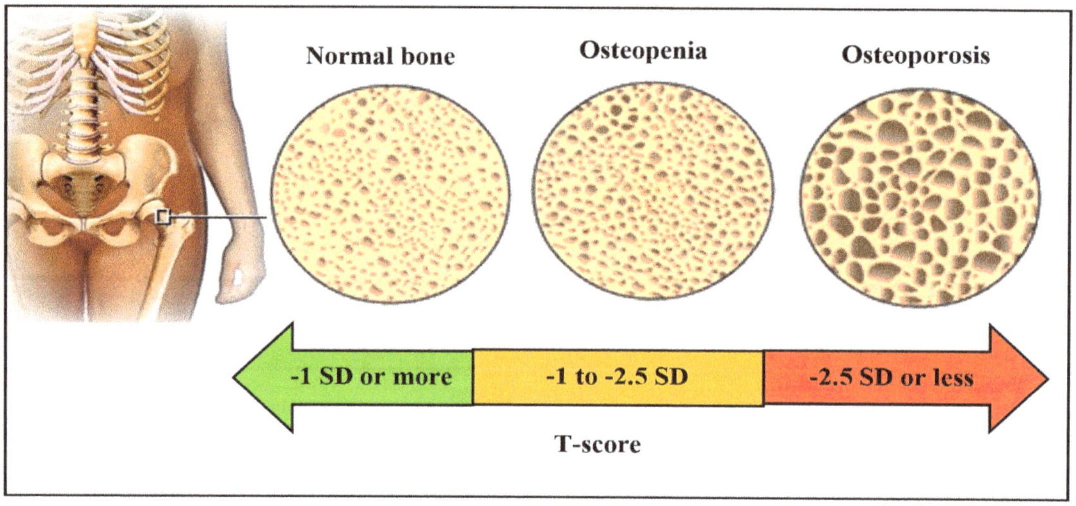

Figure 3. Comparative view of normal bone, osteopenia, and osteoporosis [26] .

3.2. Bone Cancer and Infections

Several infections and cancer also occur in bone because of unbalanced osteoclast activities, either systemically as in humoral hypercalcemia of malignancy (HHM) or regionally in bone metastasis [27]. Bone metastasis occurs when cancer cells relocate in fresh bone. Parathyroid hormone-related protein (PTHrP) increases resorption and overrides normal calcium homeostasis, leading to such diseases [28]. Bone cancer can be divided into two categories: primary bone cancer and secondary bone cancer. If cancer starts in bone cells either at its outer surface or from the center of bone, it is called primary bone cancer, while cancer that occurs in any part of body and spreads to the bone is known as secondary bone cancer [29].

3.3. Osteogenesis Imperfecta

Osteogenesis imperfecta is a rare genetic disorder that affects the connective tissues of bone, making them fragile with low bone mass. It affects the ability of the body to build stronger bones. Primarily, it occurs due to alterations in the genes (COL1A1 and COL1A2) that encrypt type I procollagen [30]. The severity of the disorder may vary with different symptoms such as blue sclera, hyperlaxity of the skin and ligaments, hearing impairment, and intrauterine fractures [31]. Osteogenesis imperfecta occurs due to the deficiency of proteins which interacts with collagen and influences its post-translational alteration [32].

3.4. Paget's Diseases of Bone

Paget's disease is a metabolic bone disorder found in elderly people age 55 and above. As the age increases, chances of Paget's diseases rise 8% in men and 5% in women above 80 years. It is a serious bone disease that occurs due to unbalanced bone remodeling [33]. Abnormal behavior during osteoclast and too much bone formation during osteoblast results in expanded and disfigured bone. Paget's disease affects various bones such as the spine, skull, hip, tibia, and ribs. In Paget's disease, the level of bone metabolism markers such as alkaline phosphatase is increased [34]. Paget's disease of bone may develop cancer in bone [35].

3.5. Osteomalacia

Bones become softer in osteomalacia. The outer surface of bone (cortex) is made up of minerals mainly including phosphate, vitamin D, and calcium, while a softer inner matrix consists of collagen fibers [36,37]. Improper mineralization and the toxic effects of drugs make the bone softer in osteomalacia [38,39]. Other various reasons such as a deficiency of vitamin D, bypass surgery of the small intestine, celiac disease, kidney, or liver disorders, tumors, and drugs can also make the bone softer [40]. Osteomalacia is also known as rickets if it occurs in childhood [41].

3.6. Osteopetrosis

Osteopetrosis is a hereditary bone disorder that makes bone abnormally dense and fragile. The bone density is increased due to unbalanced resorption by osteoclast cells. Osteopetrosis are found in three different forms: osteopetrosis tarda, osteopetrosis congenita, and marble bone. Osteopetrosis tarda is a benign form diagnosed in adulthood, while osteopetrosis congenita and marble bone are malignant variants found during infancy and childhood, respectively [42].

3.7. Fibrous Dysplasia

Fibrous dysplasia is a bone disorder in which abnormal fibrous tissues are developed in the place of normal bone. In this, osteoblast cell fails to mature and hence produces abnormal fibrous tissue, which further grows and causes weakening or a deformation of bone. However, it does not spread from one bone to another [43]. This rare bone disorder is mostly developed in children and young adults [44]. Fibrous dysplasia can affect the skull, femur, tibia, pelvis, humerus, and ribs [45]

3.8. Scoliosis

This type of bone disorder results in the deformation of bone when either the spine gets curved in sideways or it takes the form of a letter "C" or "S". It may occur in children and adolescents [46,47]. Scoliosis is a genetic disorder that may vary in intensity from mild to severe amongst individuals. There are mainly three type of scoliosis: idiopathic scoliosis is hereditary, congenital scoliosis is a rare spine abnormality detected at birth, and neuromuscular scoliosis is caused by abnormality in the muscles and nerves that support the spine [42].

3.9. Osteomyelitis

The swelling of bone tissue due to infection is known as osteomyelitis. It can be a bacterial infection of blood that may spread to bone [48]. It can affect children's long bones and adult bones of the spine [49]. It may occur due to surgery, frequent medicine injections, diabetes, and a weak immune system [50,51]. Osteomyelitis is diagnosed through bone biopsy, and treatment requires extra care with multiple surgery [52].

4. Current Diagnostic Tests for Bone Health Monitoring

Several methods are commercially available for the diagnosis of bone health.

4.1. Bone Densitometry

Bone densitometry is also known as dual-energy X-ray absorptiometry (DEXA) [53]. It was developed in the 1980s with widespread use started in 1988. Today, it is a reliable, popular, and most completely developed method in use. In this method, images of the inside bone are produced by exposing the skeletal site to two X-ray beams having different intensities of ionized radiation. Using two measurement results, the mineral content of bone is calculated through a computer. It can further be used for an analysis of osteoporosis [54]. Bone mineral density (BMD) results are useful in precisely predicting fracture risks with low ionizing radiation dose. However, the bone densitometry technique detects the bone health after the occurrence of bone loss. It cannot differentiate between osteoporosis and osteomalacia. In addition, the studies may take 2–3 years of continuous monitoring to detect significant changes in bone density [55,56].

4.2. Bone Scan

Bone scans are one of the most popular, highly sensitive diagnostic imaging techniques used for the early detection of the healing process against any bony destruction. In the case of any bony destruction originated due to traumatic, infectious, neoplastic, or benign and malignant diseases of other origin, the lytic area is surrounded by an intense osteoblastic healing process. These significant metabolic changes due to local bone remodeling are detected in a bone scan through a radiotracer that accumulates in the skeleton in proportion to local blood flow. This increased unbound radiotracer uptake is rapidly cleared from the surrounding soft tissues after intravenous injection. A bone scan may detect these significant metabolic changes much earlier than other conventional radiological images. In addition, a bone scan performs a complete skeleton examination covering a wide range of bone disorders at relatively low radiation exposure [57,58]. However, imaging devices are bulky, costlier, and need labs for assessment [59].

4.3. Bone X-ray (Radiography)

Bone X-rays have been the primary tool for imaging the stress-related bone injuries. Being relatively cheaper and widely available, they are popularly used in clinical practice worldwide. Radiographic findings are usually "normal" if obtained within the first week of pain; however, in follow-up radiography, the diagnostic findings of bone injuries are present in 30% to 70% of cases [60,61]. Only a limited part of the skeletal system can be visualized through radiography [62,63]. Bone imaging techniques have various advantages and limitations depending upon the need and clinical history of patients [64].

4.4. Calcium Blood Test

The amount of calcium in blood is determined by a calcium blood test [65]. Nearly all (99%) of calcium is stored in bone, and the remaining 1% is found in blood. If blood calcium decreases or increases, this may be a sign of bone diseases [66]. Calcium isotope measurement in blood is more sensitive to changes in bone mineral balance (BMB) when compared to existing clinical techniques. Net BMB can inherently be monitored by modeling Ca isotopes; also, Ca isotopes can detect any shift in BMB much earlier (weeks to months earlier) on occurrence when compared to radiological detection of changes in bone mineral density [67]. However, it gives very limited information related to bone health.

4.5. *Bone Biopsy*

The bone biopsy is a technique in which tissue or cells are removed by surgery and the outer layer of bone is analyzed under a microscope [68]. Needle biopsy and open biopsy are two different methods used for taking samples. Bone biopsy causes some complications such as bone fracture, discomfort, bleeding, and infection near the biopsy site [69]. Additionally, it gives information of only the tested area of infection, and it cannot identify the health loss prior to disease.

5. Biochemical Markers for Bone Health Monitoring

Biochemical markers of bone turnover are protein derivatives and collagen breakdown products released during the bone remodeling process. Bone turnover markers (BTMs) offer prognostic information of fracture risk and are found in blood and urine. Hannon et al. have reviewed the bone markers and current laboratory assays [70]. Various BTMs are briefly described below.

5.1. *Biochemical Markers for Bone Formation*

Bone biomarkers are produced during bone remodeling and are responsible for bone formation [71]. Bone specific alkaline phosphatase (BALP), procollagen I carboxyterminal propeptides (PINP), procollagen I aminio-terminal propeptide (PICP), and osteocalcin are common biomarkers used for the bone health assessment [72]. The detection of these biomarkers shows potential for the early diagnosis of bone diseases.

5.1.1. Bone-Specific Alkaline Phosphatase (BALP)

Bone-specific alkaline phosphatase (BALP) is generated by osteoblast during the bone remodeling process, and its production is related to bone formation proportion as measured by histomorphometry [72]. BALP levels remain stable in men throughout life; however, the BALP level in women increases around menopause [73].

5.1.2. Procollagen I Peptides

There are basically two types of procollagen peptides, which are described as procollagen I carboxyterminal propeptides (PICP) and procollagen I aminioterminal propeptide (PINP) [74,75]. PINP is stable at room temperature and has low diurnal variability. Its value during circulation is not affected by food intake, and hence there is no need for fasting during tests [76].

5.1.3. Osteocalcin

Osteocalcin is a biomarker produced during the osteoblast activity of bone formation [77]. It is discharged into urine by glomerular filtration [78]. The OC level is low up to middle age in men and increases thereafter; however, in women, it follows the same pattern as in BALP [79].

5.2. *Biochemical Markers of Bone Resorption*

5.2.1. Hydroxyproline (OHP)

Hydroxyproline is an impartial heterocyclic protein amino acid found in collagen [80]. During the resorption process of bone, 90% of OHP is released during collagen breakdown, and the remaining 10% releases as small polypeptide chains [81].

5.2.2. Collagen Cross-Link Molecules

Pyridinoline (PYD) and deoxypyridinoline (DPD) are two types of cross-link molecules that grow during the extracellular maturation of collagen and release into circulation after bone resorption [82]. PYD is found only in the cartilage, ligaments, and vessels of bone. However, DPD is found in bone as well as in dentin [83]. Therefore, DPD is considered a more sensitive marker as compared to PYD.

5.2.3. Hydroxylysine Glycosides

Hydroxylysine glycosides are a type I collagen that are derived from proline and produced by post-translational hydroxylation [84]. This marker is not affected by any food intake and is a more specific bone marker when compared to OHP [85].

5.2.4. Telopeptides of Type I Collagen

These telopeptides are cross-linked and derived from the carboxyterminal (CTx-I) and amino-terminal (NTx-I) during the resorption process of bone. CTx-I and NTx-I are analyzed through immunoassay in urine and serum [86]. The measurement of these two collagens from serum are more sensitive and practical as compared to those from urine [87,88].

5.2.5. Bone Sialoprotein (BSP)

The large amount of BSP is produced during osteoblasts, and a much smaller amount is produced in odontoblasts and osteoclasts. Serum is used for the analysis of BSP [89].

5.2.6. Tartrate-Resistant Acid Phosphatase (TRACP)

TRACP are enzymes found in bones, erythrocytes, platelets, spleen, and prostates released during circulation [90]. TRACP5a and TRACP5b have similar structures but different pH and carbohydrate values. TRACP5a is released from macrophages and TRACP5b is released during osteoclasts, which shows the depravity of the bone matrix. The functioning of kidney and food intake does not affect the level of TRACP5b [91].

5.2.7. Cathepsin K

Cathepsin K belongs to the cysteine proteases group and is released during bone resorption [92]. It plays a vital role in bone matrix degradation. The excessive bone loss treatment is done by cathepsin k inhibitors [93].

6. Traditional Techniques for Measurement of Bone Turnover Markers

The bone turnover markers can be analyzed with different methods such as enzyme-linked immunosorbent assay (ELISA), radioimmunoassay (RIA), and high-performance liquid chromatography (HPLC).

6.1. Enzyme-Linked Immunosorbent Assay (ELISA)

It is a plate-based assay technique for the detection of antibodies or antigens by color variation in biological fluid. The detection of target molecules depends on the antibody–antigen interaction [94]. The ELISA method is mostly used for the detection of peptide and protein. Enzyme immunoassay can be either homogeneous or heterogeneous. In the homogeneous method, enzymes become inactivated when bound with antibody, and washing is not needed, making it easier to use. However, this method is costly and less sensitive [95]. The heterogeneous method being highly sensitive is more popular comparatively. This technique relies on the formation of an antigen–antibody complex, while free antigens are removed during washing [96].

6.2. Radioimmunoassay (RIA)

Radioimmunoassay (RIA) is used for the detection of antigen and antibody. In this method, in the place of enzymes, radioisotopes are used as labels to be conjugated with antibodies or antigens [97]. The sensitivity of RIA is more than that of ELISA [98]. This test is used to measure a very less (nanograms) quantity of antigens and antibodies in serum. RIA works on the viable binding of antibody with unlabeled antigen and radiolabeled antigen [99]. There are some limitations such as costly equipment and reagents, the disposal of radioactive waste, and the short shelf-life of radiolabeled components [100].

6.3. *High-Performance Liquid Chromatography (HPLC)*

The advanced form of column liquid chromatography to separate a combination of substances into their constituents, based on their composition and molecular structure, is used in HPLC [101]. It offers several advantages in terms of the measurement technique of biochemical markers, owing to its high resolution, sensitivity, precision, low response time, and the ability to measure multiple component in single analysis [102].

Detection processes used in ELISA and RIA are highly specific and sensitive. In addition, ELISA requires minimum reagents and has no radiation hazard. HPLC has its own advantages though, as it measures accurately with high speed, sensitivity, and resolution. This automated technique can analyze multiple chemical components in a single analysis [92]. However, in ELISA, technical expertise is needed to prepare complicated samples, and results may also not be absolute, even using expensive ELISA kits. Similarly, RIA also requires technical expertise to make special arrangements for the storage and disposal of radioactive materials and avoid radiation hazards [91]. HPLC has no such limitations; however, it is expensive and uses complex equipment [94].

7. Sensors for Diagnosis of Bone Health

Two types of general sensors (physical sensors and biosensors) can be used for the diagnosis of bone health. A physical sensor is a device that measures a physical quantity (such as temperature, strain, pressure et al.) and converts it into a signal that can be read by an observer or by an instrument. A biosensor is an analytical device that is used for the detection of a chemical substance, which includes a biorecognition domain, transducer, and signal read-out system [103,104]. The following section will discuss these two types of sensors for the diagnosis of bone health.

7.1. *Physical Sensors*

Physical sensors monitor and measure force, tension, pressure, weight etc., which can be converted to a measurable signals such as electrical resistance [105]. In addition to these, physical sensors are also sensitive to the surrounding environment and temperature [106]. Thus, they primarily suffer from the limitations of non-specific analyte interactions [107]. Wen et al. shared an implantable strain gauge sensor array fabricated at microscale that can measure surface strain on a live bone. In this study, metal strain gauges encapsulated in a polydimethylsiloxane (PDMS) membrane showed more accurate strain sensing when compared to commercially available ones. This comparison is analyzed by an electromechanical test, which represents accurate strain sensing. This study reflects that the strain gauge may be implantable, and it can wirelessly perform real-time in vivo monitoring during bone remodeling [108]. In 2010, Umbrecht et al. presented wireless implantable passive strain sensors (WIPSS) to observe the disfigurement of orthopedic implants (Figure 4). The WIPSS was made from biocompatible PMMA, and an incompressible fluid was filled in the reservoir. The sensing principle of this sensor was based on amplification effect in hydromechanical systems. The strain resolution obtained was $1.70 \pm 0.2 \times 10^{-5}$ with a dynamic input frequency range of 0.1–5 Hz, while this sensor works with a signal bandwidth up to 1 Hz, since increasing the input frequency range reduces the sensor output [109].

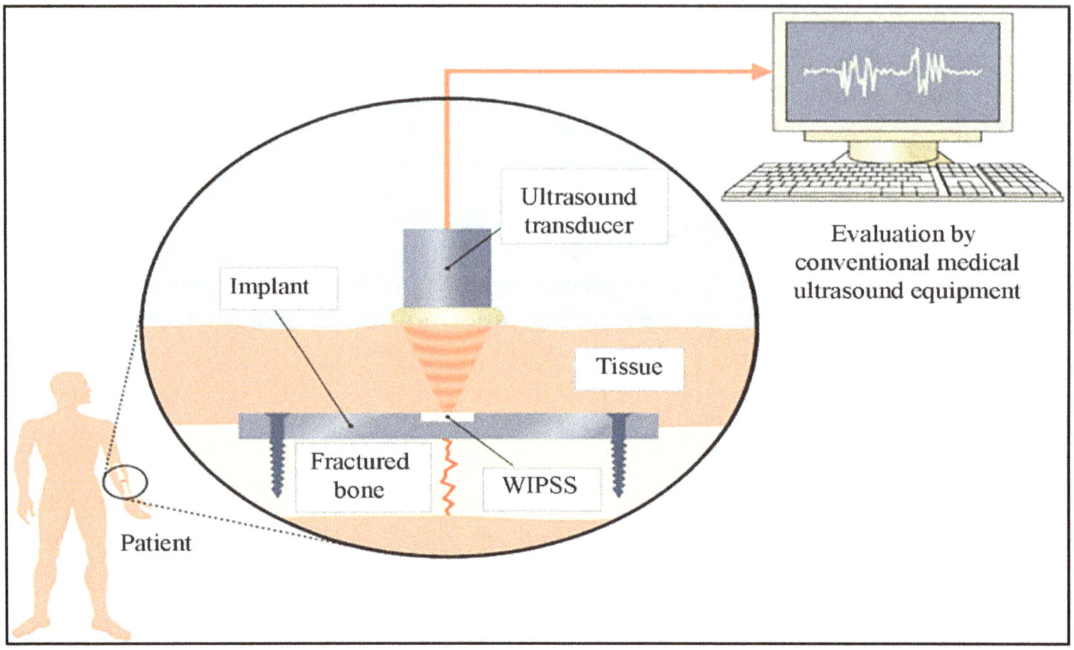

Figure 4. Schematic of the sensor concept of wireless implantable passive strain sensors (WIPSS) implant inside the body and sensor signal is detected by ultrasound waves.

In 2009, Lin et al. investigated a smart polymer hydrogel thin film used to convert tiny pressure sensors into chemomechanical sensors. The smart hydrogel was placed between a porous membrane and the diaphragm of a piezoresistive pressure transducer. The sensitivity was affected by the loading pressure and the selection of the membrane. This sensor was used in physiological monitoring [110]. The magnetoelectric (ME) effect represents the coupling of magnetic and electric properties of materials, which can be used in physical sensors to report the signal. In this type, electrical output is produced in response to the magnetic field applied [111,112]. Magnetic sensors are stable, without background noise and high sensitivity [113]. Naughton et al. disclosed in a patent the development of a magnetic biosensor for the monitoring of bone tissue growth. In this invention, they placed a magnet close to bone tissue, whereby the distance between the bone and sensing interface allows the determination of the thickness of bone tissue and in turn, the status of bone tissue degradation [114]. Physical sensors can report the optical signal as well. Singh et al. proposed a model of fiber-optic sensors (FOBs) using the micro bending technique for the measurement of bone strength. They also used an artificial neural network-based test bench for optimization of the FOBs [115]. Optical sensors are faster, having no electrical and magnetic interference with label-free detection. Two drawbacks are its low spectral resolution and bulky system, making its portability poorer [116].

Another type of physical sensors are piezoelectric sensors, which are a group of analytical devices that uses the piezoelectric effect to measure changes in force, strain, temperature, pressure, and acceleration in the form of an electrical charge. Piezoelectric biosensors offer real-time and label-free transduction [117]. Alfaro et al. designed a micro-scale implantable multi-axial bone stress sensor, as shown in Figure 5. As reported, such biosensors work on a piezoresistive pixels array, which can detect a stress between the bone and biosensor chip at an interfacial area with a pressure of around 100 Pa [13]. Piezoelectric sensors show rapid response, easy-to-use, label-free detection, low cost, and negligible phase shift with a compact size and offer output that can be directly processed by an electronic circuit. Piezoelectric sensors are also sensitive to temperature and pressure, which may also become a drawback [118].

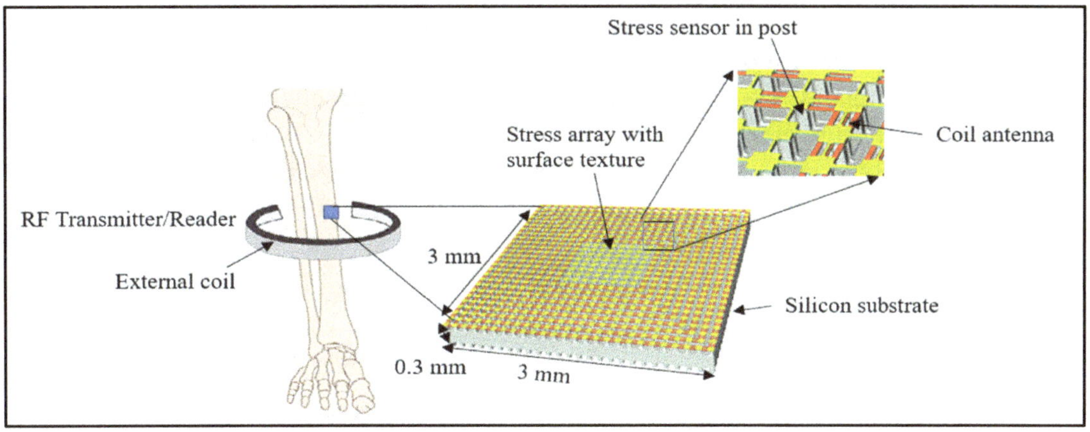

Figure 5. Schematic diagram of an implantable piezoresistive stress sensor.

The above-discussed signal (physical, magnetoelectric, piezoelectric, and optical) read-out methods used in physical sensors can also be used for biosensors [119–121]. However, so far, no biosensor using these types of signal read-out has been used for the detection of bone biomarkers to diagnose bone health.

7.2. Biosensors

In recent years, the requirement of biosensors has increased due to its fast response time, user-friendly approach, minimum cost, disposable device, and suitability for mass production. Biosensors can be very useful in bone health monitoring to timely and continuously assess issues such as fracture, the reduction of BMD, and variation in a variety of proteins [122]. Various technologies are evolving in the field of biosensors that can assess bone cells and identify the concentration of BTM in biological samples. In general, bone biosensing comprises a recognition domain that identifies the analyte that gets converted into a signal through a signal transducer, and a reader device reads this signal [123]. Advances in biosensing technology have enabled producing reliable, fast, non-invasive, real-time, and cost-effective sensors with high sensitivity that can help with precisely monitoring the bone health [124]. A bone biosensor fabrication process involves three different stages: (1) the selection of transducers; (2) fabrication of a sensing interface with recognition elements; and (3) quantitative measurements through the signal amplification and transduction element [125]. Modification of the sensing interface with nanomaterials is the attractive practice for the fabrication of a biosensor. Nanomaterials such as gold nanoparticles, carbon dots, nanorods, nanotubes, quantum dots, and nanowires-based biosensors have shown great potential in diagnostics, owing to their unique properties such as high electrical conductivity and large surface area, resulting in high sensitivity [126,127]. Based on signal read-out strategies, there are different types of biosensors such as colorimetric biosensors, fluorescence biosensors, electrochemical biosensors, et al. The following section will discuss the current biosensors that have been used for bone health studies.

7.2.1. Electrochemical Biosensors

Electrochemical biosensors can convert biological information into a measurable electrical signal using simple electronics for conditioning and read-out [128]. These biosensors are advantageous in terms of linear output, excellent repeatability, reliable, portable, accurate, and require less power [129]. On the other hand, the shelf-life, stability of biorecognition element, non-specific binding, and ultra-sensitivity to temperature are the limitations of electrochemical biosensors [130]. Ramanathan et al. developed immunosensors for the impedimetric detection of bone biomarkers (CTx-I) that can detect with a low limit (0.05 ng/mL) of detection [131]. Yun et al. developed a label-free immunosensor for detection of the C-terminal telopeptide bone turnover marker from type-1 collagen [132]. In this work, self-assembled monolayers of dithiodipropionic acid were used on the surface of gold electrodes with streptavidin immobilized, following which a biotinylated antibody was bound to the streptavidin. The different concentrations of CTx-I were measured through electrochemical impedance spectroscopy (EIS) (Figure 6). A detection limit of 50 ng/mL and a dynamic range up to 3 μg/mL was achieved. It was reported that using this method, the sensors can measure the electrical signal in just 4 h through a single step as opposed to commercially available methods such as ELISA, which takes a lot more time and a greater number of steps for analysis.

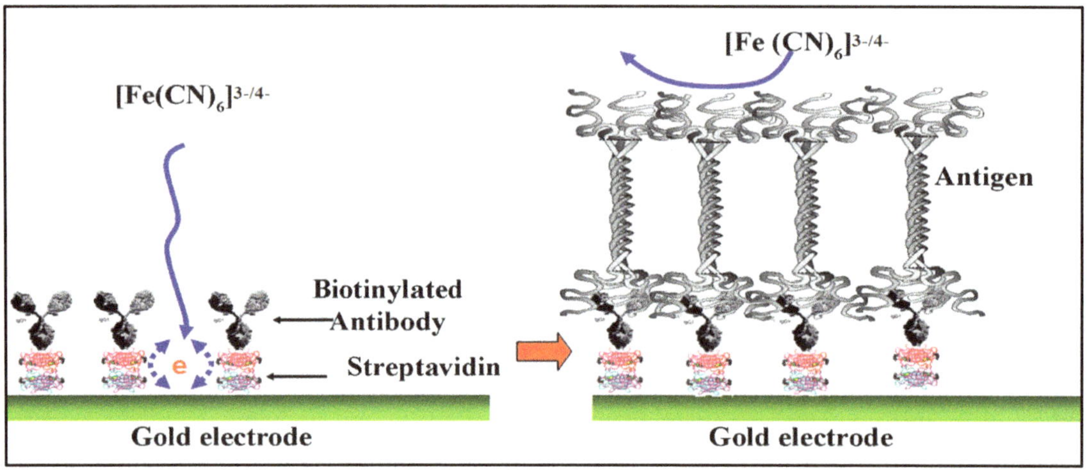

Figure 6. Schematic diagram of label-free immunobiosensor based on the detection of carboxyterminal

In 2016, Afsarimanesh et al. reported another label-free biosensing technique by monitoring the CTx-I concentration in serum [133]. The impedance variation of CTx-I at different levels was analyzed by a combination of EIS and interdigital sensor. A detection limit of 0.147 ng/mL was attained through this method, and the results were compared with ELISA for validation. In 2018, the same research team represented a new method for CTx-I detection in serum [134]. Artificial antibodies were prepared for CTx-I molecules by the molecular imprinting (MIP) technique, as shown in Figure 7. Dielectric properties of the test solution were analyzed by a combination of EIS and an interdigital capacitive sensor. The detection limit was reduced up to 0.09 ng/mL, and the results were validated using ELISA. The authors reported that this biosensor performed better as compared to ELISA.

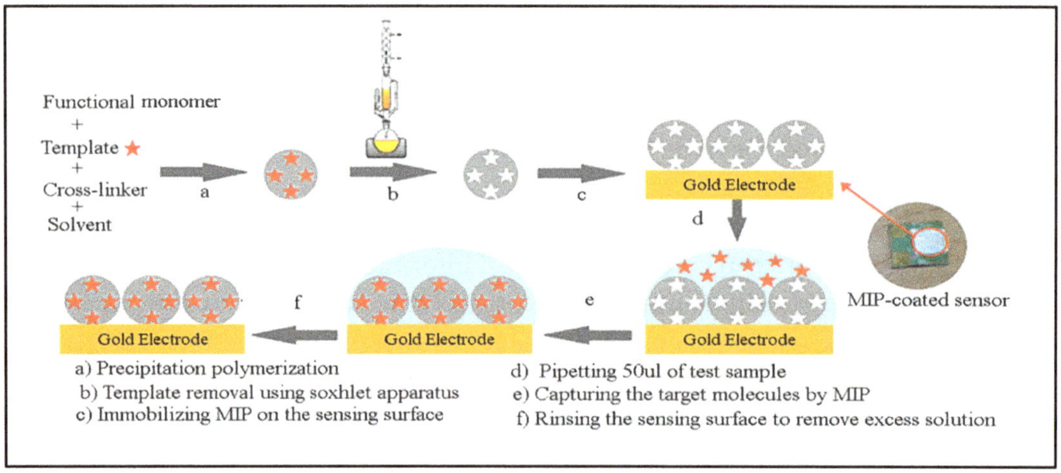

Figure 7. Process flow scheme for the preparation of molecularly imprinted polymer for CTx-I recognition

In 2019, Inal et al. developed a biosensor for the prognostic monitoring of osteoporosis by measuring osteocalcin molecules [135]. An anti-osteocalcin antibody was immobilized via the covalent immobilization method onto a gold electrode surface. Biosensor characterization and immobilization were specified by cyclic voltammetry and electrochemical impedance spectroscopy. The osteocalcin concentration was detected in 45 min with a detection range of 10–60 pg μL^{-1}. Sappia et al. developed an electrochemical biosensor, which they reported to be efficient, promising, and a simple technique for alkaline phosphatase (ALP) determination. It showed potential to be used by physicians for clinical tests requiring only 10 μL of serum even through a finger prick [136]. In 2009, Chandra et al. developed multiplexed assay for rheumatoid arthritis (RA) with more sensitivity and specificity than clinical tests [137].

7.2.2. Acoustic Biosensors

Acoustic biosensors are non-invasive in nature [138]. The emission parameters and accumulation number of recorded activities are correlated to determine the magnitude of bone damage [139]. Lentle et al. disclosed in a patent the use of acoustic biosensors to detect the osteoporosis level through acoustic sound waves by placing the sensor with skin adjacent to bone. In this invention, applied acoustic emission is detected by a biosensor, which in turn analyzes the sound waves to evaluate the extent of osteoporosis in bone [140]. Acoustic biosensors are cheaper, sensitive, provide multiplexed output, wirelessly interrogated, and able to work in liquid environment with low detection limit [141,142]. The main disadvantages of acoustic sensors are their dependence on temperature and humidity, which makes sensor replacement difficult, and the sensor sensitivity also depends on thin crystal [143].

7.2.3. Other Sensors

In addition to the popular electrochemical and acoustic biosensors, recently Liu et al. developed a portable photothermal biosensor to detect ALP enzymes on the basis of polydopamine (PDA) nanoparticle formation by using a thermometer as a read-out or temperature discoloration sticker, as indicated in Figure 8 [144]. This biosensor can work on a very low detection limit of 0.1 unit/length (U/L) for a thermometer and 1.0 U/L for a temperature discoloration sticker. As suggested, this type of biosensor can detect ALP in serum with very high sensitivity and label-free detection in real time.

Although the aforementioned examples are not exhaustive, they have demonstrated the huge potential to produce reliable, fast, non-invasive, real-time, and cost-effective biosensors with high sensitivity that can help in efficiently monitoring the bone health.

8. Conclusions and Future Trends

This paper focuses on different methods for the assessment of bone health using biochemical markers. Modeling and remodeling phenomena of bones, various bone diseases, and bone health monitoring techniques are briefly discussed. The paper highlights a variety of bone turnover markers and recent developments in this area of monitoring biochemical markers for bone health assessment. Then, the paper discusses recent bone biosensing techniques and types of biosensors, with an emphasis on electrochemical biosensors for bone health monitoring, owing to the high sensitivity and reliability.

However, it is important to note that the available sensors have certain limitations and challenges for widespread applications. Therefore, there is a critical need to further explore and develop biosensors for real-time monitoring with simpler, quicker, more cost-effective and user-friendly approaches. The majority of bone biosensors are used to detect a single biomarker of bone health. Single bone biomarker detection is not sufficient for the accurate and timely identification of bone diseases, and hence, the detection of multiple biomarkers is required to be developed. Therefore, methods for multiplex detection, which can detect multiple analytes simultaneously, are required to overcome these problems. It has been reported that multiplex assays have high sensitivity and require less sample volume.

The development of advanced biosensors that may detect multiple markers with label-free detection technique are needed to solve the ever-increasing bone health problems in the near future.

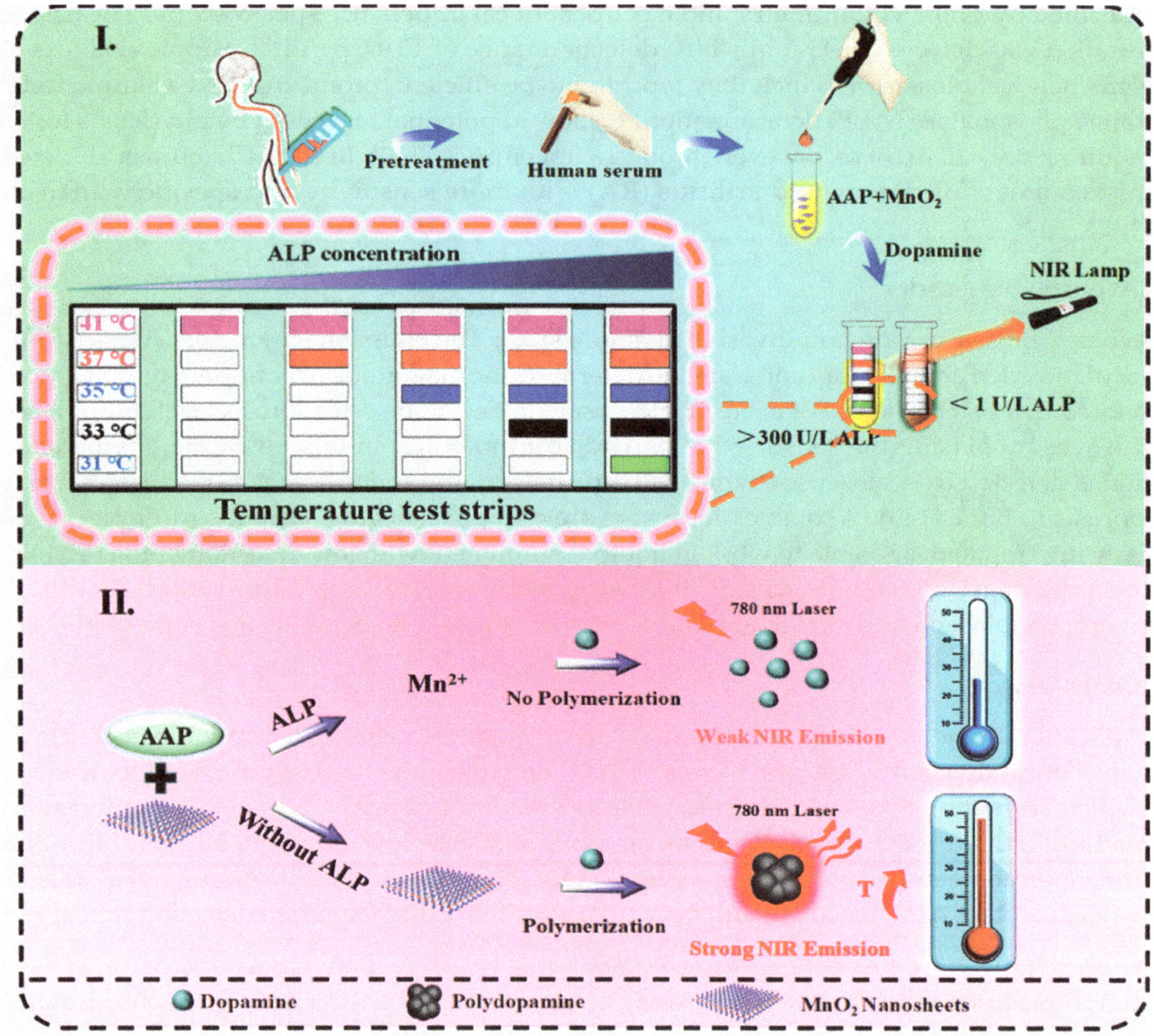

Figure 8. Photothermal biosensor for the measurement of ALP.

Author Contributions: Writing-original draft preparation, review and editing, S.R.; Conceptualization, Writing-review and editing, Funding acquisition, S.B.-G.; Writing-review and editing, S.B.G.; Conceptualization, Writing-review and editing, Funding acquisition, G.L. All authors have read and agreed to the published version of the manuscript.

Acknowledgments: Sanchita Bandyopadhyay-Ghosh, Subrata Bandhu Ghosh, and Seema Rani acknowledge Manipal University Jaipur for the funding through the Endowment research grant (EF/2017-18/QE04-07). Guozhen Liu acknowledges the Australian Research Council (ARC) for funding of the Future Fellowship (FT160100039), UNSW-CAS Bridging Grant, University of New South Wales (UNSW) for the Biomedical Engineering Seed Fund and Digital Grid Futures Institute Seed Fund.

References

1. Florencio-silva, R.; Rodrigues, G.; Sasso-cerri, E.; Simões, M.J.; Cerri, P.S.; Cells, B. Biology of Bone Tissue: Structure, Function, and Factors that Influence Bone Cells. *BioMed Res. Int.* **2015**, *2015*, 421746. [CrossRef]

2. Datta, H.K.; Ng, W.F.; Walker, J.A.; Tuck, S.P.; Varanasi, S.S. The cell biology of bone metabolism. *J. Clin. Pathol.* **2008**, *61*, 577–587. [CrossRef]
3. Robling, A.G.; Castillo, A.B.; Turner, C.H. Biomechanical and Molecular Regulation of Bone Remodeling. *Annu. Rev. Biomed. Eng.* **2006**, *8*, 455–498. [CrossRef] [PubMed]
4. Kuo, T.R.; Chen, C.H. Bone biomarker for the clinical assessment of osteoporosis: Recent developments and future perspectives. *Biomark. Res.* **2017**, *5*, 5–13. [CrossRef]
5. Chapurlat, R.D.; Confavreux, C.B. Novel biological markers of bone: From bone metabolism to bone physiologya. *Rheumatology* **2016**, *55*, 1714–1725. [CrossRef] [PubMed]
6. Ahn, J.K.; Kim, H.Y.; Lee, C.Y.; Park, K.S.; Park, H.G. Label-free and washing-free alkaline phosphatase assay using a personal glucose meter. *J. Biol. Eng.* **2019**, *13*, 1–5. [CrossRef] [PubMed]
7. Claudon, A.; Vergnaud, P.; Valverde, C.; Mayr, A.; Klause, U.; Garnero, P. New automated multiplex assay for bone turnover markers in osteoporosis. *Clin. Chem.* **2008**, *54*, 1554–1563. [CrossRef] [PubMed]
8. Clowes, J.A.; Hannon, R.A.; Yap, T.S.; Hoyle, N.R.; Blumsohn, A.; Eastell, R. Effect of feeding on bone turnover markers and its impact on biological variability of measurements. *Bone* **2002**, *30*, 886–890. [CrossRef]
9. Chang, Y.; Cho, B.; Kim, S.; Kim, J. Direct conversion of fibroblasts to osteoblasts as a novel strategy for bone regeneration in elderly individuals. *Exp. Mol. Med.* **2019**, *51*, 1–8. [CrossRef]
10. Rawadi, G.; Vayssière, B.; Dunn, F.; Baron, R.; Roman-Roman, S. BMP-2 Controls Alkaline Phosphatase Expression and Osteoblast Mineralization by a Wnt Autocrine Loop. *J. Bone Miner. Res.* **2003**, *18*, 1842–1853. [CrossRef] [PubMed]
11. Teitelbaum, S.L. Bone resorption by osteoclasts. *Science* **2000**, *289*, 1504–1508. [CrossRef] [PubMed]
12. Vasikaran, S.; Eastell, R.; Bruyère, O.; Foldes, A.J.; Garnero, P.; Griesmacher, A.; McClung, M.; Morris, H.A.; Silverman, S.; Trenti, T.; et al. Markers of bone turnover for the prediction of fracture risk and monitoring of osteoporosis treatment: A need for international reference standards. *Osteoporos. Int.* **2011**, *22*, 391–420. [CrossRef] [PubMed]
13. Alfaro, F.; Weiss, L.; Campbell, P.; Miller, M.; Fedder, G.K. Design of a multi-axis implantable MEMS sensor for intraosseous bone stress monitoring. *J. Micromech. Microeng.* **2009**, *19*, 085016. [CrossRef]
14. Heaney, R.P.; Gallagher, J.C.; Johnston, C.C.; Neer, R.; Parfitt, A.M.; Whedon, G.D. Calcium nutrition and bone health in the elderly. *Am. J. Clin. Nutr.* **1982**, *36*, 986–1013. [CrossRef] [PubMed]
15. Smith, S.M.; Heer, M.A.; Shackelford, L.C.; Sibonga, J.D.; Ploutz-Snyder, L.; Zwart, S.R. Benefits for bone from resistance exercise and nutrition in long-duration spaceflight: Evidence from biochemistry and densitometry. *J. Bone Miner. Res.* **2012**, *27*, 1896–1906. [CrossRef] [PubMed]
16. Alfaro, J.F.; Weiss, L.E.; Campbell, P.G.; Miller, M.C.; Heyward, C.; Doctor, J.S.; Fedder, G.K. BioImplantable Bone Stress Sensor. In Proceedings of the 2005 IEEE Engineering in Medicine and Biology 27th Annual Conference, Shanghai, China, 17–18 January 2006; pp. 518–521.
17. Mamtani, R.; Stern, P.; Dawood, I.; Cheema, S. Metals and disease: A global primary health care perspective. *J. Toxicol.* **2011**, *2011*, 319136. [CrossRef] [PubMed]
18. Dongre, N.N.; Suryakar, A.N.; Patil, A.J.; Hundekari, I.A.; Devarnavadagi, B.B. Biochemical effects of lead exposure on battery manufacture workers with reference to blood pressure, calcium metabolism and bone mineral density. *Indian J. Clin. Biochem.* **2013**, *28*, 65–70. [CrossRef]
19. Sánchez-Barceló, E.J.; Mediavilla, M.D.; Tan, D.X.; Reiter, R.J. Scientific Basis for the Potential Use of Melatonin in Bone Diseases: Osteoporosis and Adolescent Idiopathic Scoliosis. *J. Osteoporos.* **2010**, *2010*, 1–10. [CrossRef]
20. Liu, L.; Webster, T.J. In Situ Sensor Advancements for Osteoporosis Prevention, Diagnosis, and Treatment. *Curr. Osteoporos. Rep.* **2016**, *14*, 386–395. [CrossRef]
21. World Health Organization. IRIS (Institutional Repository for Information Sharing) Assessment of fracture risk and its application to screening for postmenopausal osteoporosis. In *Report of a WHO Study Group*; World Health Organizationh: Rome, Itly, (22 to 25 June 1992); 1994.
22. Colicino, E.; Just, A.; Kioumourtzoglou, M.; Vokonas, P.; Cardenas, A.; Sparrow, D.; Weisskopf, M.; Nie, L.H.; Hu, H.; Schwartz, J.D.; et al. Blood DNA methylation biomarkers of cumulative lead exposure in adults. *J. Expo. Sci. Environ. Epidemiol.* **2019**. [CrossRef]
23. Rodríguez, J.; Mandalunis, P.M. A review of metal exposure and its effects on bone health. *J. Toxicol.* **2018**, *2018*, 4854152. [CrossRef]

24. Khashayar, P.; Amoabediny, G.; Larijani, B.; Vanfleteren, J. Bone biosensors: Knowing the present and predicting the future. *J. Micromech. Microeng.* **2016**, *26*, 23002. [CrossRef]
25. Rachner, T.D.; Khosla, S.; Hofbauer, L.C. Osteoporosis: Now and the future. *Lancet* **2011**, *377*, 1276–1287. [CrossRef]
26. Osteopenia, Osteoporosis and Exercise. Available online: http://strongandstable.com.au/2017/10/osteopenia-osteoporosis-and-exercise/ (accessed on 17 January 2020).
27. Patel, P. Biosensors and Biomarkers: Promising Tools for Cancer Diagnosis. *Int. J. Biosens. Bioelectron.* **2017**, *3*, 1–5. [CrossRef]
28. Evola, F.R.; Costarella, L.; Pavone, V.; Caff, G.; Cannavò, L.; Sessa, A.; Avondo, S.; Sessa, G. Biomarkers of osteosarcoma, chondrosarcoma, and ewing sarcoma. *Front. Pharmacol.* **2017**, *8*, 1–14. [CrossRef] [PubMed]
29. Nugent, M. MicroRNA and bone cancer. *Adv. Exp. Med. Biol.* **2015**, *889*, 201–230. [PubMed]
30. Devogelaer, J.-P.; Coppin, C. Osteogenesis Imperfecta. *Treat. Endocrinol.* **2006**, *5*, 229–242. [CrossRef]
31. Rauch, F.; Glorieux, F.H. Osteogenesis imperfecta. *Lancet* **2004**, *363*, 1377–1385. [CrossRef]
32. Forlino, A.; Cabral, W.A.; Barnes, A.M.; Marini, J.C. New perspectives on osteogenesis imperfecta. *Nat. Rev. Endocrinol.* **2011**, *7*, 540–557. [CrossRef]
33. Gkouva, L.; Andrikoula, M. Active Paget's disease of bone with normal biomarkers of bone metabolism: A case report and review of the literature. *Clin. Rheumatol.* **2011**, *30*, 139–144. [CrossRef]
34. Siris, E.; Roodman, G.D. Paget's Disease of Bone. In *Primer on the Metabolic Bone Diseases and Disorders of Mineral Metabolism*, 7th ed.; Rosen, C.J., Compston, J.E., Bilezikian, J.P., Bouillon, R., Clemens, T., Bauer, D.C., Ebeling, P.R., Engelke, K., Goltzman, D., Guise, T., et al., Eds.; American Society for Bone and Mineral Research: Washington, DC, USA, 2009.
35. Christenson, R.H. Biochemical markers of bone metabolism: An overview. *Clin. Biochem.* **1997**, *30*, 573–593. [CrossRef]
36. Basha, B.; Rao, D.S.; Han, Z.H.; Parfitt, A.M. Osteomalacia due to vitamin D depletion: A neglected consequence of intestinal malabsorption. *Am. J. Med.* **2000**, *108*, 296–300. [CrossRef]
37. Bhan, A.; Qiu, S.; Rao, S.D. Bone histomorphometry in the evaluation of osteomalacia. *Bone Rep.* **2018**, *8*, 125–134. [CrossRef] [PubMed]
38. Sisco, M. Luiza Kerstenetzky 53. In *Abd-Elsayed A. Pain*; Springer: Cham, Switzerland, 2019; pp. 261–265.
39. Adams, J.E. Radiology of rickets and osteomalacia. In *Vitamin D*, 4th ed.; Feldman, D., Ed.; Academic Press: London, UK, 2018; Volume 1.
40. Elbossaty, W.F. Mineralization of Bones in Osteoporosis and Osteomalacia. *Ann. Clin. Lab. Res.* **2017**, *5*, 3–6. [CrossRef]
41. Noh, C.-K.; Lee, M.-J.; Kim, B.K.; Chung, Y.-S. A Case of Nutritional Osteomalacia in Young Adult Male. *J. Bone Metab.* **2013**, *20*, 51. [CrossRef]
42. Whyte, M.P. *Connective Tissue and Its Heritable Disorders: Molecular, Genetic, and Medical Aspects*, 2nd ed.; Royce, P.M., Steinmann, B., Eds.; Wiley online library: Hoboken, NJ, USA, 2002; pp. 789–807.
43. DiCaprio, M.R.; Enneking, W.F. Fibrous dysplasia: Pathophysiology, evaluation, and treatment. *J. Bone Jt. Surg. Ser. A* **2005**, *87*, 1848–1864. [CrossRef]
44. Lane, J.M.; Khan, S.N.; O'Connor, W.J.; Nydick, M.; Hommen, J.P.; Schneider, R.; Tomin, E.; Brand, J.; Curtin, J. Bisphosphonate therapy in fibrous dysplasia. *Clin. Orthop. Relat. Res.* **2001**, *382*, 6–12. [CrossRef]
45. Lustig, L.R.; Holliday, M.J.; McCarthy, E.F.; Nager, G.T. Fibrous dysplasia involving the skull base and temporal bone. *Arch. Otolaryngol. Head Neck Surg.* **2001**, *127*, 1239–1247. [CrossRef]
46. Weinstein, S.L.; Dolan, L.A.; Cheng, J.C.Y.; Danielsson, A.; Morcuende, J.A. Adolescent idiopathic scoliosis. *Lancet* **2008**, *371*, 1527–1537. [CrossRef]
47. Burwell, R.G.; Webb, J.K. Scoliosis in children and adolescents. *Curr. Paediatr.* **1991**, *1*, 137–141. [CrossRef]
48. Lombardi, G.; Akoume, M.Y.; Colombini, A.; Moreau, A.; Banfi, G. Biochemistry of adolescent idiopathic scoliosis. In *Advances in Clinical Chemistry*; Academic Press Elsevier: London, UK, 2011; Volume 54, pp. 165–182.
49. Lew, P.D.P.; Waldvogel, P.F.A. Osteomyelitis. *Lancet* **2004**, *364*, 369–379. [CrossRef]
50. Álvarez, H.C.; López, J.P.; de Rojas, L.G.; Quiroz, J.P.Y. Lumbar vertebral osteomyelitis. *Rev. Cuba. Ortop. Traumatol.* **2013**, *27*, 84–90.
51. Lazzarini, L.; Mader, J.T.; Calhoun, J.H. Osteomielitis en huesos largos. Conceptos actuales. *J. Bone Joint Surg. Am.* **2004**, *86*, 2305–2318. [CrossRef] [PubMed]

52. Sia, I.G.; Berbari, E.F. Osteomyelitis. *Best Pract. Res. Clin. Rheumatol.* **2006**, *20*, 1065–1081. [CrossRef] [PubMed]
53. Gafni, R.I.; Baron, J. Overdiagnosis of osteoporosis in children due to misinterpretation of Dual-energy x-ray absorptiometry (DEXA). *J. Pediatr.* **2004**, *144*, 253–257. [CrossRef] [PubMed]
54. Miller, P.D.; Zapalowski, C.; Kulak, C.A.M.; Bilezikian, J.P. Bone densitometry: The best way to detect osteoporosis and to monitor therapy. *J. Clin. Endocrinol. Metab.* **1999**, *84*, 1867–1871. [CrossRef] [PubMed]
55. Bartl, R.; Bartl, C. *The Osteoporosis Manual: Prevention, Diagnosis and Management*; Springer: Cham, Switzerland, 2019; pp. 67–75.
56. Cummings, S.R.; Bates, D.; Black, D.M. Clinical use of bone densitometry: Scientific review. *J. Am. Med. Assoc.* **2002**, *288*, 1889–1897. [CrossRef]
57. van den Wyngaert, T.; Strobel, K.; Kampen, W.U.; Kuwert, T.; Van der Bruggen, W.; Mohan, H.K.; Gnanasegaran, G.; Delgado-Bolton, R.; Weber, W.A.; Beheshti, M. The EANM practice guidelines for bone scintigraphy. *Eur. J. Nucl. Med. Mol. Imaging* **2016**, *43*, 1723–1738. [CrossRef]
58. Brenner, A.I.; Koshy, J.; Morey, J.; Lin, C.; Dipoce, J. The bone scan. *Semin. Nucl. Med.* **2012**, *42*, 11–26. [CrossRef]
59. Handmaker, H.; Leonards, R. The bone scan in inflammatory osseous disease. *Semin. Nucl. Med.* **1976**, *6*, 95–105. [CrossRef]
60. Kiuru, M.J.; Pihlajamaki, H.K.; Hietanen, H.J.; Ahovuo, J.A. MR imaging, bone scintigraphy, and radiography in bone stress injuries of the pelvis and the lower extremity. *Acta Radiol.* **2002**, *43*, 207–212. [CrossRef] [PubMed]
61. Handa, A.; Uchiyama, Y.; Shinpuku, E.; Watanabe, M. Comparison of three plain radiography methods for evaluating proximal humerus bone strength in women. *J. Orthop. Sci.* **2019**, *24*, 243–249. [CrossRef] [PubMed]
62. Todorović-Tirnanić, M.; Obradović, V.; Han, R.; Goldner, B.; Stanković, D.; Sekulić, D.; Lazić, T.; Djordjević, B. Diagnostic approach to reflex sympathetic dystrophy after fracture: Radiography or bone scintigraphy? *Eur. J. Nucl. Med.* **1995**, *22*, 1187–1193. [CrossRef] [PubMed]
63. Kanis, J.A.; McCloskey, E.V.; Johansson, H.; Oden, A.; Melton, L.J.; Khaltaev, N. A reference standard for the description of osteoporosis. *Bone* **2008**, *42*, 467–475. [CrossRef] [PubMed]
64. Vijayanathan, S.; Butt, S.; Gnanasegaran, G.; Groves, A.M. Advantages and Limitations of Imaging the Musculoskeletal System by Conventional Radiological, Radionuclide, and Hybrid Modalities. *Semin. Nucl. Med.* **2009**, *39*, 357–368. [CrossRef] [PubMed]
65. Eisenhauer, A.; Müller, M.; Heuser, A.; Kolevica, A.; Glüer, C.C.; Both, M.; Laue, C.; Hehn, U.; Kloth, S.; Shroff, R.; et al. Calcium isotope ratios in blood and urine: A new biomarker for the diagnosis of osteoporosis. *Bone Rep.* **2019**, *10*, 100200. [CrossRef]
66. Channon, M.B.; Gordon, G.W.; Morgan, J.L.L.; Skulan, J.L.; Smith, S.M.; Anbar, A.D. Using natural, stable calcium isotopes of human blood to detect and monitor changes in bone mineral balance. *Bone* **2015**, *77*, 69–74. [CrossRef]
67. Morgan, J.L.L.; Gordon, G.W.; Arrua, R.C.; Skulan, J.L.; Anbar, A.D.; Bullen, T.D. High-precision measurement of variations in calcium isotope ratios in urine by multiple collector inductively coupled plasma mass spectrometry. *Anal. Chem.* **2011**, *83*, 6956–6962. [CrossRef]
68. Wan-Ibrahim, W.I.; Singh, V.A.; Hashim, O.H.; Abdul-Rahman, P.S. Biomarkers for bone tumors: Discovery from genomics and proteomics studies and their challenges. *Mol. Med.* **2015**, *21*, 861–872. [CrossRef]
69. Bover, J.; Ureña-Torres, P.; Alonso, A.M.L.; Torregrosa, J.V.; Rodríguez-García, M.; Castro-Alonso, C.; Górriz, J.L.; Benito, S.; López-Báez, V.; Cora, M.J.L.; et al. Osteoporosis, bone mineral density and CKD-MBD (II): Therapeutic implications. *Nefrologia* **2019**, *39*, 227–242. [CrossRef]
70. Hannon, R.A.; Eastell, R. Bone markers and current laboratory assays. *Cancer Treat. Rev.* **2006**, *32*, 7–14. [CrossRef]
71. Nielson, C.M.; Jacobs, J.M.; Orwoll, E.S. Proteomic studies of bone and skeletal health outcomes. *Bone* **2019**, *126*, 18–26. [CrossRef]
72. Naylor, K.; Eastell, R. Bone turnover markers: Use in osteoporosis. *Nat. Rev. Rheumatol.* **2012**, *8*, 379–389. [CrossRef]

73. Sharp, C.A.; Linder, C.; Magnusson, P. Analysis of human bone alkaline phosphatase isoforms: Comparison of isoelectric focusing and ion-exchange high-performance liquid chromatography. *Clin. Chim. Acta* **2007**, *379*, 105–112. [CrossRef]
74. Burr, D.B. Bone Morphology and Organization. In *Basic and Applied Bone Biology*, 2nd ed.; Burr, D.B., Allen, M.R., Eds.; Academic Press: Indianapolis, IN, USA, 2013; pp. 3–26.
75. Eastell, R.; Garnero, P.; Audebert, C.; Cahall, D.L. Reference intervals of bone turnover markers in healthy premenopausal women: Results from a cross-sectional European study. *Bone* **2012**, *50*, 1141–1147. [CrossRef]
76. Oranger, A.; Colaianni, G.; Grano, M. Bone cells. *Imaging Prosthet. Jt. A Comb. Radiol. Clin. Perspect.* **2014**, *14*, 3–13.
77. Stella, D.; Brown, J.; Coleman, R. The role of biomarkers in the management of bone-homing malignancies. *J. Bone Oncol.* **2017**, *9*, 1–9.
78. Ivaska, K.K.; Käkönen, S.M.; Gerdhem, P.; Obrant, K.J.; Pettersson, K.; Väänänen, H.K. Urinary osteocalcin as a marker of bone metabolism. *Clin. Chem.* **2005**, *51*, 618–628. [CrossRef]
79. Ingram, R.T.; Park, Y.K.; Clarke, B.L.; Fitzpatrick, L.A. Age- and gender-related changes in the distribution of osteocalcin in the extracellular matrix of normal male and female bone. Possible involvement of osteocalcin in bone remodeling. *J. Clin. Investig.* **1994**, *93*, 989–997. [CrossRef]
80. Venkateswarlu, K.; PadmaVijayasri, A.; Rekha, P.S. Early Diagnosis of Osteoporosis in Postmenopausal Women Using Bone Markers. *IOSR J. Dent. Med. Sci.* **2015**, *14*, 102–106.
81. Swaminathan, R. Biochemical markers of bone turnover. *Clin. Chim. Acta* **2001**, *313*, 95–105. [CrossRef]
82. Lu, J.; Wang, M.; Wang, Z.; Fu, Z.; Lu, A.; Zhang, G. Advances in the discovery of cathepsi. inhibitors on bone resorption. *J. Enzyme Inhib. Med. Chem.* **2018**, *33*, 890–904. [CrossRef]
83. Robins, S.P.; Black, D.; Paterson, C.R.; Reid, D.M.; Duncan, A.; Seibel, M.J. Evaluation of urinary hydroxypyridinium crosslink measurements as resorption markers in metabolic bone diseases. *Eur. J. Clin. Investig.* **1991**, *21*, 310–315. [CrossRef]
84. Seibel, M.J. Biochemical markers of bone turnover part II: Clinical applications in the management of osteoporosis. *Clin. Biochem. Rev.* **2006**, *27*, 123–138.
85. Indumati, V.; Patil, V. Biochemical markers of bone remodeling in osteoporosis-current concepts. *J. Clin. Diagn. Res.* **2010**, *4*, 2089–2097.
86. Wu, C.H.; Chang, Y.F.; Chen, C.H.; Lewiecki, E.M.; Wüster, C.; Reid, I.; Tsai, K.S.; Matsumoto, T.; Mercado-Asis, L.B.; Chan, D.C.; et al. Consensus Statement on the Use of Bone Turnover Markers for Short-Term Monitoring of Osteoporosis Treatment in the Asia- Pacific Region. *J. Clin. Densitom.* 2019. [CrossRef]
87. Herrmann, M.; Seibel, M. The amino- and carboxyterminal cross-linked telopeptides of collagen type I, NTX-I and CTX-I: A comparative review. *Clin. Chim. Acta* **2008**, *393*, 57–75. [CrossRef]
88. Maeno, Y.; Inaba, M.; Okuno, S.; Yamakawa, T.; Ishimura, E.; Nishizawa, Y. Serum concentrations of cross-linked N-telopeptides of type I collagen: New marker for bone resorption in hemodialysis patients. *Clin. Chem.* **2005**, *51*, 2312–2317. [CrossRef]
89. Ganss, B.; Kim, R.H.; Sodek, J. Bone sialoprotein. *Crit. Rev. Oral Biol. Med.* **1999**, *10*, 79–98. [CrossRef]
90. Halleen, J.M.; Alatalo, S.L.; Suominen, H.; Cheng, S.; Janckila, A.J.; Väänänen, H.K. Tartrate-resistant acid phosphatase 5b: A novel serum marker of bone resorption. *J. Bone Miner. Res.* **2000**, *15*, 1337–1345. [CrossRef]
91. Nenonen, A.; Cheng, S.; Ivaska, K.K.; Alatalo, S.L.; Lehtimäki, T.; Schmidt-Gayk, H.; Uusi-Rasi, K.; Heinonen, A.; Kannus, P.; Sievänen, H. Serum TRACP 5b is a useful marker for monitoring alendronate treatment: Comparison with other markers of bone turnover. *J. Bone Miner. Res.* **2005**, *20*, 1804–1812. [CrossRef] [PubMed]
92. Holzer, G.; Noske, H.; Lang, T.; Holzer, L.; Willinger, U. Soluble cathepsin K: A novel marker for the prediction of nontraumatic fractures? *J. Lab. Clin. Med.* **2005**, *146*, 13–17. [CrossRef] [PubMed]
93. Nishizawa, Y.; Nakamura, T.; Ohta, H.; Kushida, K.; Gorai, I.; Shiraki, M.; Fukunaga, M.; Hosoi, T.; Miki, T.; Chaki, O.; et al. Guidelines for the use of biochemical markers of bone turnover in osteoporosis (2004). *J. Bone Miner. Metab.* **2005**, *23*, 97–104. [CrossRef] [PubMed]
94. Grange, R.D.; Thompson, J.P.; Lambert, D.G.; Mahajan, R.P. Radioimmunoassay, enzyme and non-enzyme-based immunoassays. *Br. J. Anaesth.* **2014**, *112*, 213–216. [CrossRef]
95. Engvall, E. The ELISA, enzyme-linked immunosorbent assay. *Clin. Chem.* **2010**, *56*, 319–320. [CrossRef] [PubMed]

96. Afsarimanesh, N.; Mukhopadhyay, S.C.; Kruger, M. Sensing technologies for monitoring of bone-health: A review. *Sens. Actuators A Phys.* **2018**, *274*, 165–178. [CrossRef]
97. Melkko, J.; Niemi, S.; Risteli, L.; Risteli, J. Radioimmunoassay of the carboxyterminal propeptide of human type I procollagen. *Clin. Chem.* **1990**, *36*, 1328–1332. [CrossRef]
98. Risteli, J.; Elomaa, I.; Niemi, S.; Novamo, A.; Risteli, L. Radioimmunoassay for the pyridinoline cross-linked carboxy-terminal telopeptide of type I collagen: A new serum marker of bone collagen degradation. *Clin. Chem.* **1993**, *39*, 635–640. [CrossRef]
99. Raiti, S.; Davis, W.T. The principles and application of radioimmunoassay with special reference to the gonadotropins. *Obstet. Gynecol. Surv.* **1969**, *24*, 289–310. [CrossRef]
100. Goldsmith, S.J. Radioimmunoassay: Review of basic principles. *Semin. Nucl. Med.* **1975**, *5*, 125–152. [CrossRef]
101. Afsarimanesh, N.; Mukhopadhyay, S.C.; Kruger, M. State-of-the-art of sensing technologies for monitoring of bone-health. *Smart Sens. Meas. Instrum.* **2019**, *30*, 7–31.
102. Vare, S.R.; Shelke, M.M.; Bidkar, J.S.; Dama, G.Y. HPLC: A Simple And Advance Methods Of Separation And Validation. *World J. Pharm. Res.* **2019**, *8*, 478–496.
103. Seibel, M.J.; Woitge, H.W.; Farahmand, I.; Oberwittler, H.; Ziegler, R. Automated and manual assays for urinary crosslinks of collagen: Which assay to use? *Exp. Clin. Endocrinol. Diabetes* **1998**, *106*, 143–148. [CrossRef]
104. Wingren, C.; Borrebaeck, C.A.K. Antibody Microarrays: Current Status and Key Technological Advances. *Omi. A J. Integr. Biol.* **2006**, *10*, 411–427. [CrossRef]
105. Klosterhoff, B.S.; Ghee Ong, K.; Krishnan, L.; Hetzendorfer, K.M.; Chang, Y.H.; Allen, M.G.; Guldberg, R.E.; Willett, N.J. Wireless implantable sensor for noninvasive, longitudinal quantification of axial strain across rodent long bone defects. *J. Biomech. Eng.* **2017**, *139*, 1–8. [CrossRef]
106. Luka, G.; Ahmadi, A.; Najjaran, H.; Alocilja, E.; DeRosa, M.; Wolthers, K.; Malki, A.; Aziz, H.; Althani, A.; Hoorfar, M. Microfluidics integrated biosensors: A leading technology towards lab-on-A-chip and sensing applications. *Sensors* **2015**, *15*, 30011–30031. [CrossRef]
107. Arlett, J.L.; Myers, E.B.; Roukes, M.L. Comparative advantages of mechanical biosensors. *Nat. Nanotechnol.* **2011**, *6*, 203–215. [CrossRef]
108. Wen, Y.H.; Yang, G.Y.; Bailey, V.J.; Lin, G.; Tang, W.C.; Keyak, J.H. Mechanically robust micro-fabricated strain gauges for use on bones. In Proceedings of the IEEE/EMBS Special Topic Conference on Microtechnology in Medicine and Biology, Oahu, HI, USA, 12–15 May 2005; pp. 302–304.
109. Umbrecht, F.; Wägli, P.; Dechand, S.; Gattiker, F.; Neuenschwander, J.; Sennhauser, U.; Hierold, C. Wireless implantable passive strain sensor: Design, fabrication and characterization. *J. Micromech. Microeng.* **2010**, *20*, 085005. [CrossRef]
110. Lin, G.; Chang, S.; Kuo, C.H.; Magda, J.; Solzbacher, F. Free swelling and confined smart hydrogels for applications in chemomechanical sensors for physiological monitoring. *Sens. Actuators B Chem.* **2009**, *136*, 186–195. [CrossRef]
111. Oess, N.P.; Weisse, B.; Nelson, B.J. Magnetoelastic Strain Sensor for Optimized Assessment of Bone Fracture Fixation. *IEEE Sens. J.* **2009**, *9*, 961–968. [CrossRef]
112. Bichurin, M.; Petrov, R.; Leontiev, V.; Semenov, G.; Sokolov, O. Magnetoelectric current sensors. *Sensors* **2017**, *17*, 1271. [CrossRef]
113. Hughes, S.; Dobson, J.; el Haj, A.J. Magnetic targeting of mechanosensors in bone cells for tissue engineering applications. *J. Biomech.* **2007**, *40* (Suppl. 1), 96–104. [CrossRef] [PubMed]
114. Naughton, G.K.; Mansbridge, J.N.; Horwitz, D.L.; Zeltinger, J.; Cerny, D.J. Monitorable Three-Dimensional Scaffolds And Tissue Culture Systems. International Application No. PCT/US2000/017542, 4 January 2001.
115. Singh, P.; Shrivastava, A. Optical Biosensor Based on Microbendings Technique: An Optimized Mean to Measure the Bone Strength. *Adv. Opt. Technol.* **2014**, *2014*, 1–7. [CrossRef]
116. Singh, P. SPR biosensors: Historical perspectives and current challenges. *Sens. Actuators B Chem.* **2016**, *229*, 110–130. [CrossRef]
117. Tombelli, S. Piezoelectric biosensors for medical applications. In *Biosensors for Medical Applications*; Higson, S., Ed.; Woodhead Publishing Series in Biomaterials: Cambridge, UK, 2012; pp. 41–64.
118. Pohanka, M. The piezoelectric biosensors: Principles and applications, a review. *Int. J. Electrochem. Sci.* **2017**, *12*, 496–506. [CrossRef]

119. Dey, D.; Goswami, T. Optical biosensors: A revolution towards quantum nanoscale electronics device fabrication. *J. Biomed. Biotech.* **2011**, *2011*, 1–7. [CrossRef]
120. Bunde, R.L.; Jarvi, E.J.; Rosentreter, J.J. Piezoelectric quartz crystal biosensors. *Talanta* **1998**, *46*, 1223–1236. [CrossRef]
121. Fu, Y.Q.; Luo, J.K.; Nguyen, N.T.; Walton, A.J.; Flewitt, A.J.; Zu, X.T.; Li, Y.; McHale, G.; Matthews, A.; Iborra, E. Advances in piezoelectric thin films for acoustic biosensors, acoustofluidics and lab-on-chip applications. *Prog. Mater. Sci.* **2017**, *89*, 31–91. [CrossRef]
122. Sroga, G.E.; Vashishth, D. Effects of bone matrix proteins on fracture and fragility in osteoporosis. *Curr. Osteoporos. Rep.* **2012**, *10*, 141–150. [CrossRef]
123. Hasan, A.; Nurunnabi, M.; Morshed, M.; Paul, A.; Polini, A.; Kuila, T.; Al Hariri, M.; Lee, Y.K.; Jaffa, A.A. Recent advances in application of biosensors in tissue engineering. *Biomed Res. Int.* **2014**, *2014*, 307519. [CrossRef]
124. Sabr, A.K. Biosensors. *Am. J. Biomed. Eng.* **2016**, *6*, 170–179.
125. Sirivisoot, S.; Yao, C.; Xiao, X.; Sheldon, B.W.; Webster, T.J. Developing Biosensors for Monitoring Orthopedic Tissue Growth. *MRS Online Proc. Libr. Arch.* **2006**, *950*. [CrossRef]
126. Qi, M.; Zhang, Y.; Cao, C.M.; Zhang, M.X.; Liu, S.H.; Liu, G.Z. Decoration of RGO nanosheets with aryldiazonium salt and gold nanoparticles towards a label-free amperometric immunosensor for detecting cytokine TNF-α in live cells. *Anal. Chem.* **2016**, *88*, 9614–9621. [CrossRef] [PubMed]
127. Malik, P.; Katyal, V.; Malik, V.; Asatkar, A.; Inwati, G.; Mukherjee, T.K. Nanobiosensors: Concepts and Variations. *ISRN Nanomater.* **2013**, *2013*, 1–9. [CrossRef]
128. Hammond, J.L.; Formisano, N.; Estrela, P.; Carrara, S.; Tkac, J. Electrochemical biosensors and nanobiosensors. *Essays Biochem.* **2016**, *60*, 69–80. [PubMed]
129. Batool, R.; Rhouati, A.; Nawaz, M.H.; Hayat, A.; Marty, J.L. A review of the construction of nano-hybrids for electrochemical biosensing of glucose. *Biosensors* **2019**, *9*, 46. [CrossRef]
130. Ronkainen, N.J.; Halsall, H.B.; Heineman, W.R. Electrochemical biosensors. *Chem. Soc. Rev.* **2010**, *39*, 1747–1763. [CrossRef]
131. Ramanathan, M.; Patil, M.; Epur, R.; Yun, Y.; Shanov, V.; Schulz, M.; Heineman, W.R.; Datta, M.K.; Kumta, P.N. Gold-coated carbon nanotube electrode arrays: Immunosensors for impedimetric detection of bone biomarkers. *Biosens. Bioelectron.* **2016**, *77*, 580–588. [CrossRef]
132. Yun, Y.H.; Bhattacharya, A.; Watts, N.B.; Schulz, M.J. A label-free electronic biosensor for detection of bone turnover markers. *Sensors* **2009**, *9*, 7957–7969. [CrossRef]
133. Afsarimanesh, N.; Zia, A.I.; Mukhopadhyay, S.C.; Kruger, M.; Yu, P.L.; Kosel, J.; Kovacs, Z. Smart sensing system for the prognostic monitoring of bone health. *Sensors* **2016**, *16*, 976. [CrossRef]
134. Afsarimanesh, N.; Mukhopadhyay, S.C.; Kruger, M. Molecularly imprinted polymer-based electrochemical biosensor for bone loss detection. *IEEE Trans. Biomed. Eng.* **2018**, *65*, 1264–1271. [CrossRef] [PubMed]
135. Kabala, S.I.; Yagar, H.; Ozcan, H.M. A new biosensor for osteoporosis detection. *Prep. Biochem. Biotechnol.* **2019**, *49*, 511–520. [CrossRef] [PubMed]
136. Sappia, L.; Felice, B.; Sanchez, M.A.; Martí, M.; Madrid, R.; Pividori, I. Electrochemical sensor for alkaline phosphatase as biomarker for clinical and in vitro applications. *Sens. Actuators B Chem.* **2019**, *281*, 221–228. [CrossRef]
137. Chandra, P.E.; Sokolove, J.; Hipp, B.G.; Lindstrom, T.M.; Elder, J.T.; Reveille, J.D.; Eberl, H.; Klause, U.; Robinson, W.H. Novel multiplex technology for diagnostic characterization of rheumatoid arthritis. *Arthritis Res. Ther.* **2011**, *13*, R102. [CrossRef]
138. Lee, S.; Kim, K.B.; Kim, Y.I. Love wave SAW biosensors for detection of antigen-antibody binding and comparison with SPR biosensor. *Food Sci. Biotechnol.* **2011**, *20*, 1413–1418. [CrossRef]
139. Shrivastava, S.; Prakash, R. Assessment of bone condition by acoustic emission technique: A review. *J. Biomed. Sci. Eng.* **2009**, *2*, 144–154. [CrossRef]
140. Lentle, B.C.; Aldrich, J.E.; Akhtar, A. Diagnosis of osteoporosis using acoustic emissions. U.S. Patent 6,024,711; issued, 15 February 2000.
141. Drafts, B. Acoustic wave technology sensors. *IEEE Trans. Microw. Theory Tech.* **2001**, *49*, 795–802. [CrossRef]

142. Nirschl, M.; Rantala, A.; Tukkiniemi, K.; Auer, S.; Hellgren, A.C.; Pitzer, D.; Schreiter, M.; Vikholm-Lundin, I. CMOS-integrated film bulk acoustic resonators for label-free biosensing. *Sensors* **2010**, *10*, 4180–4193. [CrossRef]
143. García-González, D.L.; Aparicio, R. Sensors: From biosensors to the electronic nose. *Grasas y Aceites* **2002**, *53*, 96–114. [CrossRef]
144. Liu, X.; Zou, L.; Yang, X.; Wang, Q.; Zheng, Y.; Geng, X.; Liao, G.; Nie, W.; Wang, K. Point-of-Care Assay of Alkaline Phosphatase Enzymatic Activity Using a Thermometer or Temperature Discoloration Sticker as Readout. *Anal. Chem.* **2019**, *91*, 7943–7949. [CrossRef]

5

Optimizing Irradiation Geometry in LED-Based Photoacoustic Imaging with 3D Printed Flexible and Modular Light Delivery System

Maju Kuriakose [1], Christopher D. Nguyen [1], Mithun Kuniyil Ajith Singh [2] and Srivalleesha Mallidi [1,*]

1 Department of Biomedical Engineering, Tufts University, Medford, MA 02155, USA; maju.kuriakose@tufts.edu (M.K.); Christopher.Nguyen@tufts.edu (C.D.N.)
2 Research and Business Development Division, CYBERDYNE INC, 3013 AK Rotterdam, The Netherlands; mithun_ajith@cyberdyne.jp
* Correspondence: Srivalleesha.Mallidi@tufts.edu

Abstract: Photoacoustic (PA) imaging–a technique combining the ability of optical imaging to probe functional properties of the tissue and deep structural imaging ability of ultrasound–has gained significant popularity in the past two decades for its utility in several biomedical applications. More recently, light-emitting diodes (LED) are being explored as an alternative to bulky and expensive laser systems used in PA imaging for their portability and low-cost. Due to the large beam divergence of LEDs compared to traditional laser beams, it is imperative to quantify the angular dependence of LED-based illumination and optimize its performance for imaging superficial or deep-seated lesions. A custom-built modular 3-D printed hinge system and tissue-mimicking phantoms with various absorption and scattering properties were used in this study to quantify the angular dependence of LED-based illumination. We also experimentally calculated the source divergence of the pulsed-LED arrays to be 58° ± 8°. Our results from point sources (pencil lead phantom) in non-scattering medium obey the cotangential relationship between the angle of irradiation and maximum PA intensity obtained at various imaging depths, as expected. Strong dependence on the angle of illumination at superficial depths (−5°/mm at 10 mm) was observed that becomes weaker at intermediate depths (−2.5°/mm at 20 mm) and negligible at deeper locations (−1.1°/mm at 30 mm). The results from the tissue-mimicking phantom in scattering media indicate that angles between 30–75° could be used for imaging lesions at various depths (12 mm–28 mm) where lower LED illumination angles (closer to being parallel to the imaging plane) are preferable for deep tissue imaging and superficial lesion imaging is possible with higher LED illumination angles (closer to being perpendicular to the imaging plane). Our results can serve as a priori knowledge for the future LED-based PA system designs employed for both preclinical and clinical applications.

Keywords: LED; photoacoustic imaging; ultrasound; 3-D printed photoacoustic probe holder; light delivery optimization; LED divergence

---

1. Introduction

Photoacoustic (PA) imaging has gained significant popularity for imaging functional and molecular information in both preclinical and clinical settings [1–5]. The technique involves sending light pulses (a few nanosecond pulse-width) into imaging planes that get absorbed by endogenous (e.g., hemoglobin) or exogenous (e.g., Indocyanine Green) tissue chromophores and generate acoustic waves, which can be detected by conventional ultrasound (US) transducers [2,6,7]. Based on the endogenous contrast provided by hemoglobin, PA imaging has shown promise in vascular functional imaging of human neonatal brains [8,9], malignant lesions [10–14], and monitoring therapies such as photodynamic therapy [1,15,16], etc. As PA imaging uniquely possesses the best properties of optical imaging (high spatial resolution, functional properties, and imaging speed) and US imaging (structural properties and penetration depth reaching tens of cm), its relevance and popularity are continuously increasing in clinical settings [2,4,17–19].

In PA phenomena, the acoustic pressure ($\mathbf{P_0}$) generated is proportional to the optical absorption coefficient (μ_a, m^{-1}) of the light absorber and locally available light fluence or radiant exposure (f_0, Jm^{-2}). This can be represented by [2,6,20,21]:

$$\mathbf{P}_0 = u_a f_0 \tag{1}$$

where, is the dimensionless, material thermal property dependent Gruneisen coefficient.

Light attenuates as it travels down through a material or tissue due to scattering and absorption. Moreover, for a limited aperture illumination, angle of illumination also plays an important role in defining local fluence (Figure 1). As a result, f_0 and thus PA signal intensity, $\mathbf{P_0}$, changes as a function of depth (distance from transducer or excitation source) and as a function of the illumination angle. Therefore, the optimization of light delivery is crucial for efficient PA imaging and obtaining high signal-to-noise (SNR) ratio at deeper penetration depths [22–26]. Specifically, for reflection mode PA imaging (transducer and light source on the same side of the sample), several studies demonstrated the dependence of irradiation angle and fiber (source)-to-transducer positioning on PA signal at various depths experimentally or through simulations [23,27–31]. Either unilateral or bilateral positioning of fiber bundles aligned with the nanosecond pulsed laser have been employed in these studies. For example, Haisch et al. utilized a mechanical setup that allowed unilateral illumination (one-side of the transducer) with 20–80 degrees range of motion [32]. The fiber bundle aperture size used in that study was shorter than the ultrasound transducer, which may hinder full aperture illumination of near field absorbers and can presumably suitable for intermediate to deep tissue imaging and is more suitable to image smaller lesions on the skin. In another study by Sivasubramanian et al., two fiber bundles were placed on either side of the transducer at a fixed angle. Change in the illumination angle would require changing the holder setup [33]. More recently, Sangha et al. designed a motorized system to change the bilateral light illumination in the 0°–60° range and concluded that the illumination geometry optimization is important to achieve high SNR at different depths [34]. All these studies point out that change in illumination geometry effects PA SNR at different depths and strongly indicate the need for a flexible handheld system that can deliver light at different angles depending on the depth of the lesions.

The light delivery optimization studies mentioned above were performed with spatially low diverging coherent laser sources. Though conventional lasers (e.g., Q-switched optical parameter oscillator (OPO)) can deliver the required pulse energy at various NIR wavelengths, their bulkiness, minimal-portability, and difficulty in operation prevent them from effortless usage in a clinical setting. Interestingly, nanosecond pulsed light-emitting diodes (LED) show promise in being an alternative to lasers, while offering cost-effectiveness and ease of operation has been recently proven to be successful in several studies [35–39]. Despite the low power of LEDs (about 3 orders of magnitude lower than the conventional Q-switched laser sources), their high pulse repetition rate (PRR) (maximum reported up to 16 kHz opposed) gives the opportunity to average several frames in real-time to achieve an SNR on par with conventional laser-based PA imaging (PAI). In addition, the large spatial divergence of LED arrays (~60°), could aid in irradiating larger sample area and potentially also provide a quasi-uniform illumination over several millimeters without a light diffuser. Given these attributes, LED-based PA systems demonstrate strong potential for clinical translation. As the use of LED's in PA imaging is still in its infancy, it is important to characterize and optimize the light delivery strategies for better SNR at various depths.

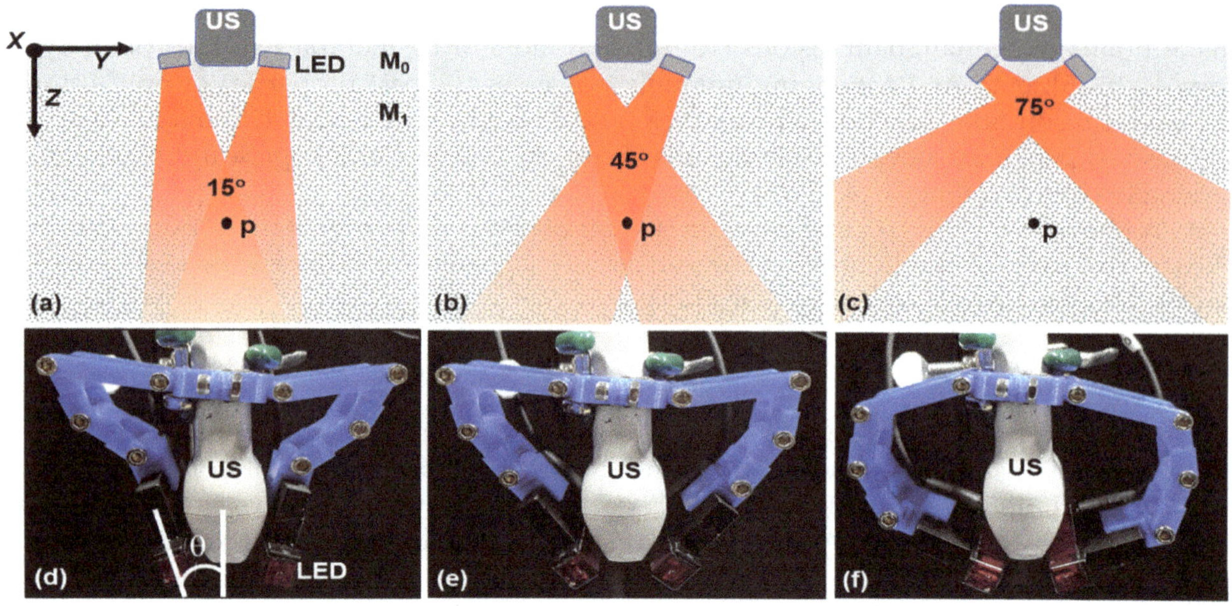

Figure 1. (**a**–**c**) Schematics of light emitting diode (LED) illumination cross-sectional view of photoacoustic (PA) setup at representative angles: 15°, 45°, and 75°, respectively, orthogonal to the imaging plane XZ, that contains a hypothetical absorber, p. M_0 is the medium that facilitates acoustic coupling between the transducer and the phantom material M_1; (**d**–**f**) Photographs of LED source pivoted at representative angles, θ = 15°, 45°, and 75°, respectively, using 3D printed modular hinge system.

LED array-based PAI studies so far have used a fixed orientation either in the reflection mode [40–42] or transmission mode [38,43]. In this study, we designed a flexible modular light delivery system for reflection mode PAI that is capable of orienting light from the LED arrays at various angles in the range of 0°–90° (Figure 1). Utilizing the flexible light delivery system, we evaluated PA image contrast in various tissue-mimicking phantoms (point targets in non-scattering and scattering liquid media, absorbing lesion under non-scattering liquid and scattering tissue such as the chicken breast) for the PA signal dependency as a function of irradiation angle and depth. We believe that our findings have an important impact on optimizing the design of LED-based PA probes and accelerate its clinical translation towards imaging both deeper and shallower lesions.

2. Materials and Methods

2.1. Photoacoustic System and Modular Arrangement for Varying Illumination Direction

2.1.1. AcousticX

An LED-based photoacoustic system (AcousticX from Cyberdyne Inc., Tsukuba, Japan) with linear US transducer (7 MHz central frequency, 128 elements, 0.315 mm pitch, and 38.4 mm aperture size, elevation focus of 15 mm) and two 850 nm LED arrays (30 to 150 ns pulse width, 4 kHz maximum repetition rate, 200 μJ pulse energy for each array, 5 mm × 40 mm aperture size, 60° divergence) on both sides of the US detector was used for the experiments [44]. PA and US raw data were sampled at 40 MHz and 20 MHz, respectively, and data was reconstructed in real-time using an inbuilt Fourier-domain reconstruction algorithm of the system. For offline analysis, both PA and US data were reconstructed using a previously reported frequency domain beamforming algorithm [45]. Radiant exposure per pulse at the LED array surface is about 100 μJ/cm^2 (200 μJ/pulse in an array area of 2 cm^2). Given the LED source divergence of 60° and ~10.5 mm distance between the US transducer and the phantom surface to accommodate LED arrays for different angles, maximum radiant exposure at the phantom surface was estimated to be about 29 μJ cm^{-2} (for an area of about 6.93 cm^2) from a single array at 0° LED illumination angle.

2.1.2. Flexible LED Holder: Modular Design for Adjusting Irradiation Direction

Two identical modular hinge systems were designed, 3D printed and used to pivot LED arrays at different illumination directions with respect to the imaging plane. The modular LED holder consisted of three parts that were designed on Autodesk and printed using polylactic acid (PLA) on a MakerBot system. All pieces were joined together with 8–32 socket head screws. (Figure 2). Each of the modules consisted of four hinges that were attached to one another. These hinges can be adjusted or pivoted to create the required angle of illumination. Modules were attached to the US transducer on its one end and the LED arrays were gripped through the heat sink of the arrays on the pivoting end of the module, as shown in the figure. The inter LED array distance (between their adjacent edges) was about 1 cm to accommodate the US transducer. Experiments were done for 0°, 15°, 30°, 45°, 60°, 75°, and 90° angles using this modular arrangement. The LED array angles were adjusted with respect to the central axis of the US transducer using a custom-made protractor as shown in Figure 1d. During the experiments, both the US transducer and sample position were unaltered and only the LED sources were adjusted, to avoid PA intensity variations due to sample motion with respect to the US transducer.

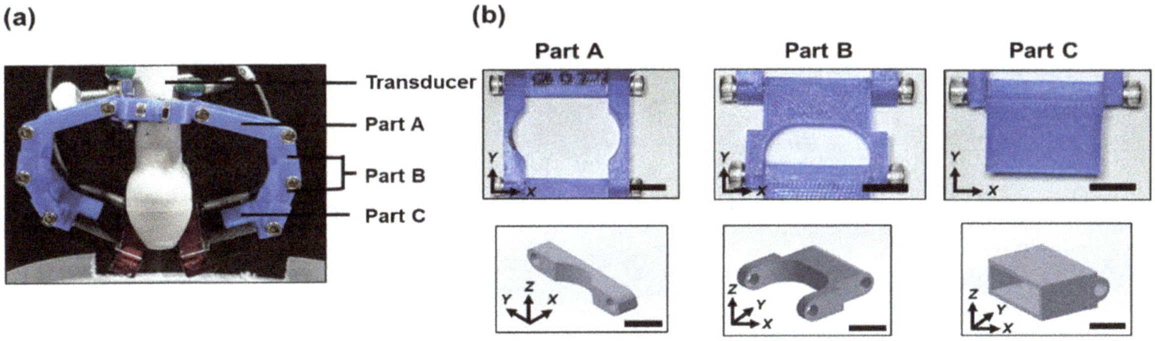

Figure 2. (**a**) Modular hinge system holding the LED arrays and attached to the US transducer. (**b**) The photographs of the individual pieces are shown in the top panel. The 3D renderings of the hinge pieces are shown on the bottom panel. Part A fits around the transducer and extends the horizontal reach of the holder to allow the LEDs to be placed at angles approaching 90°. Part B in conjunction with Part A allows precise horizontal and vertical height adjustment. The holder consists of two-part B pieces, and schematic of only one piece is shown in the panel. Part C holds the LEDs using the heat sinks and provides flexibility for any final adjustments on the LED illumination angle. Scale bar = 10 mm.

2.2. Phantoms

2.2.1. Graphite Pencil Lead Phantoms

A matrix of pencil leads (Graphite 2B 0.5 mm manufactured by June Gold, Bountiful, UT USA), arranged in 4 rows × 5 columns with a spacing of about 5 mm (columns) and 6 mm (rows), was constructed using two 3D printed plastic holders as shown in Figure 3a. The phantom construction with pencil lead is immersed in a container with water or 1% Intralipid (Sigma Aldrich Inc., Atlanta, GA, USA) solution (Figure 3b). The scattering coefficient of 1% intralipid solution is 1.8 mm^{-1} [46,47] close to the values reported for tumor tissue (1–2 mm^{-1}) [48–50]. All experiments were conducted at room temperature (22 °C).

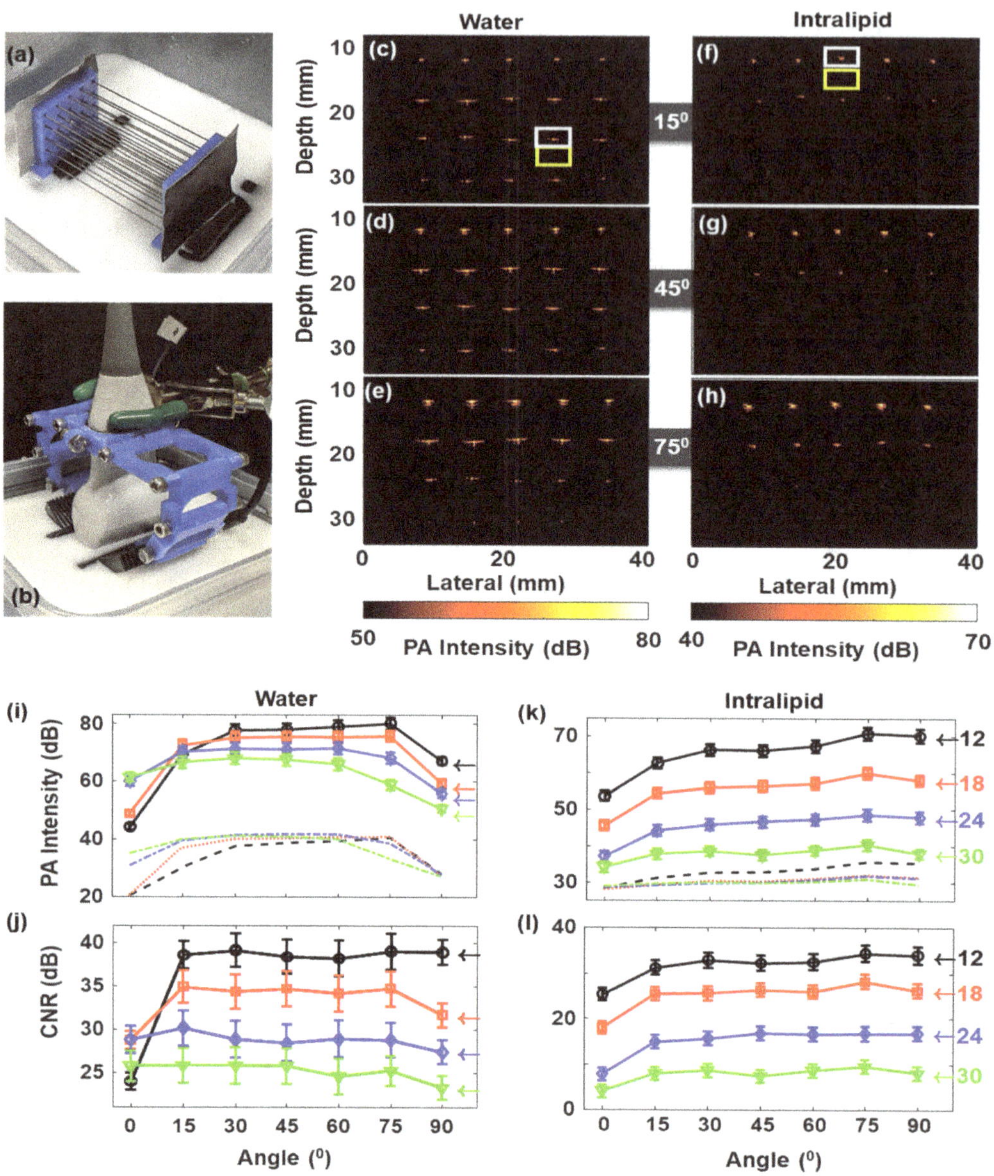

Figure 3. (**a**) Photograph of Pencil lead matrix; (**b**) photograph of an experimental arrangement using intralipid medium; (**c**–**h**) PA image acquired at representative angles 15° (**c**,**f**), 45° (**d**,**g**), and 75° (**e**,**h**) in water (**c**–**e**) and 1% intralipid (**f**–**h**); (**i**,**k**) Mean PA signal intensities and their standard deviations (of 5 lateral positions at each depth) plotted as a function of LED angles in water (**j**) and intralipid (**k**); and (**j**,**l**) corresponding contrast to noise ratios (CNRs) obtained as a function of LED angles in water (**j**) and intralipid (**l**). Different depths from the transducer are indicated by 12 mm (line with black circles), 18 mm (line with red squares), 24 mm (line with blue diamonds), and 30 mm (line with green downward triangles). The noise background levels corresponding to 12, 18, 24, and 30 mm are represented by black, red, blue, and green dash-dotted lines, respectively, in (**i**) in water and (**j**) in intralipid. The backgrounds were obtained right below from each signal regions, e.g., as indicated by the yellow rectangles in (**c**,**f**). Images for all the angles can be found in Figure S2 (for water) and Figure S3 (for intralipid).

2.2.2. Tissue Mimicking Phantom Containing Lesion with High Optical Absorbance

Tissue mimicking phantoms were prepared using agar powder (Sigma-Aldrich Inc., Atlanta, GA, USA). Titanium (IV) oxide, anatase powder (99.8%, Sigma-Aldrich Inc., Atlanta, GA, USA) was added to provide acoustic contrast and enhance the optical scattering properties of the agar. The preparation was done by slowly adding 1% wt./vol. of agar powder and 1% wt./vol. of TiO_2 powder into continually stirred deionized water at ambient conditions to avoid clumps. The final solution was then heated above 80° C, above the melting temperature of agar, and exposed to a vacuum level of about 0.1 atm for 5 min to degas the solution and cooled it down to room temperature to obtain the final phantom. A cylindrical light-absorbing lesion with acoustic scatterers was prepared in a similar aforementioned method. Additionally, 0.5% wt./vol. graphite powder (<20 µm, synthetic graphite, Sigma Aldrich Inc., Atlanta, GA, USA) and 0.5% wt./vol. TiO_2 powder were added. The concentration of the absorbing and scattering particles was chosen to mimic tumor tissue with an absorption coefficient (~0.2 cm^{-1}) and reduced scattering coefficient (~10 cm^{-1}) as previously reported in the literature [46–51].

2.3. *Signal Analysis*

2.3.1. PA Intensity & Contrast to Noise Ratio (CNR) Calculation

The PA signal intensity of each pencil lead in the phantom was calculated by taking the maximum pixel value from the region of interest (ROI) around the target (white rectangle in Figure 3c). All the five laterally positioned PA intensities were then averaged to find mean and standard deviation (σ) of PA intensities corresponding to each depth location and illumination angles. Background (Bg) was calculated from an ROI below each point target (yellow rectangle in Figure 3c). It is important to note that the noise/background values were calculated from regions close to the signal ROIs. We chose the ROIs within close proximity of the signal ROI and not from regions at the corner or with only electronic noise, including reconstruction related artifacts that may be present when changing the illumination angle. To plot PA intensity changes as a function of angle in the tissue-mimicking phantom, PA signal intensities from the lesion was obtained by choosing the median PA intensities above the Bg level. Here also, similar to the pencil phantom case, Bg and σ were chosen from a region close to the lesion ROI. PA intensity was plotted in decibel (dB) with the formula:

$$PA\ intensity\ in\ dB = 10log_{10}(PA\ intensity) \tag{2}$$

and the CNR was calculated using the formula:

$$CNR\ in\ dB = 10log_{10}\left(\frac{PA\ intensity - Bg}{\sigma}\right) \tag{3}$$

2.3.2. Divergence of the LED Source

Divergence of the LED source is an angular measure of the increase in irradiation area (and corresponding diameter or radius) with distance from the source. Laser light sources are known to have very low divergence while LED sources have high divergence. Sources with high divergence have lower radiant exposure per unit area on the target at a given depth than sources with lower divergence. These changes in radiant exposure can influence PA signal and hence it is critical to evaluate the divergence of the source and choose appropriate illumination angle to obtain maximum CNR. Assuming the LED is a line source aligned in the *X*-axis (parallel to the US transducer) while the emitted wavefronts take quasi-cylindrical shape in the imaging volume, an approximate divergence of the source in the *YZ* plane (Figure 4), in degrees can be computed using:

$$Divergence\ angle = 2 \times \left\{\tan^{-1}\left(\frac{target\ depth}{LED\ to\ Detector\ distance}\right)\right\} \tag{4}$$

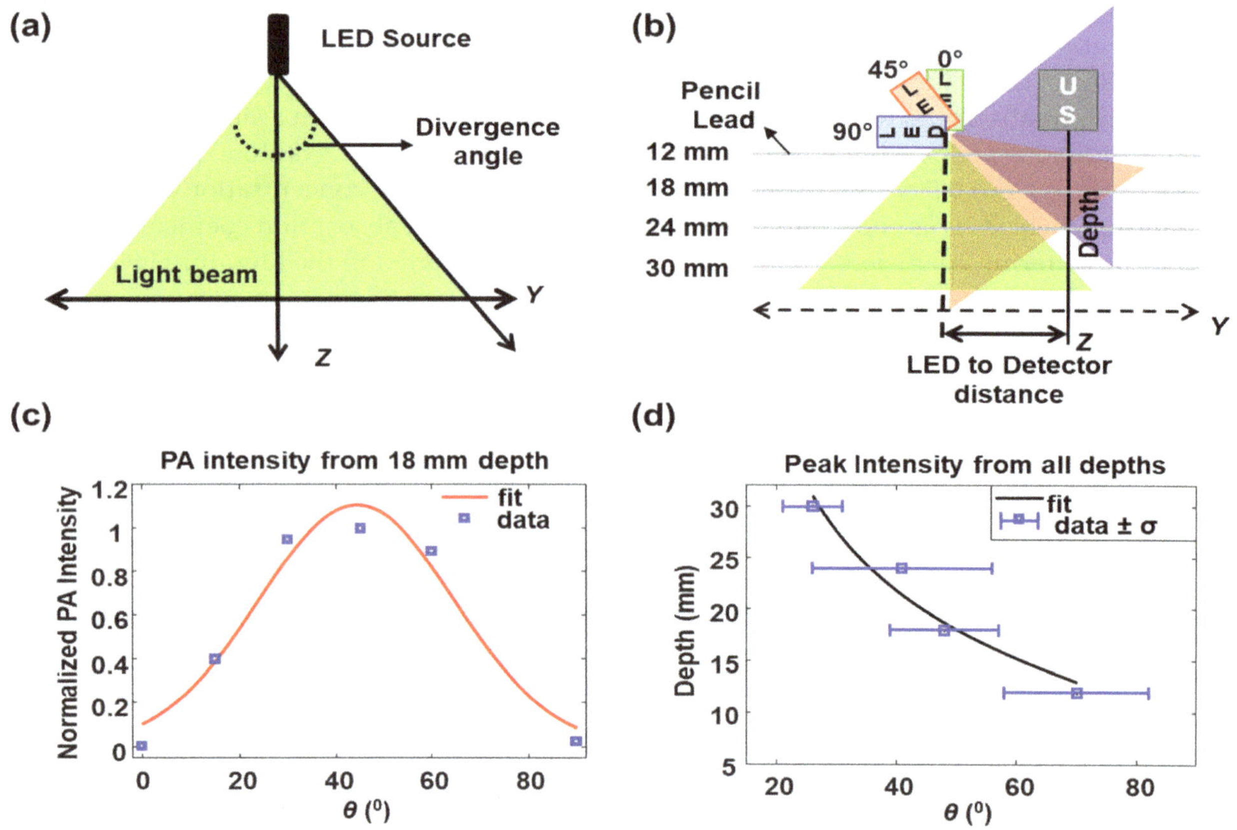

Figure 4. (**a**) Illustration of the source wavefront profile, while assuming the LED array as a line source with Gaussian profile having divergence described by Equation (4); (**b**) Source profile after pivoting LED arrays at three different angles in the imaging plane–green at 0°, red at 45°, and blue at 90°; (**c**) Normalized PA intensity obtained from 18 mm target vs. LED illumination angle, θ, is indicated in blue squares. The red solid curve shows the Gaussian fit using Equation (5), with an R-squared value of 0.95; (**d**) Blue squares with error bar show the peak PA intensity with standard deviation for each depth plotted as a function of θ for pencil lead phantom data in water. The black solid curve displays the best fit using a cotangent function ($R^2 = 0.95$).

The multiplying factor 2 is used to include both sides of the illumination plane. Target depth and LED to detector distance refer to the absorber (pencil lead) position in depth below the detector (US transducer) and its lateral distance to the source (LED array), respectively. In our experiment, the target and LED to detector distance were fixed while the source was pivoted, as shown in Figure 4b. We assume that the LED source exhibits a Gaussian spatial intensity profile and thus a Gaussian function is used to fit PA intensity vs. LED- illumination angle data to find the divergence of the LED arrays, given by

$$f(x) = a\, e^{-\left(\frac{x-b}{c}\right)^2} \tag{5}$$

where x is the source angle, a is the peak PA intensity and that corresponds to angle b, and c is the half of the angle span at which PA intensity shows half maximum (50%) or −6 dB roll-off. The divergence can then be calculated by multiplying c by two, resulting in the full width of the angle at half maximum of the PA intensity (FWHM). The model can be fitted using a least-squares minimization method to obtain best-fit parameters. Moreover, the position of the peak intensity for a chosen depth can be described by

$$d = m + n\cdot \cot(\theta) \tag{6}$$

where θ is the LED illumination angle (Figure 1), m is the offset of imaging plane in depth, n is the separation between LED and detector, and d is the imaging depth.

3. Results

Experiments were conducted in two different phantom environments: liquid and chicken tissue. The first phantom consisted of pencil lead (point source) as absorbing targets (Figure 3) in water or 1% intralipid media. The second tissue-mimicking phantom consisted of an absorbing cylindrical lesion made of graphite powder (Figure 5), which was placed on top of a chicken breast tissue arranged obliquely to the imaging plane, while the top layer was interchanged between water or chicken breast tissue. The experiments were designed to probe the phantom at all depths simultaneously for each angle of choice, thereby reducing experimental uncertainties.

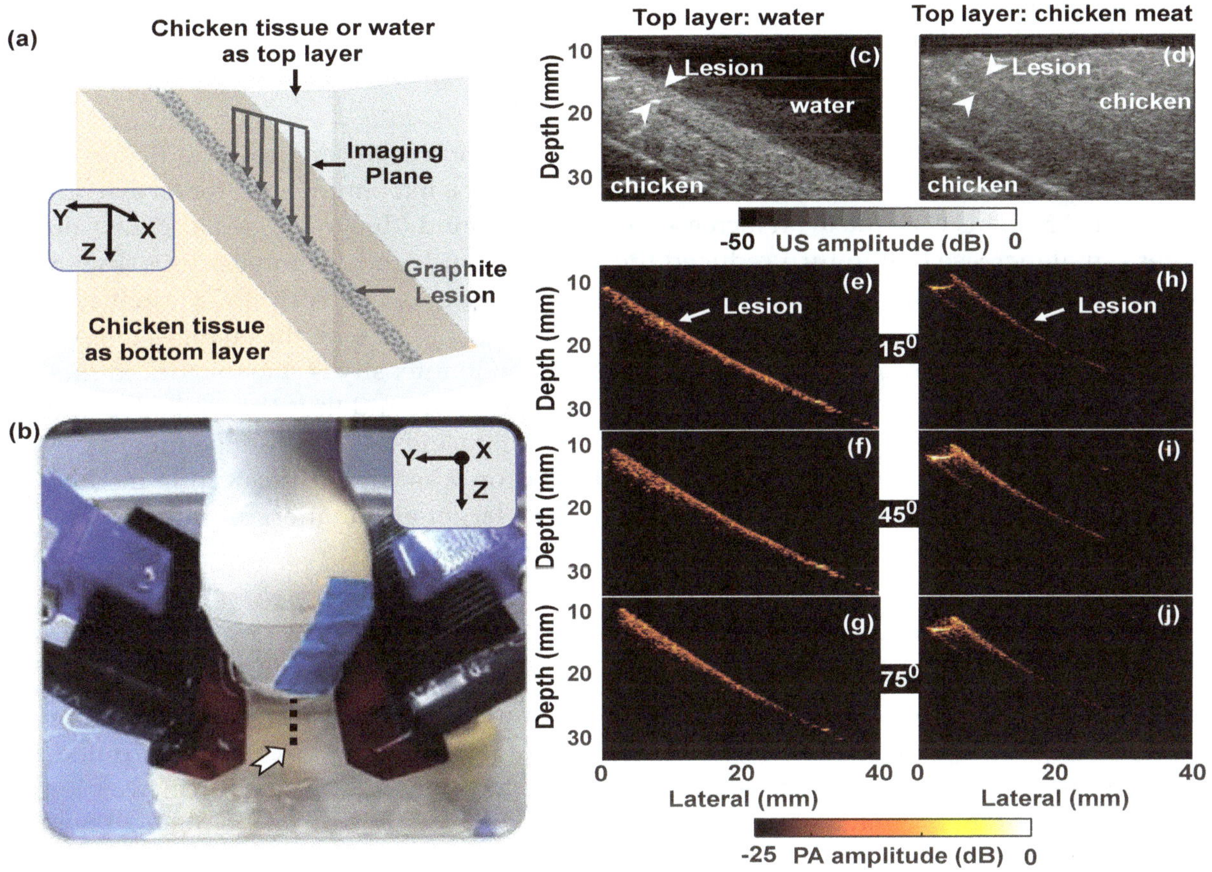

Figure 5. (**a**) Schematic of the tissue-mimicking phantom: Absorbing lesion (cylindrical in shape, 2 mm in diameter) placed on chicken tissue and arranged obliquely in the *XZ* plane. (**b**) Photograph of the experiment. The dotted line indicated by arrowhead shows the projection of lesion to the *x*-axis; (**c**,**d**) US image of the sample showing water top layer (**c**) or chicken layer (**d**) lesion and bottom chicken tissue in both cases; (**e**–**j**) PA intensity images captured using water as the top layer (**e**–**g**) or chicken tissue as the top layer (**h**–**j**), by choosing LED array directions: 15° (**e**,**h**), 45° (**f**,**i**), and 75° (**g**,**j**) with respect to the imaging plane.

3.1. Pencil Lead Phantom Experiments

3.1.1. Pencil Lead in Scattering and Non-Scattering Media Shows Weak Dependency on the LED Illumination Angle

Initially, PA intensities were monitored as a function of the illumination angle using a 4 × 5 pencil-lead matrix (as detailed previously) aligned orthogonal to the imaging axis to form point targets at defined locations. LED directions were varied from 0° to 90° in steps of 15°, as shown in Figure 1. Figure 3a,b shows the photographs of the lead matrix and an experimental arrangement in intralipid, respectively. PA intensity images (in dB scale) obtained at three representative angles: 15°, 45°, and 75°

in water and 1% intralipid medium are shown in Figure 3c–e, Figure 3f–h, respectively. PA images from all the angles between 0° and 90° can be found in Figure S2 (for water) and Figure S3 (for intralipid). Angle dependent PA intensities and CNR were calculated for four depths (approximately at 12 mm, 18 mm, 24 mm, and 30 mm) as described in Section 2.3 and plotted in Figure 3i, Figure 3k, Figure 3j, Figure 3l, respectively. An approximate gap of 10.5 mm from the US transducer to the sample was kept avoiding near field reconstruction errors and also to allow room for LED adjustments. For non-scattering media (water), the PA signal intensity increased as LED illumination angle increased from parallel orientation (0°), and then reached a maximum value at intermediate angles and finally decreased in its strength as the angle approached 90° (LED illumination perpendicular to the transducer). It is obvious from the plots that the angles corresponding to the maximum PA intensity value were in an inverse relation to the target depth, by showing a maximum value at a steeper angle for the 12 mm target and a maximum value at a shallower angle corresponding for the 30 mm target.

Figure 3j demonstrates CNR obtained in water as a function of the angle of irradiation. It reveals that the PA contrast did not change significantly after reaching a maximum level for an extended angle range of 15° to 75°. This was due to an increase in the background (due to various artifacts) along with the target signal increase that in turn reduced the angle dependency. PA intensities using intralipid (Figure 3k,l) showed a similar trend as water, especially for angles between 15° to 75°. In the cases of 0° and 90°, even though the trend was similar to that of the water phantom, the changes in PA intensity were less for intralipid phantom as expected. This reduction in intensity is due to reduced fluence due to optical scattering that reduces the incoming light directionality (and thus the angle dependency) as opposed to the case of non-scattering water medium. Comparing the depth-dependent CNR within the quasi angle-independent regime (15°–75°), the total drop was larger in scattering media (~30 dB) than in the water phantom (~15 dB). This can be due to a larger attenuation promoted by increased light scattering.

3.1.2. LED Source Divergence and Optimum Illumination Angle from Pencil Lead Targets in Water

Knowing the target location in depth and its lateral separation from the illumination plane, the source divergence (Figure 4) orthogonal to the illumination plane (Y) can be computed. In our experiments, the center of the light source (approximated here as a line source) was located at 10.5 ± 2 mm away from the imaging plane (imaging axis of the US transducer). Utilizing Equation (5), the divergence of the LED source was calculated to be 58 ± 8° at FWHM from the Gaussian fit of PA intensities from pencil lead target at 18 mm depth (Figure 4c). The experimentally derived divergence value is in good agreement with the manufacturer's data (60°, from Cyberdyne Inc., Tsukuba, Japan). The peak PA intensity (coefficient b in Equation (5)) at 18 mm depth was observed at 44° ± 3°. We further analyzed the data in Figure 3i to infer the angle at which maximum PA intensity could be obtained as a function of depth (Figure 4d) using the coefficient b in Equation (5). The black solid curve in Figure 4d shows the cotangent fit (Equation (6)) to the data shown in blue squares with a goodness of fit (R-squared) value equal to 0.95. Fitting was done by choosing m (depth offset) and n (separation of LED to the detector) as free fit parameters. Best fits (and 95% confidence interval bounds) obtained for, m is 9 mm (−0.6, 18.6 mm) and n is 10.7 mm (3, 18 mm). A large offset value might be due to the experimental error coming from the spatial width of the LED array, which takes up ~10.5 mm below the US transducer, in the imaging plane, at its steepest angle (90°). The value of n matched well to our experimentally set approximate value of 10.5 mm. From the fit, maximum PA signal intensity value at 12 mm can be obtained with a LED illumination angle of 74° while 27° can be used to image lesions at 30 mm depth. It should be noted that there exists a strong dependency of the illumination angle at superficial regions (slope of −5°/mm at 10 mm), which weakens as it goes to deeper locations (−2.5°/mm at 20 mm and −1.1°/mm at 30 mm) due to the nature of the cotangent function. The diameter of the projected beam onto the imaging plane, Z, at a given θ is estimated to be about 11.2 mm (θ = 84.5°) and 11.8 mm (θ = 27°) at 10 mm and 30 mm depths, respectively. Interestingly, less than 4% variation in the beam diameter in the imaging range is observed with different LED illumination angle. So, the large source divergence of about 11–12 mm overcomes the strong angle dependencies and can be used to lower the number of illumination angles for imaging lesions at various depths as is the case with Laser illumination. The LED illumination angle effects are even less notable in scattering medium, where deep tissue imaging can be achieved with smaller LED illumination angles (closer to being parallel to the imaging plane) and superficial lesion imaging is possible with larger LED illumination angles (closer to being perpendicular to the imaging plane).

3.2. *Effect of Surrounding Media and Illumination Direction on PA Signal from Tumor Mimicking Lesion*

A second set of experiments were conducted using tumor mimicking light-absorbing lesion placed obliquely in the imaging plane on top of chicken breast tissue (backing layer) while using water (Figure 5a) or scattering chicken tissue as the top layer (Figure 5b). This phantom study aimed to simulate superficial or deep-seated tumor lesions filled with blood vessels or contrast agents. US images corresponding to experiments using a top water layer (Figure 5c) and top chicken layer (Figure 5d) show the lesion placement and surrounding layers for comparison with corresponding PA images. The PA images using water as the top layer or chicken tissue as the top layer at LED source angles 15°, 45°, and 75° are shown in Figure 5e–g, Figure 5h–j, respectively. An apparent lateral shift in lesion positions between the images generated with water and chicken top layers was due to a change in imaging transducer placement about 2 mm in the horizontal axis, between the experiments (Figure 5h–j), which had negligible or no effects in our depth-dependent analysis.

Experiments with the top water layer show PA signals from the lesion for the entire imaging depth (Figure 5e–g), which can be associated with the negligible light scattering in water, opposed to chicken tissue (Figure 5h–j). Angle dependent PA intensity variations were also visible in both cases, where deeper tissue illumination was achieved at lower incident angles while increased PA intensity in the detector vicinity was observed for higher illumination angles. These results are very similar to those observed in Figure 3 using pencil lead phantom in water and intralipid. For a detailed analysis of depth-dependent PA intensity variation, Figure 6 was presented with analyses from three depth locations at 12 mm, 20 mm, and 28 mm, in which PA signals were plotted as a function of illumination angle, for the tissue-mimicking phantom with the top water and chicken layers. The white parallelograms in Figure 6a indicate the selected ROI from where the median PA intensity was calculated and the yellow parallelogram ROIs were considered for the background. Calculated PA intensities and CNRs as a function of angle for different depths are shown, respectively, in Figure 6b,c while using water as the top layer, and Figure 6d,f for chicken breast as the top layer. In the case of water as the top layer, the illumination angle parallel to the imaging plane, i.e., 0°, produced highest PA intensity (~23 dB) at the bottom (28 mm) than at the top regions; at 12 mm, the intensity dropped to ~17 dB as demonstrated in Figure 6b. On the other hand, experiment with the chicken top layer (Figure 6d) showed almost equal but low PA intensity (~17 dB) for all depths at 0°. It is interesting to note that the PA signal from 12 mm was quasi-constant for all angles from 30° and above. For the intermediate depth (20 mm), the intensities showed an increase up to 15°, then stayed almost unchanging until 60° and showed a slight decrease in the mean value with further increase in angle from 75° and above. It should also be noted that the signal from 28 mm depth while using chicken top layer was very close to the background level (CNR is less than 5 dB), which shows the maximum penetration depth achieved within our experimental limits.

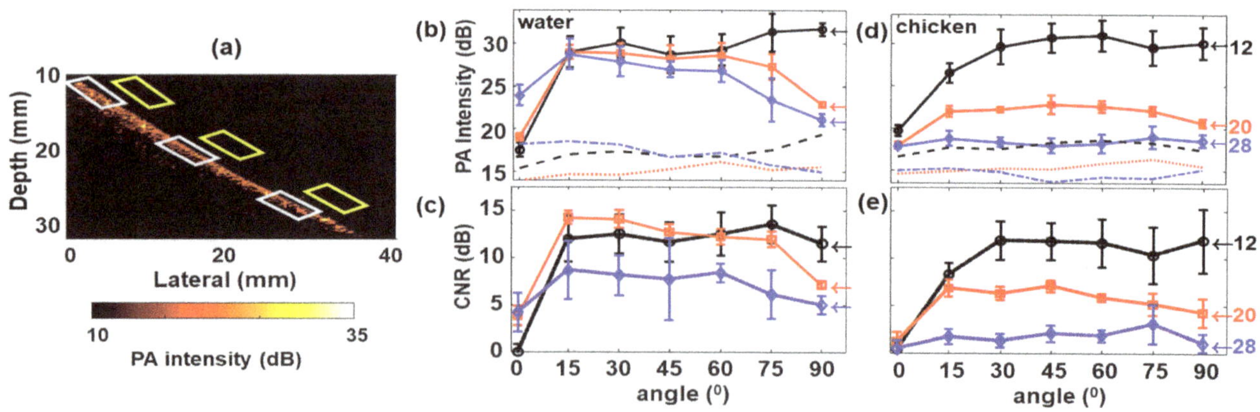

Figure 6. (**a**) PA image of a sample containing absorbing lesion (2 mm diameter) with the top water layer. White parallelograms indicate the regions selected for PA intensity and yellow for the background; (**b**,**d**) PA signal intensity plotted as a function of LED angles for selected depths in mm as labeled by numbers with the corresponding color, right next to each plot. Black circle with line corresponds to 12 mm, red squares with line corresponds to 20 mm and blue diamond with line indicates 28 mm. The black dotted lines, red dash-dotted lines, and blue dashed lines represent the background levels for 12, 20, and 28 mm depths (from the transducer) respectively; a gap of 10.5 mm exists between the transducer and the phantom surface. (**c**) CNR of the lesion under water; (**e**) CNR of the lesion under chicken breast. The error bars represent the standard deviation.

4. Discussion

The dependence of image contrast on irradiation parameters such as the angle of irradiation relative to the transducer, wavelength of the light irradiation, and distance between the transducer and the light source is undisputed. In this paper, we studied the dependence of signal intensity and contrast in PA images generated by an LED light source at various illumination angles. The 3D modular hinge design gave extreme flexibility to adjust the illumination angle as well as the transducer to LED-array distance. In the current work, the distance between the LED light source and transducer was relatively constant with the LED array positioned very close to the transducer (Figure 1). Studies addressing different separation distances between the transducer and the LED array can potentially give complementary information to our results. With respect to the 3D modular hinge system itself (Figure 2), several design criteria could be improved. Currently, the footprint of the modular system is large (11.5 cm at its widest dimension). Though the complete probe is lightweight due to lack of any heavy motors or metallic pieces, it is still larger than the other 3D printed fixed angle holders, e.g., by Sivasubramanian et al. [33]. The hinge system can be further modified with computer-controlled micro-hinges, can be adapted to any fiber bundles irrespective of their shape or size and can also be integrated with any laser or pulsed diode-based systems.

In all our results, it is evident that the background signal is also increasing along with the PA signal of interest (Figure S1), resulting in less impact on CNR when the illumination angle is increased beyond a certain limit. We believe that the background signal may be affected by various artifacts like reflection artifacts, out-of-plane clutter, and side lobes. For example, it is well known that more reflection artifacts are caused by high PA signal from tissue/phantom surface reflecting off acoustically dense structures when the illumination angle is steep and the fluency is high just beneath the US probe. These reverberation type of reflection artifacts are visible in our results too (Figure 3 and Figure S1) and would have impacted the CNR calculation. At lower illumination angle setups, light can scatter outside the imaging plane, get absorbed by different features, and generate out-of-plane artifacts and this also may have an impact in the CNR [52]. We strongly believe that it is also important to consider these common artifacts in the CNR analysis hence we chose a region very close to the target of interest for the calculations, instead of choosing a blank image (image generated with no light) or electronic noise. Furthermore, we used 850 nm irradiation, a wavelength at which there is relatively high penetration depth in tissue. The utility of other illumination wavelengths will impact the PA signal intensity and CNR based on the absorption properties of lesions at those wavelengths. Our future studies will involve evaluating these observations especially in an in vivo situation with both subcutaneous (superficial lesions) and orthotopic tumors (deep lesions).

A recent study by Agarwal et al. demonstrated that single-shot laser-based PAI and LED-based PAI achieved the same SNR from lesions 2–3 cm deep in chicken tissue. Though high frame averaging (2560 frames) was performed in LED-based PAI, they achieved real-time imaging due to the high pulse repetition frequency of LED sources [53]. The utility of LED-based PAI systems has been extensively reviewed by Zhu et al. [37] and one of the key factors currently hindering the clinical translation of LED-based photoacoustic imaging systems regardless of demonstrated promise in multiple preclinical and clinical imaging applications is the optical output power of the LED arrays [37,54]. It is of paramount importance to improve the optical output power of LEDs to enhance its usage in a wide range of deep-tissue imaging applications, and thus accelerate the clinical translation. The pulse repetition rate of LEDs is several-fold higher than pulsed LASER systems and it is feasible to average multiple image frames to improve SNR without compromising on real-time imaging capability. However, averaging N frames can improve SNR by only $\sqrt{N}$, and thus this approach has its limitations. Recently several developments in beamforming methodologies are made to improve the CNR and SNR of the LED-based PA systems [55,56]. We believe that the improvement of optical pulse energy and the development of novel image reconstruction and enhancement algorithms will be critical to accelerate the clinical translation of LED-based PAI [54].

5. Conclusions

Our results show that the optical excitation using an LED source behaves differently than the laser excitation due to a large source divergence of LED arrays, which we calculated to be 58° ± 8°. This in turn reduces the source direction dependency of PA signal at different depths. Our analysis in the non-scattering medium shows a strong dependence of illumination angle vs. depth at near field regions (−5°/mm at ~10 mm) and weak dependence at deeper locations (−2.5°/mm at 20 mm; −1.1°/mm at 30 mm). On the other hand, results from tissue-mimicking phantom in scattering media showed significantly weaker angle dependence of PA signal intensity than the phantom in water. So, utilizing an LED-based system (or a source with similar divergence) for either deep tissue lesions or superficial lesions would be less cumbersome in terms of source alignment by offering the freedom to choose a wide range of irradiation angles without losing CNR in the images. In contrast, spatially coherent sources would require stringent alignment strategies for illuminating lesions at various depths [57,58]. The modular light delivery system and results presented in this study can serve as a priori knowledge for future LED-based PA system designs and aid in further catapulting its utility in both preclinical and clinical applications.

Author Contributions: Conceptualization, M.K., M.K.A.S., and S.M.; methodology, M.K., C.D.N., and S.M.; software, M.K.; validation, M.K. and C.D.N.; formal analysis, M.K.; investigation, M.K.; resources, S.M.; data curation, M.K. and C.D.N.; writing—original draft preparation, M.K. and S.M.; writing—review and editing, M.K., M.K.A.S., C.D.N., and S.M.; visualization, M.K. and S.M.; supervision, S.M.; project administration, S.M.; funding acquisition, S.M. All authors have read and agreed to the published version of the manuscript.

Acknowledgments: The authors would like to thank Michael D. Kennedy, Department of Biomedical Engineering, Tufts University, Medford, MA, USA, for 3D printing the modular holder for LED arrays.

References

1. Hester, S.C.; Kuriakose, M.; Nguyen, C.D.; Mallidi, S. Role of Ultrasound and Photoacoustic Imaging in Photodynamic Therapy for Cancer. *Photochem. Photobiol.* **2020**, *96*, 260–279. [CrossRef]
2. Beard, P. Biomedical photoacoustic imaging. *Interface Focus* **2011**, *1*, 602–631. [CrossRef]
3. Brown, E.; Brunker, J.; Bohndiek, S.E. Photoacoustic imaging as a tool to probe the tumour microenvironment. *Dis. Model Mech.* **2019**, *12*, dmm039636. [CrossRef]
4. Steinberg, I.; Huland, D.M.; Vermesh, O.; Frostig, H.E.; Tummers, W.S.; Gambhir, S.S. Photoacoustic clinical imaging. *Photoacoustics* **2019**, *14*, 77–98. [CrossRef]
5. Zackrisson, S.; van de Ven, S.; Gambhir, S.S. Light in and sound out: Emerging translational strategies for photoacoustic imaging. *Cancer Res.* **2014**, *74*, 979–1004. [CrossRef]
6. Liu, G. Theory of the photoacoustic effect in condensed matter. *Appl. Opt.* **1982**, *21*, 955–960. [CrossRef] [PubMed]
7. Wang, L.V. Tutorial on Photoacoustic Microscopy and Computed Tomography. *IEEE J. Sel. Top. Quantum Electron.* **2008**, *14*, 171–179. [CrossRef]
8. Craig, B.; Sussman, C.R.; Zhang, Q.; Jiang, H.; Zheng, T.; Steindler, D.; Young, L.; Weiss, M.D. Photoacoustic tomography can detect cerebral hemodynamic alterations in a neonatal rodent model of hypoxia-ischemia. *Acta Neurobiol. Exp.* **2012**, *72*, 253–263.
9. Wang, X.; Chamberland, D.L.; Xi, G. Noninvasive reflection mode photoacoustic imaging through infant skull toward imaging of neonatal brains. *J. Neurosci. Methods* **2008**, *168*, 412–421. [CrossRef]
10. Lin, L.; Hu, P.; Shi, J.; Appleton, C.M.; Maslov, K.; Li, L.; Zhang, R.; Wang, L.V. Single-breath-hold photoacoustic computed tomography of the breast. *Nat. Commun.* **2018**, *9*, 2352. [CrossRef]
11. Dogra, V.S.; Chinni, B.K.; Valluru, K.S.; Moalem, J.; Giampoli, E.J.; Evans, K.; Rao, N.A. Preliminary results of ex vivo multispectral photoacoustic imaging in the management of thyroid cancer. *AJR Am. J. Roentgenol.* **2014**, *202*, W552–W558. [CrossRef] [PubMed]
12. Yang, M.; Zhao, L.; He, X.; Su, N.; Zhao, C.; Tang, H.; Hong, T.; Li, W.; Yang, F.; Lin, L.; et al. Photoacoustic/ultrasound dual imaging of human thyroid cancers: An initial clinical study. *Biomed. Opt. Express* **2017**, *8*, 3449–3457. [CrossRef] [PubMed]
13. Mallidi, S.; Luke, G.P.; Emelianov, S. Photoacoustic imaging in cancer detection, diagnosis, and treatment guidance. *Trends Biotechnol.* **2011**, *29*, 213–221. [CrossRef] [PubMed]
14. Valluru, K.S.; Wilson, K.E.; Willmann, J.K. Photoacoustic Imaging in Oncology: Translational Preclinical and Early Clinical Experience. *Radiology* **2016**, *280*, 332–349. [CrossRef]
15. Mallidi, S.; Watanabe, K.; Timerman, D.; Schoenfeld, D.; Hasan, T. Prediction of tumor recurrence and therapy monitoring using ultrasound-guided photoacoustic imaging. *Theranostics* **2015**, *5*, 289–301. [CrossRef]
16. Moore, C.; Jokerst, J.V. Strategies for Image-Guided Therapy, Surgery, and Drug Delivery Using Photoacoustic Imaging. *Theranostics* **2019**, *9*, 1550–1571. [CrossRef]
17. Kim, J.; Park, S.; Jung, Y.; Chang, S.; Park, J.; Zhang, Y.; Lovell, J.F.; Kim, C. Programmable Real-time Clinical Photoacoustic and Ultrasound Imaging System. *Sci. Rep.* **2016**, *6*, 35137. [CrossRef] [PubMed]
18. Schellenberg, M.W.; Hunt, H.K. Hand-held optoacoustic imaging: A review. *Photoacoustics* **2018**, *11*, 14–27. [CrossRef]
19. Upputuri, P.K.; Pramanik, M. Photoacoustic imaging in the second near-infrared window: A review. *J. Biomed. Opt.* **2019**, *24*, 1–20. [CrossRef]
20. Xu, M.; Wang, L.V. Photoacoustic imaging in biomedicine. *Rev. Sci. Instrum.* **2006**, *77*, 041101. [CrossRef]
21. Oraevsky, A.A.; Karabutov, A.A. Optoacoustic Tomography. In *Biomedical Photonics Handbook*; Vo-Dinh, T., Ed.; CRC: Boca Raton, FL, USA, 2003; Chapter 34.
22. Sivasubramanian, K.; Pramanik, M. High frame rate photoacoustic imaging at 7000 frames per second using clinical ultrasound system. *Biomed. Opt. Express* **2016**, *7*, 312–323. [CrossRef]

23. Sowers, T.; Yoon, H.; Emelianov, S. Investigation of light delivery geometries for photoacoustic applications using Monte Carlo simulations with multiple wavelengths, tissue types, and species characteristics. *J. Biomed. Opt.* **2020**, *25*, 1–16. [CrossRef]
24. Wang, Y.; Lim, R.S.A.; Zhang, H.; Nyayapathi, N.; Oh, K.W.; Xia, J. Optimizing the light delivery of linear-array-based photoacoustic systems by double acoustic reflectors. *Sci. Rep.* **2018**, *8*, 13004. [CrossRef]
25. Wang, Z.; Ha, S.; Kim, K. A new design of light illumination scheme for deep tissue photoacoustic imaging. *Opt. Express* **2012**, *20*, 22649–22659. [CrossRef]
26. Yang, G.; Amidi, E.; Nandy, S.; Mostafa, A.; Zhu, Q. Optimized light delivery probe using ball lenses for co-registered photoacoustic and ultrasound endo-cavity subsurface imaging. *Photoacoustics* **2019**, *13*, 66–75. [CrossRef] [PubMed]
27. Carles, G.; Zammit, P.; Harvey, A.R. Holistic Monte-Carlo optical modelling of biological imaging. *Sci. Rep.* **2019**, *9*, 15832. [CrossRef] [PubMed]
28. Flock, S.T.; Patterson, M.S.; Wilson, B.C.; Wyman, D.R. Monte Carlo modeling of light propagation in highly scattering tissue–I: Model predictions and comparison with diffusion theory. *IEEE Trans. Biomed. Eng.* **1989**, *36*, 1162–1168. [CrossRef]
29. Held, K.G.; Jaeger, M.; Ricka, J.; Frenz, M.; Akarcay, H.G. Multiple irradiation sensing of the optical effective attenuation coefficient for spectral correction in handheld OA imaging. *Photoacoustics* **2016**, *4*, 70–80. [CrossRef] [PubMed]
30. Watte, R.; Aernouts, B.; Van Beers, R.; Herremans, E.; Ho, Q.T.; Verboven, P.; Nicolai, B.; Saeys, W. Modeling the propagation of light in realistic tissue structures with MMC-fpf: A meshed Monte Carlo method with free phase function. *Opt. Express* **2015**, *23*, 17467–17486. [CrossRef] [PubMed]
31. Held, G.; Preisser, S.; Akarcay, H.G.; Peeters, S.; Frenz, M.; Jaeger, M. Effect of irradiation distance on image contrast in epi-optoacoustic imaging of human volunteers. *Biomed. Opt. Express* **2014**, *5*, 3765–3780. [CrossRef]
32. Haisch, C.; Eilert-Zell, K.; Vogel, M.M.; Menzenbach, P.; Niessner, R. Combined optoacoustic/ultrasound system for tomographic absorption measurements: Possibilities and limitations. *Anal. Bioanal. Chem.* **2010**, *397*, 1503–1510. [CrossRef]
33. Sivasubramanian, K.; Periyasamy, V.; Wen, K.K.; Pramanik, M. Optimizing light delivery through fiber bundle in photoacoustic imaging with clinical ultrasound system: Monte Carlo simulation and experimental validation. *J. Biomed. Opt.* **2017**, *22*, 41008. [CrossRef]
34. Sangha, G.S.; Hale, N.J.; Goergen, C.J. Adjustable photoacoustic tomography probe improves light delivery and image quality. *Photoacoustics* **2018**, *12*, 6–13. [CrossRef]
35. Jo, J.; Xu, G.; Zhu, Y.; Burton, M.; Sarazin, J.; Schiopu, E.; Gandikota, G.; Wang, X. Detecting joint inflammation by an LED-based photoacoustic imaging system: A feasibility study. *J. Biomed. Opt.* **2018**, *23*, 1–4. [CrossRef] [PubMed]
36. Leskinen, J.; Pulkkinen, A.; Tick, J.; Tarvainen, T.; Ntziachristos, V.; Zemp, R. Photoacoustic tomography setup using LED illumination. In Proceedings of the Opto-Acoustic Methods and Applications in Biophotonics IV, Munich, Germany, 24–25 June 2019.
37. Zhu, Y.; Feng, T.; Cheng, Q.; Wang, X.; Du, S.; Sato, N.; Kuniyil Ajith Singh, M.; Yuan, J. Towards Clinical Translation of LED-Based Photoacoustic Imaging: A Review. *Sensors* **2020**, *20*, 2484. [CrossRef]
38. Agrawal, S.; Fadden, C.; Dangi, A.; Yang, X.; Albahrani, H.; Frings, N.; Heidari Zadi, S.; Kothapalli, S.R. Light-Emitting-Diode-Based Multispectral Photoacoustic Computed Tomography System. *Sensors* **2019**, *19*, 4861. [CrossRef]
39. Xia, W.; Kuniyil Ajith Singh, M.; Maneas, E.; Sato, N.; Shigeta, Y.; Agano, T.; Ourselin, S.; J West, S.; E Desjardins, A. Handheld real-time LED-based photoacoustic and ultrasound imaging system for accurate visualization of clinical metal needles and superficial vasculature to guide minimally invasive procedures. *Sensors* **2018**, *18*, 1394. [CrossRef]
40. Zhu, Y.; Xu, G.; Yuan, J.; Jo, J.; Gandikota, G.; Demirci, H.; Agano, T.; Sato, N.; Shigeta, Y.; Wang, X. Light Emitting Diodes based Photoacoustic Imaging and Potential Clinical Applications. *Sci. Rep.* **2018**, *8*, 9885. [CrossRef]
41. Jo, J.; Xu, G.; Cao, M.; Marquardt, A.; Francis, S.; Gandikota, G.; Wang, X. A Functional Study of Human Inflammatory Arthritis Using Photoacoustic Imaging. *Sci. Rep.* **2017**, *7*, 15026. [CrossRef]

42. Hariri, A.; Lemaster, J.; Wang, J.; Jeevarathinam, A.S.; Chao, D.L.; Jokerst, J.V. The characterization of an economic and portable LED-based photoacoustic imaging system to facilitate molecular imaging. *Photoacoustics* **2018**, *9*, 10–20. [CrossRef]
43. Joseph Francis, K.; Boink, Y.E.; Dantuma, M.; Ajith Singh, M.K.; Manohar, S.; Steenbergen, W. Tomographic imaging with an ultrasound and LED-based photoacoustic system. *Biomed. Opt. Express* **2020**, *11*, 2152–2165. [CrossRef]
44. Toshitaka Agano, M.K.A.S.; Nagaoka, R.; Awazu, K. Effect of light pulse width on frequency characteristics of photoacoustic signal—An experimental study using a pulse-width tunable LED-based photoacoustic imaging system. *Int. J. Eng. Technol.* **2018**, *7*, 4300–4303.
45. Jaeger, M.; Schüpbach, S.; Gertsch, A.; Kitz, M.; Frenz, M. Fourier reconstruction in optoacoustic imaging using truncated regularized inversek-space interpolation. *Inverse Probl.* **2007**, *23*, S51–S63. [CrossRef]
46. Driver, I.; Feather, J.W.; King, P.R.; Dawson, J.B. The optical properties of aqueous suspensions of Intralipid, a fat emulsion. *Phys. Med. Biol.* **1989**, *34*, 1927. [CrossRef]
47. Pogue, B.W.; Patterson, M.S. Review of tissue simulating phantoms for optical spectroscopy, imaging and dosimetry. *J. Biomed. Opt.* **2006**, *11*, 041102. [CrossRef] [PubMed]
48. Van Leeuwen-van Zaane, F.; Gamm, U.A.; van Driel, P.B.A.A.; Snoeks, T.J.A.; de Bruijn, H.S.; van der Ploeg-van den Heuvel, A.; Mol, I.M.; Löwik, C.W.G.M.; Sterenborg, H.J.C.M.; Amelink, A.; et al. In vivo quantification of the scattering properties of tissue using multi-diameter single fiber reflectance spectroscopy. *Biomed. Opt. Express* **2013**, *4*, 696–708. [CrossRef] [PubMed]
49. Elena Vladimirovna, S.; Brian, J.; John, N.; Anna, N.Y. Optical properties of normal and cancerous human skin in the visible and near-infrared spectral range. *J. Biomed. Opt.* **2006**, *11*, 1–9.
50. Vogt, W.C.; Jia, C.; Wear, K.A.; Garra, B.S.; Joshua Pfefer, T. Biologically relevant photoacoustic imaging phantoms with tunable optical and acoustic properties. *J. Biomed. Opt.* **2016**, *21*, 101405. [CrossRef]
51. Bohndiek, S.E.; Bodapati, S.; Van De Sompel, D.; Kothapalli, S.R.; Gambhir, S.S. Development and Application of Stable Phantoms for the Evaluation of Photoacoustic Imaging Instruments. *PLoS ONE* **2013**, *8*, e75533. [CrossRef]
52. Nguyen, H.N.Y.; Steenbergen, W. Three-dimensional view of out-of-plane artifacts in photoacoustic imaging using a laser-integrated linear-transducer-array probe. *Photoacoustics* **2020**, *19*, 100176. [CrossRef]
53. Sumit, A.; Mithun Kuniyil Ajith, S.; Xinyi, Y.; Hussain, A.; Ajay, D.; Sri-Rajasekhar, K. Photoacoustic imaging capabilities of light emitting diodes (LED) and laser sources: A comparison study. In Proceedings of the SPIE 11240, Photons Plus Ultrasound: Imaging and Sensing 2020, San Francisco, CA, USA, 17 February 2020.
54. Kuniyil Ajith Singh, M.; Sato, N.; Ichihashi, F.; Sankai, Y. Clinical Translation of Photoacoustic Imaging—Opportunities and Challenges from an Industry Perspective. In *LED-Based Photoacoustic Imaging: From Bench to Bedside*; Kuniyil Ajith Singh, M., Ed.; Springer: Singapore, 2020; pp. 379–393. [CrossRef]
55. Miri Rostami, S.R.; Mozaffarzadeh, M.; Ghaffari-Miab, M.; Hariri, A.; Jokerst, J. GPU-accelerated Double-stage Delay-multiply-and-sum Algorithm for Fast Photoacoustic Tomography Using LED Excitation and Linear Arrays. *Ultrason. Imaging* **2019**, *41*, 301–316. [CrossRef] [PubMed]
56. Farnia, P.; Najafzadeh, E.; Hariri, A.; Lavasani, S.N.; Makkiabadi, B.; Ahmadian, A.; Jokerst, J.V. Dictionary learning technique enhances signal in LED-based photoacoustic imaging. *Biomed. Opt. Express* **2020**, *11*, 2533–2547. [CrossRef]
57. Alijabbari, N.; Alshahrani, S.S.; Pattyn, A.; Mehrmohammadi, M. Photoacoustic Tomography with a Ring Ultrasound Transducer: A Comparison of Different Illumination Strategies. *Appl. Sci.* **2019**, *9*, 94. [CrossRef] [PubMed]
58. Luo, H.; Yang, G.; Zhu, Q. Fiber endface illumination diffuser for endo-cavity photoacoustic imaging. *Opt. Lett.* **2020**, *45*, 632–635. [CrossRef] [PubMed]

6

An Automatic Unmixing Approach to Detect Tissue Chromophores from Multispectral Photoacoustic Imaging

Valeria Grasso [1,2], Joost Holthof [1] and Jithin Jose [1,*]

1 FUJIFILM VisualSonics, 1114 AB Amsterdam, The Netherlands; valeria.grasso@fujifilm.com (V.G.); joost.holthof@fujifilm.com (J.H.)

2 Institute for Animal Science, Hannover Medical School, 30625 Hannover, Germany

* Correspondence: jithin.jose@fujifilm.com

Abstract: Multispectral photoacoustic imaging has been widely explored as an emerging tool to visualize and quantify tissue chromophores noninvasively. This modality can capture the spectral absorption signature of prominent tissue chromophores, such as oxygenated, deoxygenated hemoglobin, and other biomarkers in the tissue by using spectral unmixing methods. Currently, most of the reported image processing algorithms use standard unmixing procedures, which include user interaction in the form of providing the expected spectral signatures. For translational research with patients, these types of supervised spectral unmixing can be challenging, as the spectral signature of the tissues can differ with respect to the disease condition. Imaging exogenous contrast agents and accessing their biodistribution can also be problematic, as some of the contrast agents are susceptible to change in spectral properties after the tissue interaction. In this work, we investigated the feasibility of an unsupervised spectral unmixing algorithm to detect and extract the tissue chromophores without any a-priori knowledge and user interaction. The algorithm has been optimized for multispectral photoacoustic imaging in the spectral range of 680–900 nm. The performance of the algorithm has been tested on simulated data, tissue-mimicking phantom, and also on the detection of exogenous contrast agents after the intravenous injection in mice. Our finding shows that the proposed automatic, unsupervised spectral unmixing method has great potential to extract and quantify the tissue chromophores, and this can be used in any wavelength range of the multispectral photoacoustic images.

Keywords: photoacoustic; optoacoustic; spectral imaging; blind source separation; unsupervised unmixing

---

1. Introduction

The accurate detection and quantification of tissue chromophores is vital in molecular imaging, as it can facilitate the early detection, prediction, and monitor the disease conditions. In recent years, multispectral photoacoustic imaging has emerged as a noninvasive tool to visualize the tissue chromophores [1–4]. The underlying principle of photoacoustic (PA) imaging is based on the conversion of absorbed nanosecond laser pulses into acoustic waves that can be detected just as conventional ultrasound [5,6]. Based on this approach, PA images combine the peculiar optical absorption contrast of the tissue chromophores and the spatial resolution of ultrasound imaging (US). Being a hybrid imaging modality of ultrasound and optical, this multimodal imaging technology can provide anatomical, functional, and molecular information several centimeters deep in the tissues with a resolution up to tens of micrometers. The potential of PA imaging has been demonstrated in various preclinical applications, such as tumor progression and the prediction of tumor recurrence, therapy monitoring, imaging of vasculature, and the biodistribution of the contrast agents [7–13].

Apart from the preclinical applications, PA imaging is also used in clinical research. In addition to breast cancer monitoring [14,15] and sentinel lymph node imaging [16,17], the PA approach is also used to examine inflammatory bowel disease (IBD) [18] and the temporal arteries in patients with suspected giant cell arteritis (GCA) [19]. To expedite the clinical applications of PA imaging, recently, there has been a lot of focus on developing affordable light sources and the use of this technology in low-resource settings. Xia et al. demonstrated the feasibility of a Light-Emitting Diode (LED) based PA imaging system for the visualization of superficial vasculatures and needle guidance for minimally invasive procedures [20]. Zhu et al. used the LED-based approach to explore more clinical applications, such as diagnosing inflammatory arthritis and assessing peripheral microvascular function in patients [21–23].

Although there has been a lot of emphasis on PA hardware development, in the field of affordable settings, data analysis and reconstruction algorithms also play a crucial role in increasing the utility of the technology. Multiwavelength acquisition and spectral image processing is one of the commonly used techniques in PA. Since the optical absorption coefficient of the tissue chromophores varies over the spectrum, multispectral image processing approach can be applied to distinguish and characterize the molecules present in the tissues [24].

In general, the pixel intensity of the multispectral photoacoustic image is proportional to the absorption value of the respective tissue at a specific wavelength. In reality, due to the finite dimension of the pixel (partial volume effect) and the presence of instrumental noise, each spectrum can be a combination of different tissue chromophores. Therefore, it is a challenging task to unmix these signals spectrally and estimate their concentrations. The most common solution to detect the tissue chromophores from multispectral PA imaging is the supervised unmixing [25]. Although this technique yields acceptable results, it requires user interaction to provide the expected source spectral curves as an input to unmix the signals. For translational research with patients, these types of supervised spectral unmixing can be challenging, as the spectral signature of the tissues differs with respect to the disease condition. Imaging exogenous contrast agents and accessing their biodistribution can also be problematic, as some of the contrast agents are susceptible to change in spectral properties after the tissue interaction; thus, the algorithm can forfeit the sensitivity and specificity of imaging.

Hence, an unsupervised unmixing algorithm that can automatically detect the tissue chromophores, without any a-priori knowledge and user interaction, will be optimal, as this can facilitate and improve sensitivity and specificity. Generally, this class of algorithms is referred to as blind source separation (BSS) algorithms, as no a-priori information is required. The study reported by Glatz et al. [26] demonstrated the potential of these approaches to "blindly" extract the oxygenated and deoxygenated hemoglobin absorption spectra from the multispectral photoacoustic images. In the study, they evaluated different unsupervised algorithms, such as multivariate curve resolution analysis (MCR), principal component analysis (PCA), and independent component analysis (ICA) [27–31]. PCA yields an orthogonal transformation that decorrelates the variables. This approach relies upon the hypothesis that the source components are uncorrelated. On the other hand, ICA is based on a different assumption that the source components are maximally independent and non-Gaussian. Recently, Arabul et al. [32] used a similar approach to explore human carotid plaques, in which the ICA blind unmixing approach was constrained non-negatively. Although these approaches demonstrated the potential to detect the tissue chromophores, they suffer from limitations related to the interpretability of the mixed-sign values of their outcomes. Indeed, these aim to fit the training data well but often do not generalize the real and positive data sets.

In this paper, we investigated the possibility of using another blind source separation approach, which is based on non-negative matrix factorization (NNMF) [33]. The concept of NNMF has been widely used in a variety of applications, such as image recognition [34], text classification [35,36], and recommender systems [37]. This approach uses only the non-negative matrices to estimate the prominent components and their spatial distribution, from a linear mixture model. Montcuquet et al. [38] used this approach for in-vivo fluorescent imaging and demonstrated that the positivity condition enhances the convergence and, thus, improves the sensitivity of spectral unmixing [39].

Here, we examine the performance of non-negative matrix factorization (NNMF) to unmix tissue chromophores from multispectral PA images. The algorithm has been optimized to extract the tissue chromophores in the wavelength range of 680–900 nm. We tested the NNMF on synthetic data and on experimental data that mimic the blood vessels. Further, we validated the potential of the approach on an in-vivo study to detect and quantify the endogenous absorbers and exogenous contrast agent accumulation. To our knowledge, this is the first time the NNMF algorithm has been used for PA imaging.

2. Non-Negative Matrix Factorization (NNMF)

NNMF is a data decomposition approach, and it is based on the linear mixing model [40]. In this algorithm, the acquired mixed pixel spectra are differentiated into a collection of constituent spectra (called endmembers) and a set of fractional abundance maps. The endmembers represent the pure molecule absorption spectra present in the imaged sample, and these are extracted from the mixed pixel spectra. The maps of abundance at each pixel represent the percentage of each endmember present in that pixel.

Since the acquired spectral images are known, and the rest has to be estimated, the mixed data (multispectral PA images) can be arranged as a matrix $\boldsymbol{X} \in \mathbb{R}^{n \times m}$, where $\boldsymbol{n}$ represents the number of observations (pixels), and $\boldsymbol{m}$ corresponds to the number of variables per object (different wavelengths). In particular, the unmixing problem can be formulated as a matrix factorization:

$$X \approx WS \tag{1}$$

where X represents the mixed multispectral PA images, W the abundance maps, and S the source spectra. The dimensions of the matrices W and S are $\boldsymbol{n} \times \boldsymbol{k}$ and $\boldsymbol{k} \times \boldsymbol{m}$, respectively, where $\boldsymbol{k}$ is the hyperparameter which represents the number of prominent components.

The NNMF constrained cost function of the optimization problem can be formulated as follows:

$$[W, S] = \min_{W,S} \frac{1}{2} \parallel X - WS \parallel_F^2 \tag{2}$$

$$W_{ij} \geq 0, \;\; S_{ij} \geq 0 \tag{3}$$

where, in Equation (2), the defined cost function considers a Frobenius distance between the acquisition X and the model WS [33]. W and S are iteratively obtained until both matrices satisfy Equation (1), where the distance defined in the cost function (2) is constrained non-negatively (3). The NNMF learns a parts-based representation of the data, and the whole image is formed as a combination of additive components. The non-negativity constraint is computationally expensive to implement but it can lead to more interpretable data.

To solve the iterative optimization, the multiplicative update rules [41] can be used, and the steps can be defined as:

$$S\,(p+1) = S(p) \otimes \frac{\left(W^T \cdot X\right)}{\left(W^T W \cdot S\right)} \tag{4}$$

$$W(p+1) = W(p) \otimes \frac{\left(X \cdot S^T\right)}{\left(W \cdot S \cdot S^T\right)} \tag{5}$$

where $\boldsymbol{p}$ is the iteration step, and the operations of $\otimes$ and division in (4) and (5) are considered element by element. Each component is estimated only up to a multiplying scale factor. Hence, the factorization problem does not have a unique solution, where WS is a lower-rank approximation of X.

3. Experimental Methods

3.1. Simulated Multispectral PA Images

To evaluate the performance of the NNMF algorithm, simulation studies were performed by using a synthetic data set. The synthetic data set contains implemented photoacoustic spectral images within the wavelength range of 680–900 nm, with a step size of 5 nm. Each image at the respective wavelength contains 400 × 600 pixels. From the photoacoustic signal generation, it is evident that the PA signal is not only proportional to the absorption coefficient but also depends on the local fluence. The light fluence generally decreases with depth, and thus degrades the image uniformity, causing spatial fluence variations within the tissue. Consequently, the fluence compensation is significant for quantitative spectral imaging. Since the main focus of the simulation was to test the unmixing algorithm and its accuracy to detect the spectral signature of the prominent components, in this study, the local fluence was assumed to be constant.

Figure 1a depicts the schematic of the 2-dimensional (2-D) data set with six homogeneous inclusions. The inclusions mimic the cross section of blood vessels with different concentrations of oxyhemoglobin and deoxyhemoglobin. The inclusions 1, 2, and 3 contain oxyhemoglobin at 100%, 70%, and 30% of the intensity, respectively. Conversely, the inclusions 4, 5, and 6 include deoxyhemoglobin at 30%, 70%, and 100% of the intensity. Figure 1b shows the theoretical absorption spectra [42] expected from these inclusions, in addition to the background tissue absorption. To mimic the experimental conditions, a positive Gaussian distribution of noise ($mean = 0.04$; $std = 0.1\%$; $SNR = 30$ dB) was also added to the respective data set.

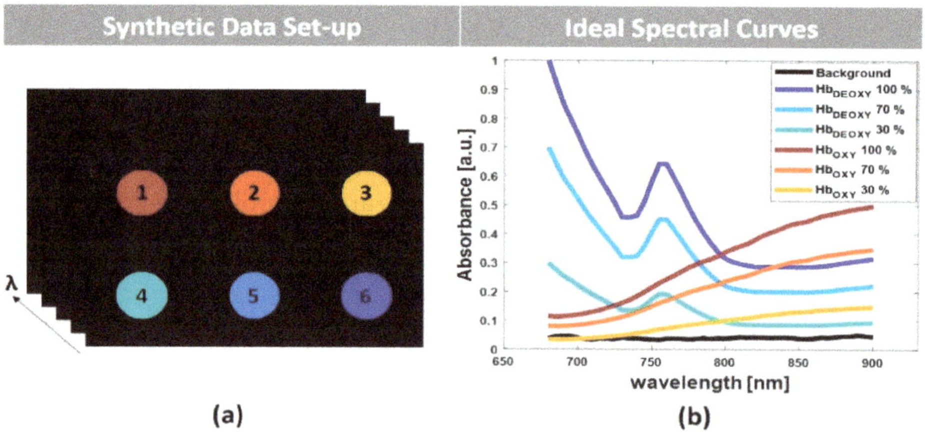

Figure 1. (**a**) Schematic representation of the simulated multispectral photoacoustic (PA) images with six inclusions, (**b**) ideal spectral curves of the inclusions.

3.2. Experimental Set-Up and Tissue-Mimicking Vessel Phantom

In addition to the simulation studies, experiments were performed by using Vevo LAZR-X photoacoustic image technology (FUJIFILM VisualSonics, Inc., Toronto, ON, Canada), as described elsewhere [43]. Vevo Phantom (FUJIFILM VisualSonics, Inc., Toronto, ON, Canada) containing two capillary tubes filled with Indocyanine Green (ICG, PULSION Verwaltungs, GmbH) and Methylene Blue (MB, Sigma-Aldrich), was used to mimic the blood vessels in the tissue. Transparent polyethylene (PE) tubes (SAI Infusion Technologies, Lake Villa, IL, USA), with an inner diameter of 15 μm and an outer diameter of 33 μm, were used. The tubes were positioned at a reciprocal distance of 6 mm and fixed at the same depth of 14 mm from the surface of the transducer. Demineralized water was used as a coupling medium, and the multispectral PA images were obtained in the wavelength range of 680–900 nm, with a step size of 5 nm. Figure 2a shows the schematic of the phantom and the experimental set-up. A 256-element linear array transducer with a central frequency of 21 MHz (MX250), including the integrated light delivery fibers from the sides of the transducer, was used to acquire the PA images. The transducer was aligned perpendicular to the capillary tubes, and the cross-sectional image of the tubes was acquired throughout the wavelength range. 3-Dimensional (3-D) data sets were also collected by linearly translating the transducer with a stepper motor over the capillary tubes while capturing cross-sectional 2-D slices. Figure 2b shows the photoacoustic spectra measured from the capillary tubes by using the Spectro-Mode in the VevoLab software (FUJIFILM VisualSonics, Inc., Toronto, ON, Canada). In the measurement tool, the system allows the user to select the region of interest (ROI) and calculate the average intensity of the photoacoustic signal at different wavelengths. Although this is not quantitative and the values are in arbitrary units, it can provide the spectral absorption trend of the agents in the respective wavelength range.

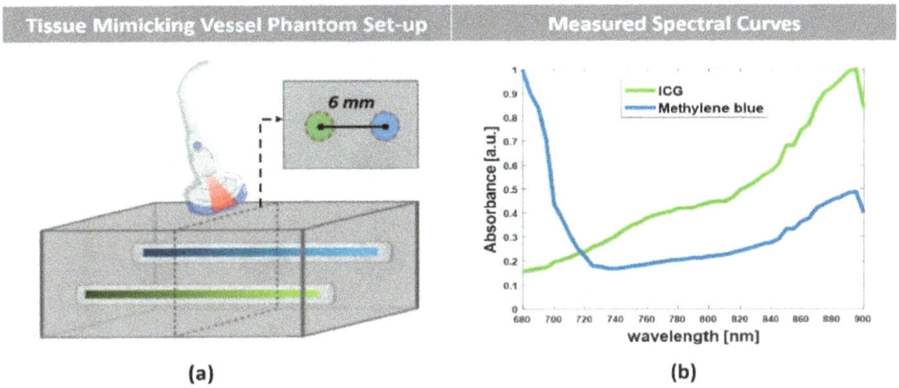

Figure 2. (**a**) Schematic of the tissue-mimicking vessel phantom. (**b**) The PA absorbance spectral graph of the agents measured by using VevoLab.

3.3. *In-Vivo Study*

Further, in-vivo animal experiments were performed to evaluate the feasibility of the NNMF data analysis on multispectral PA Imaging. The animal experiments were performed at the FUJIFILM Sonosite/VisualSonics facility in Amsterdam. The animal protocols used in this work were evaluated and approved by the Animal Use and Ethics Committee (CEUA) of The Netherlands (Protocol AVD2450020173644). They are in accordance with FELASA guidelines and the National Law for Laboratory Animal Experimentation (Law No. 18.611). The experiments were performed by using the same apparatus (Vevo LAZR-X) used for the phantom studies. A CD-1 female mouse model (Envigo, Horst, the Netherlands) was used for the experiments. The animal was anesthetized with isoflurane and placed on the animal imaging platform of the Vevo LAZR-X system, where temperature, heart rate, and respiration rate were monitored in real time. During the experiments, anesthesia was maintained using a vaporized isoflurane (1 L/min of oxygen and 0.75% isoflurane) gas system. The animal was positioned in right lateral recumbency, and the transducer was aligned perpendicularly. The kidney–spleen area of the animal was imaged before and after the intravenous injection of ICG. To obtain a concentration of 800 μM, 25-mg vial of ICG (PULSION Verwaltungs, GmbH) was resuspended in sterile water. With the help of an infusion pump (flowrate of 15 μL/sec), 80 μL of ICG was injected into the tail vein, and multispectral PA images were acquired in the wavelength range of 680–900 nm.

4. Results and Discussion

4.1. *Simulated Multispectral PA Images*

Figure 3 shows the main component spectra (a) and the respective abundance maps (b, c, and d) extracted from the synthetic PA data set by using the NNMF algorithm. The obtained spectral graphs (Figure 3a) show that the prominent absorbers present within the inclusions consist of two different endmembers: oxyhemoglobin and deoxyhemoglobin. As expected from the synthetic data, the oxyhemoglobin is mainly distributed on the first row of inclusions, with decreasing intensity from left to right (Figure 3c). The deoxyhemoglobin is present in the second row of inclusions, with increasing intensity from left to right (Figure 3b). Figure 3d displays the spatial distribution of the detected third component (named as background in Figure 3a), which is principally present in the region around the inclusions.

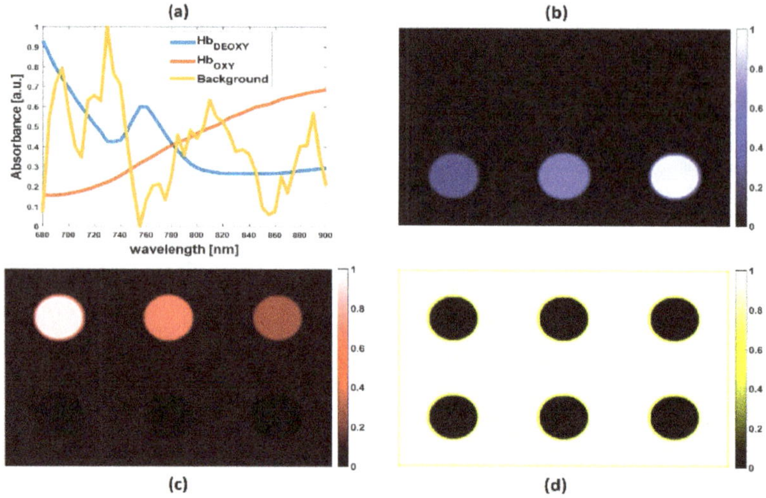

Figure 3. (**a**) Source spectra of oxyhemoglobin, deoxyhemoglobin, and background extracted by the non-negative matrix factorization (NNMF) algorithm. Abundance maps of (**b**) deoxyhemoglobin, (**c**) oxyhemoglobin, and (**d**) background.

NNMF appears to be an accurate method, yielding an explicit unmixing of specific tissue biomarkers, such as oxyhemoglobin and deoxyhemoglobin, and extracting the respective spectral signatures. The calculated Pearson correlation coefficient between the ideal spectra of the oxy and deoxyhemoglobin, and the extracted spectra was equal to 1 (Table 1). This confirms that NNMF can provide encouraging results on extracting tissue chromophores from multispectral PA images.

Table 1. Correlation values between the extracted source components by using the NNMF unmixing approach, and the respective absorption spectral curves used as a reference.

Data Set-Up	Chromophores	Correlation Value
Synthetic data	Oxyhemoglobin	1
	Deoxyhemoglobin	1
Vessel mimicking phantom	ICG	0.9943
	Methylene Blue	0.8344

Further, we investigated the performance of the NNMF approach to quantify the extracted prominent components. Figure 4a shows a graph with the quantitation of the source components (oxyhemoglobin, deoxyhemoglobin) per each circular inclusion of the synthetic data. Considering the synthetic data: inclusions 1, 2, and 3 present approximatively a decreasing content of oxyhemoglobin, and the regions 4, 5, and 6 present an increasing content of deoxyhemoglobin. In the graph, the variations are in the range of zero to one, and it is evident that these normalized intensities are matching the expected proportion of the components. Figure 4b shows the overlapped abundance maps of oxyhemoglobin and deoxyhemoglobin, and it also confirms the expected distribution of the prominent components.

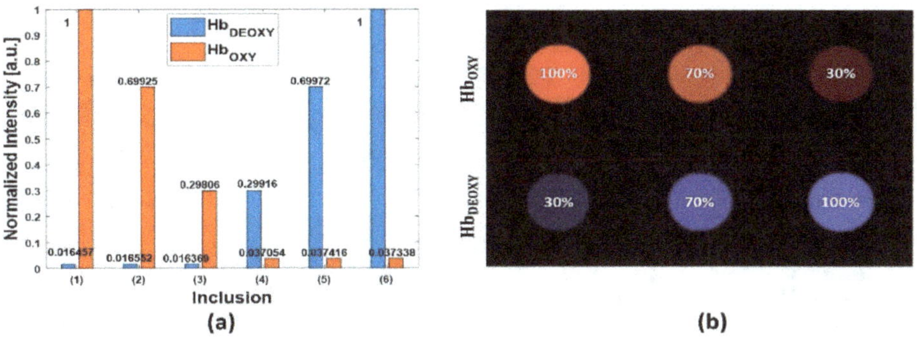

Figure 4. (**a**) Quantitative evaluation of the prominent source components (oxyhemoglobin and deoxyhemoglobin), per each circular region of the synthetic phantom. (**b**) Overlapped abundance maps of oxyhemoglobin and deoxyhemoglobin.

4.2. Tissue-Mimicking Vessel Phantom

Figure 5 shows the prominent spectral curves (a) and the abundance maps of the dyes in the capillary tubes, obtained by using the NNMF algorithm. The abundance maps overlapped in Figure 5b correspond to the 2-D spatial distribution of the contrast agents (ICG in green and MB in blue). Figure 5c shows the unmixing of the capillary tubes in 3-D, where the total imaged range was 6.5 mm with a step size of 200 µm. The Pearson correlation coefficient was evaluated between the extracted spectral curves, by using the NNMF, and the spectra measured by using the Spectro-Mode in the VevoLab.

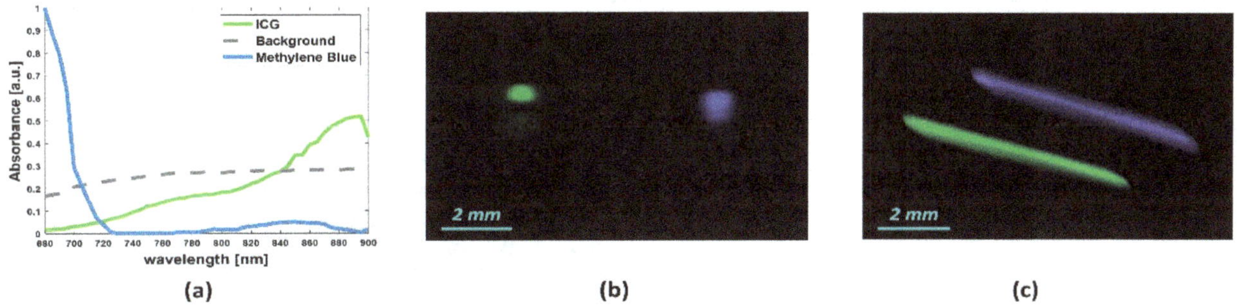

Figure 5. (**a**) Spectral absorption curves of the detected source components by NNMF, from 2-D spectral PA images of the tissue-mimicking vessel phantom. The overlapped abundance 2-D maps (**b**) and 3-D maps (**c**) of the detected source components: ICG and MB.

Table 1 reports the correlation coefficients measured for the ICG and methylene blue. The correlation value obtained for the methylene blue was 0.8344, and it was comparatively lower to the value obtained for the ICG, which was 0.9943. This could be due to the experimental conditions, as the tubes are located adjacently, into the phantom chamber. Hence, due to the short distance, the ICG that has an absorption peak at around 880 nm could influence the absorption spectrum of the MB. The graph reported in Figure 2b supports this assumption, as the MB spectrum shows an additional peak at around 880 nm. This may entail that measured spectral curves in Figure 2b are not the pure agent spectra. On the other hand, the spectra extracted by using NNMF are in accordance with the expected spectral signatures, and it shows promising unmixing performance.

4.3. In-Vivo Study

Figure 6a shows a high-resolution ultrasound (US) image of the kidney–spleen region and (b) is the PA image obtained at 880 nm. Figure 6c shows the oxygen saturation (SO_2) map, obtained before the contrast agent injection. To obtain the oxygen saturation map, we have followed the algorithm reported by Needles et al. [5], where the pixel values of the image are in the range of 0% (lower oxygenation) to 100% (higher oxygenation).

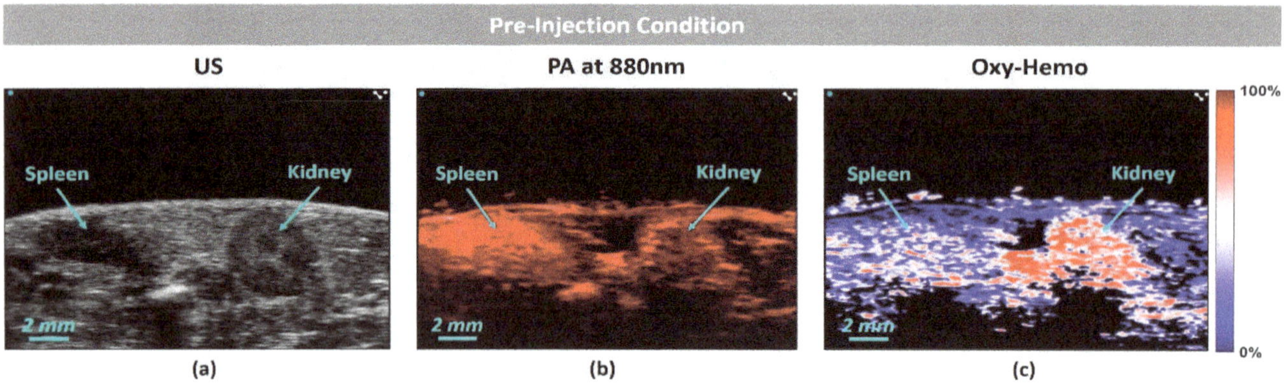

Figure 6. Pre-injection conditions: (**a**) ultrasound (US) image of the kidney–spleen view; respectively (**b**) photoacoustic (PA) image obtained at 880nm, and (**c**) SO_2 map.

Figure 7 shows the post-ICG injection condition. Figure 7a displays the source absorption spectra extracted by the NNMF approach. As expected, in the post-injection condition, the NNMF extracted the typical absorption spectral curve of the ICG, in addition to the endogenous chromophores such as oxy and deoxyhemoglobin spectra. The extracted spectrum of the ICG appears slightly different than the vessel mimicking phantom. Although the peak absorption was at 880 nm, the ICG spectrum at the lower wavelengths was altered. This could be due to the ICG interaction with other chromophores within the tissues. Figure 7 also shows the abundance maps of deoxyhemoglobin (b), oxyhemoglobin (c), and ICG (d). In the ICG map, it is evident that the dye is mostly accumulated in the spleen region. This is in accordance with the biodistribution of the ICG, as the kinetic of the kidney is much faster than the spleen [44].

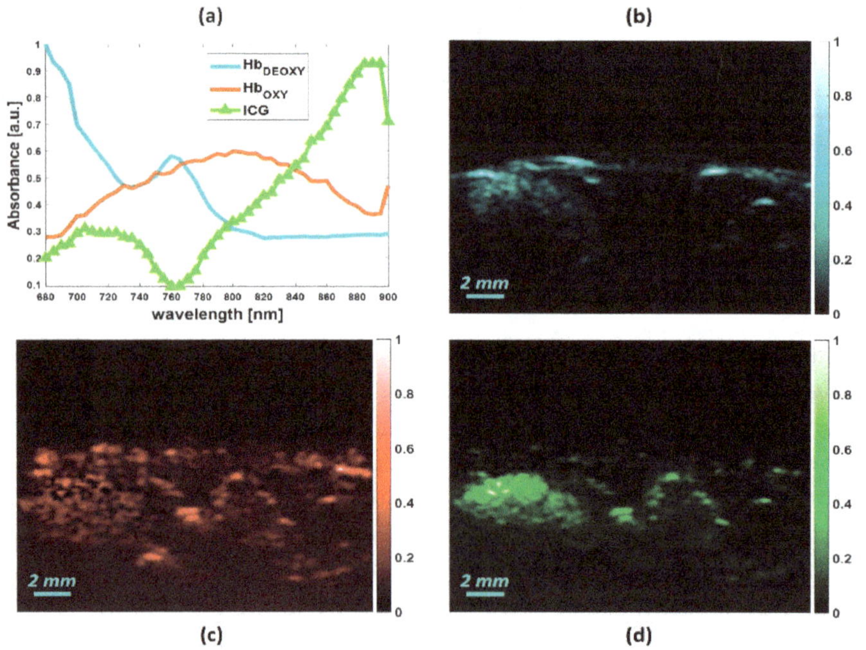

Figure 7. Post-injection conditions: (**a**) spectral signature of the endmembers obtained by using NNMF and abundance distribution maps of (**b**) deoxyhemoglobin, (**c**) oxyhemoglobin, and (**d**) ICG.

5. Conclusions

In summary, we investigated the spectral decomposition of various tissue biomarkers from multispectral PA images. In particular, we have explored the performance of an unsupervised spectral unmixing algorithm, NNMF, in the wavelength range of 680–900 nm. Considering the evidence obtained from the initial results, the NNMF can extract both endogenous and exogenous agents from the multispectral PA data. The unmixing results obtained from the simulation studies performed on synthetic data revealed a high correlation with the expected spectra, and also yielded the quantification of the chromophores. The experiment performed on the tissue-mimicking phantom also supported the results obtained on the synthetic data. Indeed, the NNMF showed promising unmixing performance, allowing the accurate detection of ICG and MB, by eliminating the spectral influence of the other dyes. The in-vivo experiments in the animal model showed the detection of a contrast agent signature, accounting for the spectral variations that may ensue due to tissue–dye interactions. The NNMF can also provide the maps of abundance distribution of contrast agents in different anatomical targets, facilitating in-vivo biodistribution and kinetics studies. Since the algorithm facilitates the automatic unmixing of the tissue chromophores, without any a-priori knowledge about the source components and user interactions, it is easy to adapt, and promising for data-driven studies in multispectral photoacoustic imaging.

In the current algorithm, we have used the time gain compensation (TGC) approach to overcome the PA signal attenuation through depth. Although the approach is not quantitative, it gives improved results. Recent studies demonstrate that taking into account the fluence variance [45,46] can overcome the quantification limits of photoacoustic imaging. Therefore, in future studies, we will investigate the corruption effects of the fluence variation, the finite size, and band-limited frequency response of the detectors, to consider the respective changes on the absorption spectra. Besides, we will expand the current wavelength range of 680–900 nm to the far infrared (FIR), as this may entail the detection of less prominent tissue chromophores, such as melanin, lipids, and collagens.

In conclusion, to the best of our knowledge, this would be the first time that NNMF was used for unmixing multispectral PA imaging. The obtained results confirmed that the NNMF algorithm automatically and accurately detects the component spectra. This proves that the imposed positivity constraints, to the source spectra and abundance distribution maps, are appropriate requirements to unmix tissue chromophores from multispectral PA images.

Author Contributions: Conceptualization, V.G. and J.J.; Methodology, V.G., J.H. and J.J.; Software, V.G.; Validation, V.G. and J.J.; Investigation, J.J.; Resources, J.J.; Data curation, V.G., J.H. and J.J.; Writing—original draft preparation, V.G.; Writing—review and editing, V.G. and J.J.; Visualization, V.G. and J.J.; Supervision, J.J.; Project administration, J.J.; Funding acquisition, J.J. All authors have read and agreed to the published version of the manuscript.

Acknowledgments: This publication is part of a project that has received funding from the European Union's Horizon 2020 research and innovation program under the Marie Skłodowska-Curie grant, agreement No 811226.

References

1. Cox, B.; Laufer, J.G.; Arridge, S.R.; Beard, P.C. Quantitative spectroscopic photoacoustic imaging: A review. *J. Biomed. Opt.* **2012**, *17*, 061202. [CrossRef] [PubMed]
2. Razansky, D.; Vinegoni, C.; Ntziachristos, V. Multispectral photoacoustic imaging of fluorochromes in small animals. *Opt. Lett.* **2007**, *32*, 2891. [CrossRef] [PubMed]
3. Buchmann, J.; Kaplan, B.; Powell, S.; Prohaska, S.; Laufer, J. Quantitative PA tomography of high resolution 3-D images: Experimental validation in a tissue phantom. *Photoacoustics* **2020**, *17*, 100157. [CrossRef] [PubMed]
4. Jnawali, K.; Chinni, B.; Dogra, V.; Rao, N. Automatic cancer tissue detection using multispectral photoacoustic imaging. *Int. J. Comput. Assist. Radiol. Surg.* **2020**, *15*, 309–320. [CrossRef]
5. Needles, A.; Heinmiller, A.; Sun, J.; Theodoropoulos, C.; Bates, D.; Hirson, D.; Yin, M.; Foster, F. Development and initial application of a fully integrated photoacoustic micro-ultrasound system. *IEEE Trans. Ultrason. Ferroelectr. Freq. Control* **2013**, *60*, 888–897. [CrossRef]
6. Xu, M.; Wang, L.V. Photoacoustic imaging in biomedicine. *Rev. Sci. Instrum.* **2006**, *77*, 041101. [CrossRef]
7. Diot, G.; Metz, S.; Noske, A.; Liapis, E.; Schroeder, B.; Ovsepian, S.V.; Meier, R.; Rummeny, E.; Ntziachristos, V. Multispectral Optoacoustic Tomography (MSOT) of human breast cancer. *Clin. Cancer Res.* **2017**, *23*, 6912–6922. [CrossRef]

8. Wilson, K.E.; Wang, T.Y.; Willmann, J.K. Acoustic and photoacoustic molecular imaging of cancer. *J. Nucl. Med.* **2013**, *54*, 1851–1854. [CrossRef]
9. Heijblom, M.; Piras, D.; van den Engh, F.M.; van der Schaaf, M.; Klaase, J.M.; Steenbergen, W.; Manohar, S. The state of the art in breast imaging using the Twente Photoacoustic Mammoscope: Results from 31 measurements on malignancies. *Eur. Radiol.* **2016**, *26*, 3874–3887. [CrossRef]
10. Bauer, D.R.; Olafsson, R.; Montilla, L.G.; Witte, R.S. 3-D photoacoustic and pulse echo imaging of prostate tumor progression in the mouse window chamber. *J. Biomed. Opt.* **2011**, *16*, 026012. [CrossRef]
11. Margolis, R.; Wessner, C.; Stanczak, M.; Liu, J.B.; Li, J.; Nam, K.; Forsberg, F.; Eisenbrey, J.R. Monitoring Progression of Ductal Carcinoma In Situ Using Photoacoustics and Contrast-Enhanced Ultrasound. *Transl. Oncol.* **2019**, *12*, 973–980. [CrossRef] [PubMed]
12. Gargiulo, S.; Albanese, S.; Mancini, M. State-of-the-Art Preclinical Photoacoustic Imaging in Oncology: Recent Advances in Cancer Theranostics. *Contrast Media Mol. Imaging* **2019**, *2019*, 5080267. [CrossRef] [PubMed]
13. Jose, J.; Manohar, S.; Kolkman, R.G.M.; Steenbergen, W.; Leeuwen, T.G. Van Imaging of tumor vasculature using Twente photoacoustic systems. *J. Biophotonics* **2009**, *717*, 701–717. [CrossRef] [PubMed]
14. Manohar, S.; Dantuma, M. Current and future trends in photoacoustic breast imaging. *Photoacoustics* **2019**, *16*, 100134. [CrossRef] [PubMed]
15. Rao, A.P.; Bokde, N.; Sinha, S. Photoacoustic imaging for management of breast cancer: A literature review and future perspectives. *Appl. Sci.* **2020**, *10*, 767. [CrossRef]
16. Liu, S.; Wang, H.; Zhang, C.; Dong, J.; Liu, S.; Xu, R.; Tian, C. In Vivo Photoacoustic Sentinel Lymph Node Imaging Using Clinically-Approved Carbon Nanoparticles. *IEEE Trans. Biomed. Eng.* **2019**. [CrossRef]
17. Jose, J.; Grootendorst, D.J.; Vijn, T.W.; van Leeuwen, T.G.; Steenbergen, W.; Manohar, S.; Wouters, M.; Ruers, T.J.; van Boven, H. Initial results of imaging melanoma metastasis in resected human lymph nodes using photoacoustic computed tomography. *J. Biomed. Opt.* **2011**, *16*, 096021. [CrossRef]
18. Alaeian, M.; Orlande, H.R.B.; Machado, J.C. Temperature estimation of inflamed bowel by the photoacoustic inverse approach. *Int. J. Numer. Methods Biomed. Eng.* **2020**, *36*, e3300. [CrossRef]
19. Sheikh, R.; Cinthio, M.; Dahlstrand, U.; Erlov, T.; Naumovska, M.; Hammar, B.; Zackrisson, S.; Jansson, T.; Reistad, N.; Malmsjo, M. Clinical Translation of a Novel Photoacoustic Imaging System for Examining the Temporal Artery. *IEEE Trans. Ultrason. Ferroelectr. Freq. Control* **2019**, *66*, 472–480. [CrossRef]
20. Xia, W.; Singh, M.K.A.; Maneas, E.; Sato, N.; Shigeta, Y.; Agano, T.; Ourselin, S.; West, S.J.; Desjardins, A.E. Handheld real-time LED-based photoacoustic and ultrasound imaging system for accurate visualization of clinical metal needles and superficial vasculature to guide minimally invasive procedures. *Sensors* **2018**, *18*, 1394. [CrossRef]
21. Zhu, Y.; Lu, X.; Dong, X.; Yuan, J.; Fabiilli, M.L.; Wang, X. LEd-based photoacoustic imaging for monitoring angiogenesis in fibrin scaffolds. *Tissue Eng. Part C Methods* **2019**, *25*, 523–531. [CrossRef] [PubMed]
22. Jo, J.; Xu, G.; Zhu, Y.; Burton, M.; Sarazin, J.; Schiopu, E.; Gandikota, G.; Wang, X. Detecting joint inflammation by an LED-based photoacoustic imaging system: A feasibility study. *J. Biomed. Opt.* **2018**, *23*, 110501. [CrossRef] [PubMed]
23. Zhu, Y.; Xu, G.; Yuan, J.; Jo, J.; Gandikota, G.; Demirci, H.; Agano, T.; Sato, N.; Shigeta, Y.; Wang, X. Light emitting diodes based photoacoustic imaging and potential clinical applications. *Sci. Rep.* **2018**, *8*, 1–12. [CrossRef] [PubMed]
24. Razansky, D.; Distel, M.; Vinegoni, C.; Ma, R.; Perrimon, N.; Köster, R.W.; Ntziachristos, V. Multispectral opto-acoustic tomography of deep-seated fluorescent proteins in vivo. *Nat. Photonics* **2009**, *3*, 412–417. [CrossRef]
25. Cox, B.T.; Arridge, S.R.; Beard, P.C. Estimating chromophore distributions from multiwavelength photoacoustic images. *JOSA A* **2009**, *26*, 443–455. [CrossRef]
26. Glatz, J.; Deliolanis, N.C.; Buehler, A.; Razansky, D.; Ntziachristos, V. Blind source unmixing in multi-spectral optoacoustic tomography. *Opt. Express* **2011**, *19*, 3175. [CrossRef]
27. Bartholomew, D.J. Principal components analysis. *Int. Encycl. Educ.* **2010**, 374–377.
28. Hyvärinen, A. Independent component analysis: Recent advances. *Philos. Trans. R. Soc. A Math. Phys. Eng. Sci.* **2013**, *371*, 20110534. [CrossRef]

29. Le, Q.V.; Karpenko, A.; Ngiam, J.; Ng, A.Y. ICA with reconstruction cost for efficient overcomplete feature learning. In *Advances in Neural Information Processing Systems*; Neural Information Processing Systems Foundation, Inc.: San Diego, CA, USA, 2011; pp. 1017–1025.
30. Ngiam, J.; Koh, P.W.; Chen, Z.; Bhaskar, S.; Ng, A.Y. Sparse filtering. In *Advances in Neural Information Processing Systems*; Neural Information Processing Systems Foundation, Inc.: San Diego, CA, USA, 2011; pp. 1125–1133.
31. Wang, P.; Wang, P.; Wang, H.-W.; Cheng, J.-X. Mapping lipid and collagen by multispectral photoacoustic imaging of chemical bond vibration. *J. Biomed. Opt.* **2012**, *17*, 0960101. [CrossRef]
32. Arabul, M.U.; Rutten, M.C.M.; Bruneval, P.; van Sambeek, M.R.H.M.; van de Vosse, F.N.; Lopata, R.G.P. Unmixing multi-spectral photoacoustic sources in human carotid plaques using non-negative independent component analysis. *Photoacoustics* **2019**, *15*, 100140. [CrossRef]
33. Lee, D.D.; Seung, H.S. Learning the parts of objects by non-negative matrix factorization. *Nature* **1999**, *401*, 788–791. [CrossRef] [PubMed]
34. Lil, S.; Hou, X.; Zhangl, H.; Cheng, Q. Learning Spatially Localized, Parts-B ased Representation. In Proceedings of the 2001 IEEE Computer Society Conference on Computer Vision and Pattern Recognition. CVPR 2001, Kauai, HI, USA, 8–14 December 2001.
35. Buciu, I. Non-negative matrix factorization, a new tool for feature extraction: Theory and applications. *Int. J. Comput. Commun. Control* **2008**, *3*, 67–74.
36. Li, L.; Yang, J.; Xu, Y.; Qin, Z.; Zhang, H. Documents clustering based on max-correntropy nonnegative matrix factorization. *Proc. Int. Conf. Mach. Learn. Cybern.* **2014**, *2*, 850–855.
37. Luo, X.; Zhou, M.; Xia, Y.; Zhu, Q. An efficient non-negative matrix-factorization-based approach to collaborative filtering for recommender systems. *IEEE Trans. Ind. Inform.* **2014**, *10*, 1273–1284.
38. Montcuquet, A.-S.; Herve, L.; Garcia, F.P.N.Y.; Dinten, J.-M.; Mars, J.I. Nonnegative matrix factorization: A blind spectra separation method for in vivo fluorescent optical imaging. *J. Biomed. Opt.* **2010**, *15*, 56009.
39. Lipovetsky, S. PCA and SVD with nonnegative loadings. *Pattern Recognit.* **2009**, *42*, 68–76. [CrossRef]
40. Keshava, N.; Mustard, J.F. Spectral unmixing. *IEEE Signal Process. Mag.* **2002**, *19*, 44–57. [CrossRef]
41. Lee, D.D.; Seung, H.S. Algorithms for non-negative matrix factorization. In *Advances in Neural Information Processing Systems*; The MIT Press: Cambridge, MA, USA, 2001; pp. 556–562.
42. Prahl, S. Tabulated Molar Extinction Coefficient for Hemoglobin in Water. Available online: https://omlc.org/index.html (accessed on 5 June 2020).
43. Toumia, Y.; Cerroni, B.; Trochet, P.; Lacerenza, S.; Oddo, L.; Domenici, F.; Paradossi, G. Performances of a Pristine Graphene—Microbubble Hybrid Construct as Dual Imaging Contrast Agent and Assessment of Its Biodistribution by Photoacoustic Imaging. *Part. Part. Syst. Charact.* **2018**, *35*, 1800066. [CrossRef]
44. Song, W.; Tang, Z.; Zhang, D.; Burton, N.; Driessen, W.; Chen, X. RSC Advances Comprehensive studies of pharmacokinetics and biodistribution of indocyanine green and liposomal indocyanine green by multispectral optoacoustic. *RSC Adv.* **2014**, *5*, 3807–3813. [CrossRef]
45. Gröhl, J.; Kirchner, T.; Adler, T.; Maier-Hein, L. Estimation of blood oxygenation with learned spectral decoloring for quantitative photoacoustic imaging (LSD-qPAI). *arXiv* **2019**, arXiv:1902.05839.
46. Brochu, F.M.; Joseph, J.; Tomaszewski, M.; Bohndiek, S.E. Light fluence correction for quantitative determination of tissue absorption coefficient using multi-spectral optoacoustic tomography. In Proceedings of the European Conference on Biomedical Optics 2015, Munich, Germany, 21–25 June 2015; p. 95390Z.

7

A Novel Efficient FEM Thin Shell Model for Bio-Impedance Analysis

Jiawei Tang [1], Mingyang Lu [1], Yuedong Xie [2,3] and Wuliang Yin [1,*]

1 School of Electrical and Electronics Engineering, The University of Manchester, Manchester M13 9PL, UK; jiawei.tang@postgrad.manchester.ac.uk (J.T.); mingyang.lu@manchester.ac.uk (M.L.)
2 School of Instrumentation and Optoelectronic Engineering, Beihang University, Beijing 100036, China; yuedongxie@buaa.edu.cn
3 Beijing Advanced Innovation Center for Big Data-based Precision Medicine, Beihang University, Beijing 100036, China
* Correspondence: wuliang.yin@manchester.ac.uk

Abstract: In this paper, a novel method for accelerating eddy currents calculation on a cell model using the finite element method (FEM) is presented. Due to the tiny thickness of cell membrane, a full-mesh cell model requires a large number of mesh elements and hence intensive computation resources and long time. In this paper, an acceleration method is proposed to reduce the number of mesh elements and therefore reduce the computing time. It is based on the principle of replacing the thin cell membrane with an equivalent thicker structure. The method can reduce the number of mesh elements to 23% and the computational time to 17%, with an error of less than 1%. The method was verified using 2D and 3D finite element methods and can potentially be extended to other thin shell structures. The simulation results were validated by measurement and analytical results.

Keywords: finite element method; thin shell model; β dispersion; Maxwell–Wagner effect; bio-impedance spectroscopy

1. Introduction

β-dispersion analysis has been widely investigated for medical [1,2] and industrial [3,4] applications. For example, it has been proposed for the detection of tumours [5,6] and cerebral stroke [7], and it has been applied to the quality inspection of food such as meat, fruit and vegetables [3]. The mechanism of β-dispersion was first described by Schwan [8,9]. β-dispersion takes place at radio frequency, mainly from hundreds of hertz to megahertz. This dispersion is caused by Maxwell–Wagner effect, an interfacial polarisation of cell membrane blocking the ion-flow of intra and extracellular dielectrics.

Analytical solutions are well developed to calculate the β dispersion [10–12]. However, the analytical solution is only designed to analyze the models with a regular shape (i.e., spherical cell model) [13,14]. In reality, most cell shapes are anomalous. The finite element method is a methodology that discretises an entire continuous domain into discrete domains. An irregular cell shape can be simulated in a high accuracy using the finite element method. Therefore, FEM is a feasible and effective way to simulate the dielectric dispersions for models with irregular shapes [15,16].

The difficulty of FEM is that the number of meshing elements is significantly large due to the tiny thickness of the cell membrane; it takes a long time to compute with numerous meshing elements. In this paper, a novel FEM acceleration method was proposed to simulate β dispersion. The acceleration method is to reduce the number of meshing elements and computing time by replacing the full-mesh cell membrane model with an equivalent reduced-mesh model. In this paper, the FEM acceleration method was used to simulate the spherical and oval cell model in two-dimensional and three-dimensional versions.

2. Materials and Methods

2.1. Single Spherical Cell Model

The full-mesh cell model is the single shell spherical model introduced by Asami [15]. The spherical cell model is shown in Figure 1. The parameters of the cell model are $k_m = 10^{-7}$ S/m, $k_a = k_c = 1$ S/m. $\varepsilon_c = \varepsilon_a = 80$, $\varepsilon_m = 5$, R = 5000 nm, $d_m = $ 5nm. k_m is the conductivity of the cell membrane. k_a and k_c are the conductivity of the extracellular and intracellular fluid, respectively. ε_c and ε_a are the relative permittivity of the intracellular and extracellular fluid, respectively. ε_m is the relative permittivity of the cell membrane. R is the radius of the cell. d_m is the cell membrane thickness [10,17,18].

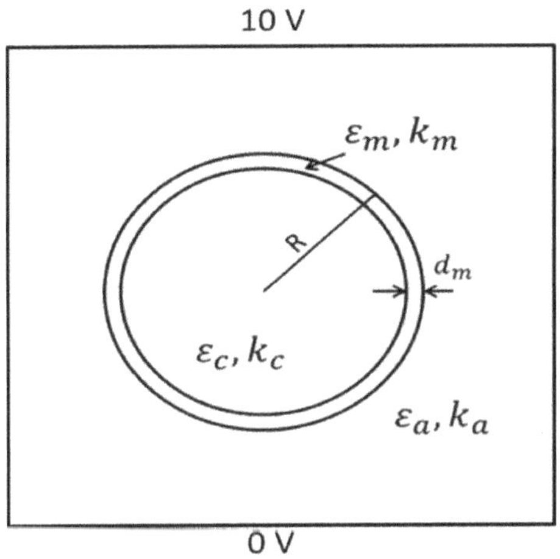

Figure 1. Spherical cell model.

The two-dimensional simulation model is a single cell model, as shown in Figure 1. The spherical cell is put in a suspension with an applied alternating electric field. The voltage of the upper electrode was set to be 10 V, and the voltage of the lower electrode was set to be 0 V [14]. The intracellular and extracellular fluid were conductive while the cell membrane blocked current flow between intracellular and extracellular fluid at low frequency. Dielectric relaxation describes a phenomenon that the permittivity decreases when the frequency of applied electric field increases at a certain range. The relaxation occurs when the electric dipoles are not able to reverse at the same rate with the frequency of the applied field. β-dispersion was observed from 10 kHz to 1 MHz. The dispersion was described by Schwan and could be explained by Maxwell–Wagner effect [8]. The effect occurs at the boundary of layered or inhomogeneous dielectrics. Applying an electric field would build up charges at the boundaries created by different dielectrics. The double-layer dielectrics system can be represented by one capacitance in parallel with one another. Applying a static electric field would charge both capacitances and creates charges at the boundary of the dielectrics. This phenomenon is also called interfacial polarisation.

The equivalent complex relative permittivity of the cell model in Figure 1 can be calculated according to Asami [12]:

$$\varepsilon_p^* = \varepsilon_m^* \frac{2(1-v)\varepsilon_m^* + (1+2v)\varepsilon_c^*}{(2+v)\varepsilon_m^* + (1-v)\varepsilon_c^*} \tag{1}$$

where $v = \left(1 - \frac{d_m}{R}\right)^n$, d_m is the cell membrane thickness, R is the radius of the cell, and n stands for the factor of dimension. When n = 2, the equation is applied to the two-dimension model. When n = 3, the equation is applied to three-dimension model. ε_p^* is the complex relative permittivity of the cell model, ε_m^* is the complex relative permittivity of the cell membrane and ε_c^* is the complex relative permittivity of cytoplasm; then the complex relative permittivity of the suspension can be calculated by Wagner's equation:

$$\varepsilon^* = \varepsilon_a^* \frac{2(1-P)\varepsilon_a^* + (1+2P)\varepsilon_p^*}{(2+P)\varepsilon_a^* + (1-P)\varepsilon_p^*} \tag{2}$$

where P is the volume fraction, ε^* is the complex relative permittivity of cell suspension, ε_a^* is the complex relative permittivity of the external medium.

The conductivity of the suspension can be derived:

$$\varepsilon^* = \frac{\sigma^*}{j\omega\varepsilon_0} = \frac{\sigma_r + j\omega\varepsilon_r\varepsilon_0}{j\omega\varepsilon_0} \tag{3}$$

where σ_r and ε_r are the conductivity and permittivity of the suspension, respectively. σ^* is the complex conductivity of the suspension, ε_0 is the permittivity of vacuum, $\omega = 2\pi f$ where f is the frequency of the applied field and j is the imaginary unit.

According to Schwan [9], when $\frac{d_m}{R} \ll 1$, $k_m \ll k_a = k_c$, the dielectric relaxation of the cell suspension can be represented by the Debye relaxation model:

$$\varepsilon^* = \varepsilon_h + \frac{\varepsilon_l - \varepsilon_h}{1 + j\omega\tau} + \frac{k_l}{j\omega\varepsilon_0} \tag{4}$$

where ε_h and ε_l are the high-frequency limit and low-frequency limit of the relative permittivity, τ is the relaxation time and k_l is the low-frequency limit of the conductivity.

2.2. D FEM Simulation

Normally, the finite element problems could be solved by two kinds of methods which are Galerkin's method and Ritz's method [19]. In this paper, Galerkin's method is used to build up simulations.

According to the Gaussian equation,

$$\nabla \cdot D = \rho \tag{5}$$

where $\vec{D} = \varepsilon\vec{E}$, $\vec{D}$ is the electric flux density, $\vec{E}$ is the electrical field intensity, $\varepsilon = \varepsilon_r\varepsilon_0$, ε_r is the relative permittivity of the material, ρ is the quantity of electric charge, which is zero in the cell model. So the equation could be rewritten as:

$$\nabla \cdot (\sigma + j\omega\varepsilon)\vec{E} = \nabla \cdot (\sigma + j\omega\varepsilon)\nabla U = 0 \tag{6}$$

where σ is the conductivity of the material and $\varepsilon = \varepsilon_r\varepsilon_0$. ε_r is the relative permittivity of the material. ε_0 is the permittivity of vacuum. U is the electric potential which is the objective value to be solved [20]. To obtain the equivalent conductivity of the total cell suspension, we calculate the total current flowing through the cell suspension from the top electrode to the bottom electrode [15]. According to Kirchhoff's current law, the current flow through any plane, which is in parallel with the electrodes is the same with the total current flow through the cell suspension. So the current I flow through a chosen plane in parallel with electrodes can be calculated as:

$$I = \sum j^{(i)} = \sum \sigma^{(i)} \vec{E}^{(i)} \tag{7}$$

where $j^{(i)}$ is the current density of the element on the chosen plane, $\sigma^{(i)}$ is the conductivity of the element on the chosen plane, $\vec{E}^{(i)}$ is the background electrical field on the chosen plane. Then the complex conductivity of the cell suspension can be calculated as:

$$\sigma^* = \frac{1}{\rho^*} = \frac{L}{S} * \frac{I}{U} \quad (8)$$

where σ^* and ρ^* are the complex conductivity and resistivity, respectively. L is the distance between the top electrode and the bottom electrode. S is the area of the electrodes.

2.3. D FEM Simulation

An induction model was built for the three-dimension FEM simulation. As shown in Figure 2, the cylinder stands for the cell suspension, and the spherical model stands for the cell. Imaginary transmitter and receiver coils are put on the top of the suspension to provide an alternating magnetic field as an exciting signal and detect induced secondary magnetic field. The single-cell model in a three-dimension situation is shown in Figure 2b. The applied field is a magnetic field excited by the transmitter in Figure 2a. The radius of the sphere cell model is R and the cell membrane thickness of the sphere cell model is d_m. All the electric parameters of the sphere cell model are set to be the same with the parameters in Figure 1. The Mxwell–Wagner effect can be calculated by calculating the eddy current distribution induced by the applied magnetic field.

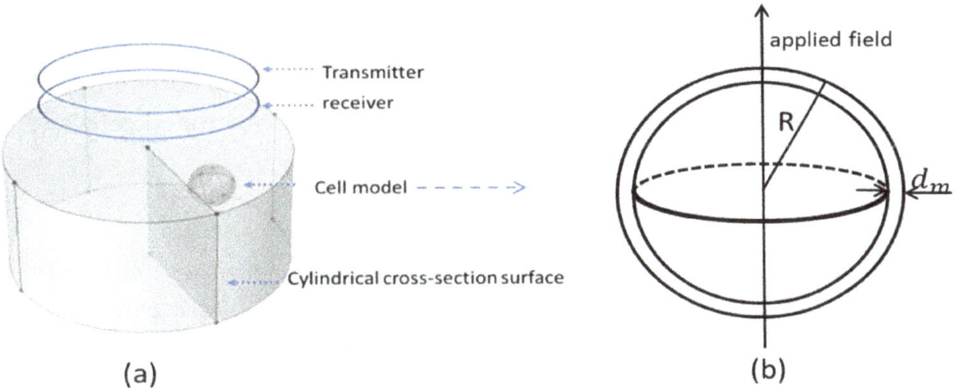

Figure 2. (**a**) 3D suspension model, (**b**) 3D single cell model.

According to Oszkar Biro [21], the basic formulas for the three-dimension edge elements simulation of eddy current problems, Galerkin's equation is shown as following:

$$\begin{aligned} &\int_{\Omega_c} \nabla \times N_i \cdot v \nabla \times A^{(n)} d\Omega + \int_{\Omega_c} j\omega\sigma N_i \cdot A^{(n)} d\Omega + \int_{\Omega_c} \sigma N_i \cdot \nabla V^{(n)} d\Omega \\ &= \int_{\Omega_c} \nabla \times N_i \cdot v_0 \nabla \times A_s d\Omega \quad i = 1, 2, \ldots, 6 \end{aligned} \quad (9)$$

$$\int_{\Omega_c} j\omega\sigma\nabla L_i \cdot A^{(n)} d\Omega + \int_{\Omega_c} \sigma\nabla L_i \cdot \nabla V^{(n)} d\Omega = 0 \quad i = 1, 2, \ldots, 4 \quad (10)$$

where L_i is the elemental interpolation of ith node corresponding to the nth element of it; N_i stands for the vector interpolation of ith edge relating to the nth edge element of it; $A^{(n)}$ stands for the excited edge vector potential of the nth element; A_s represents the original edge vector potential of the nth element; $V^{(n)}$ represents the electrical potential excited by the nth element on the receiving coil; v stands for the reluctivity of the model; v_0 is the reluctivity of the air; σ is the conductivity of the model [22–24].

The eddy current density is:

$$J^{(i)} = \sigma^{(i)} E^{(i)} \quad (11)$$

where $E^{(i)}$ denotes the vector sum of the electrical field on all the edges of each tetrahedral element, $\sigma^{(i)}$ is the complex conductivity parameter of the of each tetrahedral element.

The model is shown in Figure 2. Assuming there is an equivalent model with uniform dielectric and the background suspension has exactly the same shape with the simulation model in Figure 2. Since the normal component of the electrical field relative to each cross-section surface of suspension (shown in Figure 2) is identical, then

$$\sum \vec{n}\cdot E^{(i)} = \sum \vec{n}\cdot E_s^{(i)} \tag{12}$$

where, $E_s^{(i)}$ denotes the background electrical field of the of each tetrahedral element; $\vec{n}$ is the normal unit vector relative to the surface of target;

Since the equivalent model is uniform, the electrical background field $E_s^{(i)}$ is always vertical to every cylindrical cross-section surface of the suspension model shown in Figure 2. Then the equivalent complex conductivity of the original suspension (as shown in Figure 2) can be derived from (8) and (9) that

$$\sigma_s = \frac{\sum J_s^{(i)}}{\sum \vec{n}\cdot \frac{J^{(i)}}{\sigma^{(i)}}} \tag{13}$$

$\sigma^{(i)}$ is the complex conductivity of each tetrahedral element, $J_s^{(i)}$ is the eddy current density through each cylindrical cross-section of equivalent suspension model, $J^{(i)}$ is the eddy current density through each cylindrical cross-section of the original suspension model with arranged cells and $\vec{n}$ is the current flow direction.

2.4. Acceleration Method

The complicated calculation progress and the long computing time are caused by a large number of meshing elements around the thin cell membrane. The number of meshing elements could be reduced by enlarging the cell membrane thickness. However, changing the cell membrane thickness affects the conductivity spectrum of the cell suspensions. The aim of the proposed acceleration method is to keep the accuracy of the simulation result while enlarging the cell membrane thickness (reducing the number of elements). This acceleration method replaces the full-mesh model with an equivalent thicker cell membrane (reduce-mesh model) with an equivalent complex conductivity, as shown in Figure 3. The M_1 in Figure 3 is the full-mesh model cell membrane with normal thickness l_1. The M_2 in Figure 3 is the enlarged part of the reduce-mesh model cell membrane with thickness l_2, R is the radius of the cell model. The electrical parameter of the cell membrane M_2 is exactly the same with the intracellular fluid. The cell membrane M_1 and M_2 combine as one thicker equivalent cell membrane (reduce-mesh model cell membrane), and the thickness of the reduce-mesh model cell membrane is $l_1 + l_2$. The number of meshing elements is reduced due to a thicker equivalent cell membrane. In this case, the factor $v = \left(1 - \frac{d_m}{R}\right)^n$ in Equation (1) can be rewritten as $v = \left(1 - \frac{(l_1+l_2)}{R}\right)^n$ to describe the Maxwell–Wagner effect in the equivalent model. According to the Maxwell–Wagner Equation (2), as the parameter P and ε_a^* of the equivalent model are fixed, the dielectric behaviour of the suspension model ε^* only depends on the dielectric property of the cell model ε_p^*. According to Equation (1), ε_p^* is determined by ε_m^* and the factor v. In order to retain the dielectric behaviour of the suspension model, the equivalent dielectric parameters of the equivalent cell membrane ε_m^* can be calculated by Equations (14)–(18). With the equivalent complex conductivity, the behaviour of Maxwell–Wagner effect, which leads to β-dispersion remains the same.

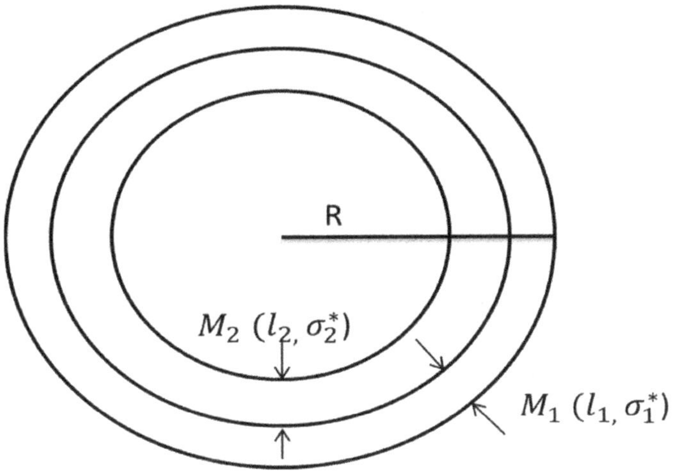

Figure 3. Equivalent cell membrane model.

The parameters of the cell membrane M_1 and M_2 in Figure 3 are:

$$\sigma_1^* = \sigma_1 + j\omega\varepsilon_1\varepsilon_0 \tag{14}$$

$$\sigma_2^* = \sigma_2 + j\omega\varepsilon_2\varepsilon_0 \tag{15}$$

where σ_1^* and σ_2^* are the complex conductivity of M_1 cell membrane and M_2 cell membrane in Figure 3, respectively. σ_1 and σ_2 are the conductivity of cell membrane M_1 and cell membrane M_2 in Figure 3, respectively. ε_1 and ε_2 are the relative permittivity of the cell membrane M_1 and cell membrane M_2, respectively. Considering the two cell membranes M_1 and M_2 are connected as two electrolytes in series. The total impedance Z is:

$$Z = Z_1 + Z_2 = \frac{l_1}{\sigma_1^* S_1} + \frac{l_2}{\sigma_2^* S_2} \tag{16}$$

where Z_1 and Z_2 are the impedance of the cell membrane M_1 and M_2, respectively. σ_1^* and σ_2^* are the complex conductivity of cell membrane M_1 and M_2 respectively. l_1 and l_2 are the thickness of the cell membrane M_1 and the cell membrane M_2 in Figure 3, respectively. S_1 and S_2 are the area of cell membrane M_1 and the cell membrane M_2, respectively. As l_1 and l_2 are negligible comparing with radius R, the area $S_1 = S_2$.

Then the equivalent complex conductivity can be derived as:

$$Z = \frac{l_1}{\sigma_1^* S_1} + \frac{l_2}{\sigma_2^* S_2} = \frac{l_1\sigma_2^* + l_2\sigma_1^*}{\sigma_1^*\sigma_2^*}\frac{1}{S_1} = \frac{(l_1 + l_2)}{\sigma_e^*}\frac{1}{S_1} \tag{17}$$

$$\sigma_e^* = \frac{(l_1 + l_2)\sigma_1^*\sigma_2^*}{l_1\sigma_2^* + l_2\sigma_1^*} \tag{18}$$

σ_e^* is the complex conductivity of the equivalent cell membrane (reduce-mesh model cell membrane).

The replacement of the thin cell membrane with an equivalent thicker structure appears to have reflected an equivalent Maxwell–Wagner effect from the computation results. Theoretically, less contrasting EM properties between the boundary of two materials cause less Maxwell–Wagner effect (i.e., less charge building-up). At the same time, thicker materials between the two charged surfaces would mean the equivalent capacitance is smaller. These two effects would mean the electric field E = Q/C would be kept to a constant; this is possibly the reason why we can use the replacement to carry out the calculation of the dispersion caused by the MW effect. Equations (17) and (18) considered the complex conductivity, and therefore, the physics would be masked to a certain degree, but the principle can be explained as above.

2.5. Meshing Details

The suspension model shown in Figure 1 was discretised into three regions, cell membrane and intra and extracellular fluid, for meshing. The commercial software Comsol 5.0 was used for meshing. The convergent criterion was accelerated BICGS with an optimal precondition. The initial precondition was based on optimised initial guess: the final solution from the previous frequency [25–30]. As shown in Table 1, the minimum and maximum element sizes are set to be the same to maintain the meshing accuracy. The maximum element growth rate controls the maximum changing rate of the dimension of the element among the adjacent subdomains. The narrow factor controls the mesh density on the narrow region. Increasing the cell membrane thickness reduces the narrow regions. Therefore, the meshing density is larger in the cell model with smaller cell membrane thickness. Table 2 shows the number of meshing element in each specific region, including total suspension, cell membrane, intracellular fluid and extracellular fluid. In addition, a specific region surrounding the cell membrane was created to obtain the number of meshing elements around the cell membrane. It is obvious from Table 2 that the most meshing elements concentrate at the region around the cell membrane. The narrow region is reduced when the cell membrane thickness is enlarged, thus, the number of meshing elements is decreased when increasing cell membrane thickness.

Table 1. Meshing information for acceleration model.

	Original Model Meshing Information	**Acceleration Model Meshing Information** ($l_1 : l_2 = 1:1$)
Maximum element size (μm)	0.1	0.1
Minimum element size (μm)	0.01	0.01
Maximum element growth rate	1.20	1.20
Narrow factor	1	1

Table 2. The number of meshing element in different regions.

Regions	**Original Model**	**Acceleration Model** ($l_1 : l_2 = 1:1$)
Extracellular fluid	32,814	15,668
Intracellular fluid	30,566	14,748
Cell membrane	9712	4856
Region around cell membrane	70,528	33,620
Total suspension	73,092	35,272

3. Results and Discussion

3.1. D Single Spherical Cell Model

The full-mesh model cell membrane thickness is 5 nm. There are two simulations with equivalent thicker cell membrane (reduce-mesh model) thickness of 10 nm and 20 nm, respectively. The ratio between the full-mesh model cell membrane (cell membrane M_1 in Figure 3) thickness and the enlarged part of reduce-model cell membrane (cell membrane M_2 in Figure 3) thickness is 1:1 and 1:3, respectively. The simulation results are the progress of β-dispersion which reflects dispersions on relative permittivity and conductivity, as shown in Figures 4 and 5. The main characteristics of β-dispersion are the dispersion frequency range and the magnitude of the relative permittivity and conductivity [27,30,31]. As shown in Figure 4, the dispersion frequency is ranging from 100 kHz to 10 MHz. The magnitude of relative permittivity at low frequency and high frequency are 960 and 80, respectively. The magnitude of conductivity at low frequency and high frequencies were 0.925 S/m and 1.04 S/m, respectively. This work was aimed at accelerating the computing progress with high accuracy,

15 sample points are selected in Figure 4 to describe the main feature of an entire β -dispersion and verify the accuracy of the acceleration method. The results of acceleration models are validated by the full-mesh model to verify the accuracy of the acceleration method. The errors between the acceleration model and full-mesh model at each point in Figures 4 and 5 have been calculated. The calculated error and computing time for acceleration model and full-mesh model are shown in Table 3.

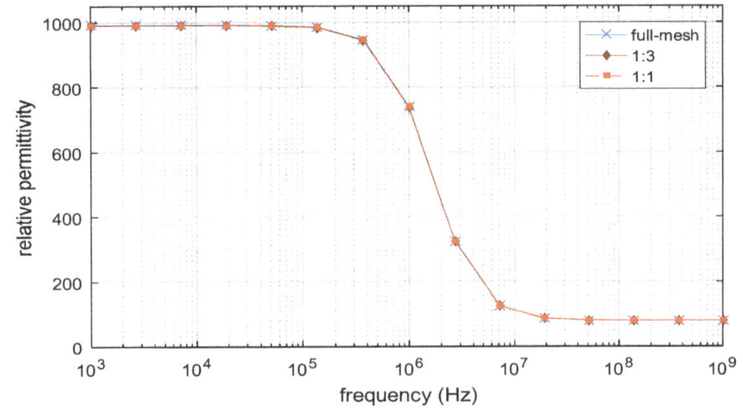

Figure 4. Permittivity of 2D single spherical cell model.

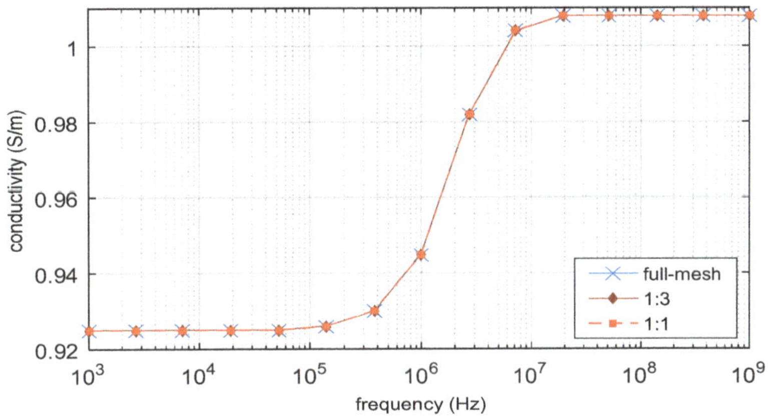

Figure 5. Of 2D single spherical cell model.

Table 3. Results of the 2D spherical cell model.

Thickness Ratio (M_1/M_2)	Number of Elements	Error	Computing Time (Minutes)
Original model	73,092	N/A	73
1:1	35,272	0.07%	28
1:3	17,342	0.2%	13

As shown Table 3, the number of elements of the full-mesh model can be reduced to 24% when the equivalent cell membrane (reduce-mesh model) is four times as the thickness of the full-mesh model cell membrane (M_1 cell membrane to M_2 cell membrane thickness ratio is 1:3). The computing time was reduced from 73 min to 13 min, with only a 0.2% error on the simulation result. The computing time of the reduce-mesh model is 18% of the full-mesh model. The spectroscopy of conductivity and relative permittivity is shown in Figures 4 and 5, the results of the reduce-model and full-mesh model show the same magnitude over the same frequency range with an error less than 0.2%. The β dispersion of reduce-model and full-mesh model both starts at 100 kHz and both ends at 10 MHz. This shows that the reduce-mesh model can significantly accelerate the computing progress with only a tiny error on the result in the 2D-FEM spherical model simulation.

3.2. D Cell Deformation Model

This simulation is to verify that the acceleration method not only works on spherical cell model but also works on the deformation model (oval model).

The deformation model is an oval model in order to simulation the cell deformation [28]. The electrical parameters of the oval model are the same as that of the custom spherical model. The model is shown in Figure 6, where a and b are the length of the semi-major and semi-minor axis, respectively. The length of the semi-major axis is set to be a = 12 μm and the length of the semi-minor axis is set to be b = 2 μm, k_a and k_c are the conductivity of the extracellular and intracellular fluid, respectively, ε_c and ε_a are the relative permittivity of the intracellular and extracellular fluid respectively, ε_m is the relative permittivity of cell membrane, d_m is the cell membrane thickness. The full-mesh model cell membrane thickness is still 5 nm and the electrical properties are calculated using equation 18. The simulation result of β dispersion is shown in Figure 7, Figure 8 and the parameters of the computing time and error are shown in Table 4.

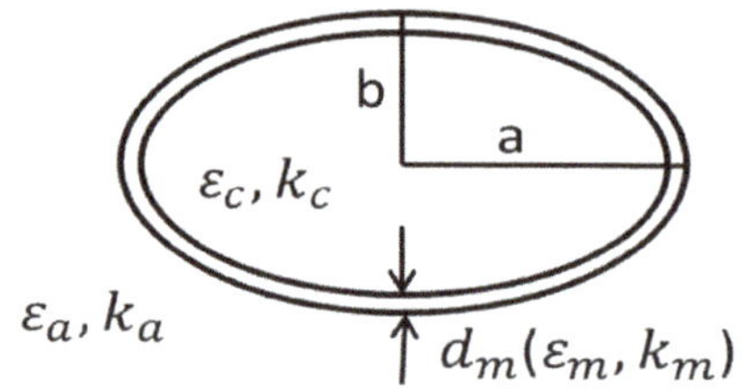

Figure 6. Deformation model.

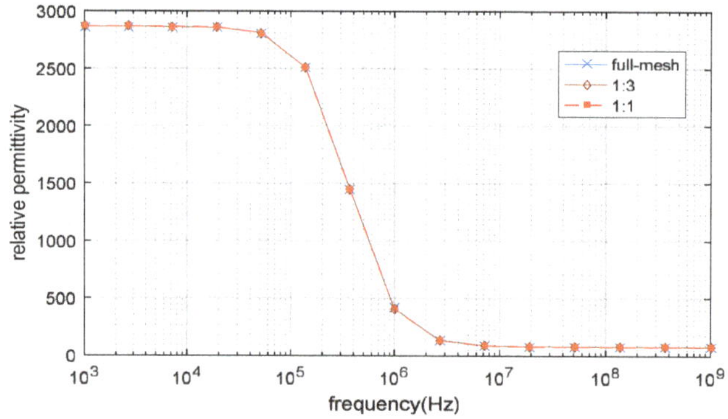

Figure 7. The relative permittivity of the 2D single deformation cell model.

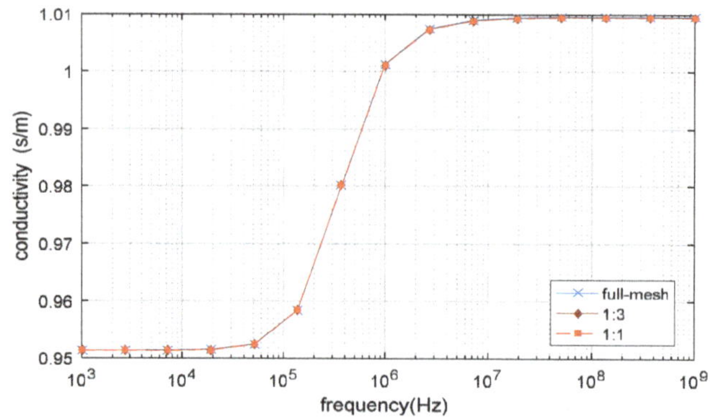

Figure 8. The conductivity of 2D single deformation cell model.

Table 4. Results of 2D Deformation Cell Model.

Thickness Ratio (M_1/M_2)	Number of Elements	Error	Computing Time
Original (a = 12, b = 2)	133,184	N/A	2 h 24 min
1:1	64,600	0.04%	62 min
1:3	32,097	0.11%	25 min

The number of elements of full-mesh model can be reduced to 24.1% as shown in Table 4 and the computing time is reduced from 2h 24mins to 25mins. The simulation error between reduce-mesh model and full-mesh model is only 0.11%. As shown in Figures 7 and 8, the results of the full-mesh model and reduce-mesh model exhibits β dispersion with tiny error in the same frequency range. The results show that the acceleration method is feasible to simulate not only the spherical model but also deformation model (oval model). The computing time is significantly reduced with acceptable error.

3.3. D Spherical Cell Model

The simulation model used for 3D FEM simulation is shown in Figure 2. 3-D single sphere cell model is used. The radius of the cell model is set to be 5 μm, and the cell membrane thickness is 5 nm. The top view of eddy current distributions at lower frequency 1 kHz and higher frequency 10 MHz are shown in Figure 9. The single-cell model blocks eddy currents at a lower frequency and becomes conductive at a higher frequency which meets the expectations of maxwell–wagner effect and other published works [9,11,15,29].

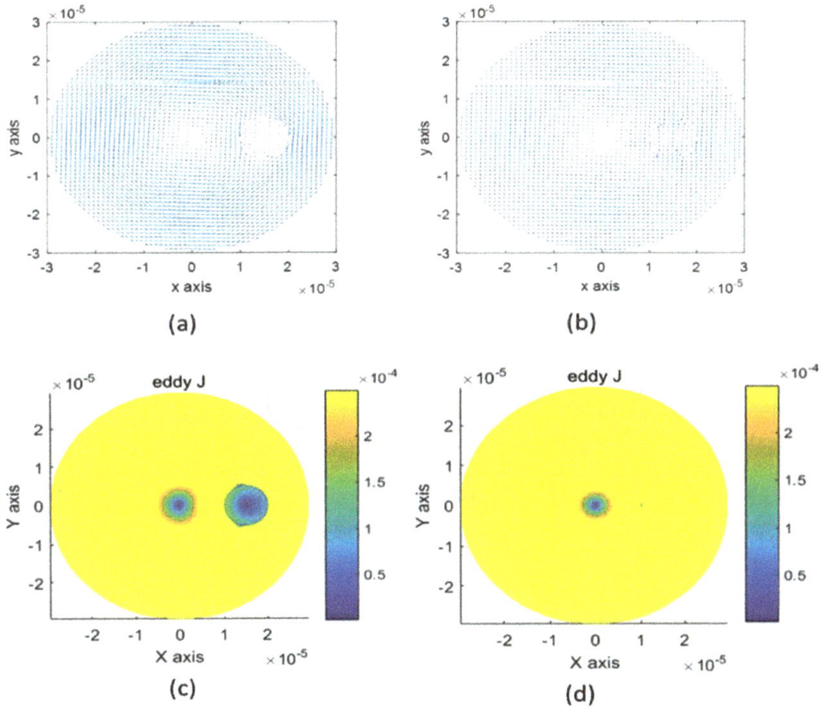

Figure 9. (**a**) Eddy current flow at low frequency 1 kHz. (**b**) Eddy current flow at high frequency 10 MHz. (**c**) Eddy current density at low frequency 1 kHz. (**d**) Eddy current density at high frequency 10 MHz.

The full-mesh model cell membrane thickness is 5 nm. There are two reduce-models with equivalent thicker cell membrane (reduce-mesh model) thickness of 10 nm and 20 nm, respectively. The ratio between the full-mesh model cell membrane thickness and the reduce-mesh cell membrane thickness is 1:1 and 1:3, respectively. The relative permittivity and conductivity result are shown in Figures 10 and 11. β dispersion can be observed from Figures 10 and 11. The β dispersion of the full-mesh model and reduce-mesh model has an error of 2% on the magnitude. The frequency range of the β dispersion of full-mesh model and reduce-mesh model are the same, ranging from 100 kHz to 10 MHz. The results, including the number of elements, the computing time and error of full-mesh model and reduce-mesh model, are shown in Table 5. The number of elements of the full-mesh model can be reduced to 28%, as shown in Table 5, and the computing is reduced from 4 h 37 min to 71 min. The simulation error between reduce-mesh model and full-mesh model is 2%. The error is larger than the two-dimensional simulation result, but it is acceptable for β-dispersion simulations. The results show that the acceleration method is feasible to simulate a three-dimensional spherical model. The computing time is significantly reduced with acceptable error.

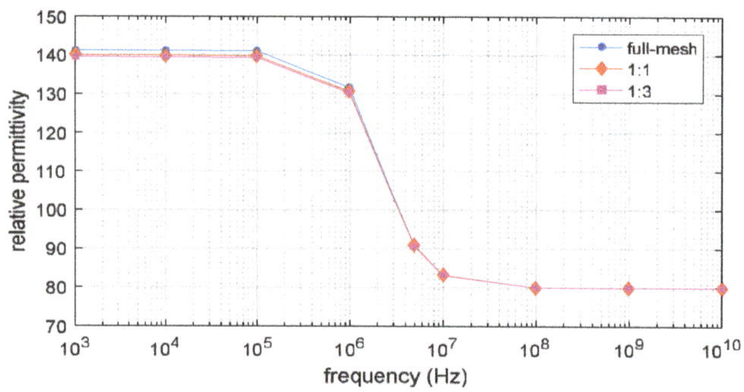

Figure 10. The relative permittivity of the 3D single spherical cell model.

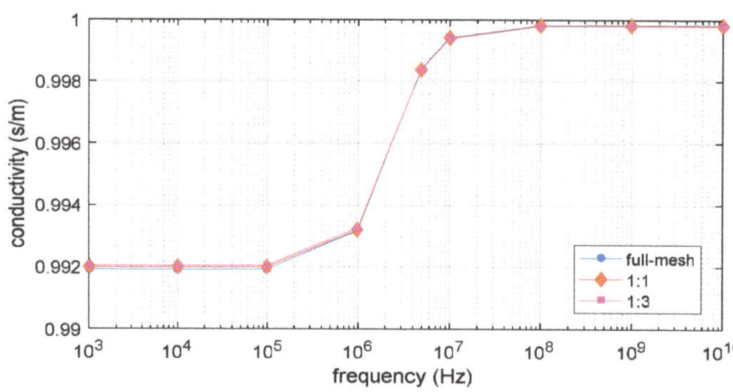

Figure 11. The conductivity of 3D single spherical cell model.

Table 5. Result of 3D Spherical Cell Model.

Thickness Ratio (M_1/M_2)	Number of Elements	Error	Computing Time
Original model	205,604	N/A	4 h 37 min
1:1	141,870	0.4%	3 h 5 min
1:3	57,934	2%	1 h 11 min

3.4. Experimental Validation by Contact-Electrode Measurement

The four-electrode measurement system is used to measure the impedance spectroscopy of biological samples. The electrode is contacted directly to the samples to measure the impedance over the samples using an impedance analyser. The measurement system work in the following way: the electrodes generate an input signal which applies an alternating electric field and current in the samples. By measuring the current and voltage across the samples, the conductivity and permittivity of the samples can be calculated. The impedance analyser used in this work is Solatron 1260, which is efficient and accurate over the frequency ranging from hundreds of hertz to 32 MHz. The effective area of the measurement electrodes is fixed to $S = 2\text{ cm} * 3\text{ cm} = 6\text{ cm}^2$, and the distance between the electric field measuring electrodes is fixed to L = 6.6 cm. The conductivity can then be calculated by $\sigma = 1/\rho = L/RS$. R is the real part of the measured impedance, ρ is the resistivity. The measurement sample is fresh potato (obtained from a local market). This measurement is to validate the FEM simulation result. All FEM simulation parameters are set to be the realistic value obtained from the measurement.

In Figure 12, the FEM and measurement results show similar β -dispersion with the same dispersion frequency range. There is some error on the magnitude of the conductivity between the measurement result and the simulation result. However, the error is acceptable for the simulation approach of the measurement result. The conductivity of measurement and simulation result is low at a lower frequency, and the dispersion starts at around 50 kHz. The dispersion ends at around 2 MHz and the conductivity of measurement and simulation result is increased to 0.15 S/m. The spectroscopy curve is flat over the higher frequency range. The measurement result validated the full-mesh and reduce-mesh FEM simulation result and agreed with other published works [9,13,15,21,25,32].

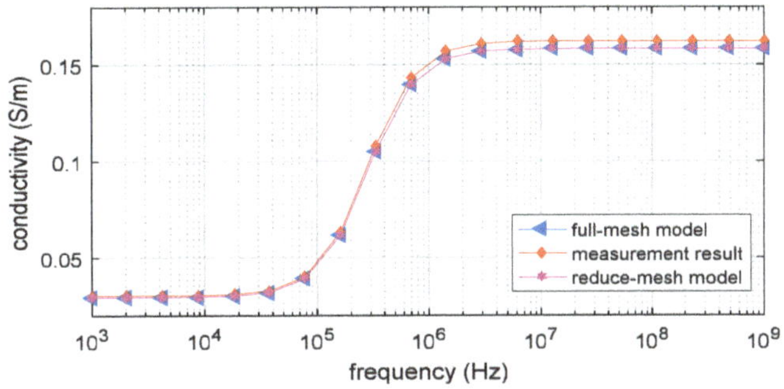

Figure 12. Impedance spectroscopy of FEM and measurement result.

3.5. Verification by Analytical Result

The analytical result can be calculated according to Maxwell–Wagner Equations (1) and (2). The analytical result is compared with the 3D finite element simulation result. So the factor v in equation (1) is defined as $v = \left(1 - \frac{d_m}{R}\right)^3$. According to Schwan [9], the impedance spectroscopy of the cell model can be described by Debye relaxation based on Equation (4). In Figures 13 and 14, both analytical and FEM results show the same magnitude and frequency range of beta dispersion with an error less than 0.1%. The volume fraction of the cell is set to be the same as P = 3.5%. The magnitude and frequency range of β-dispersion on the full-mesh model and reduce-mesh model agree with the analytical result. The result validates that the three-dimension FEM simulation on cell suspension is accurate and the improved acceleration method is also validated. The proposed acceleration method can be applied to further FEM simulations on irregular shape cell models and thin shell models.

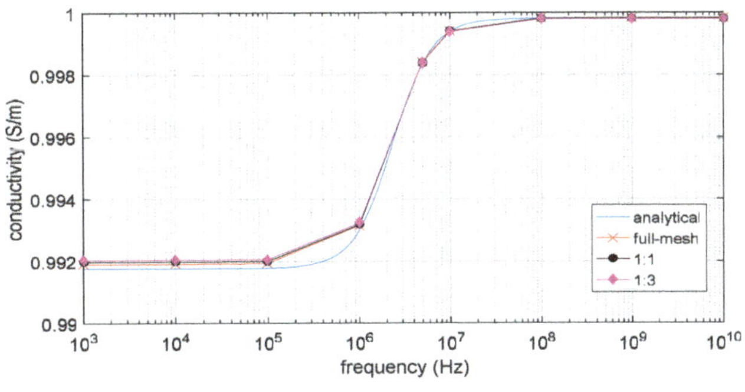

Figure 13. Calculated conductivity of the analytical solution and FEM simulation.

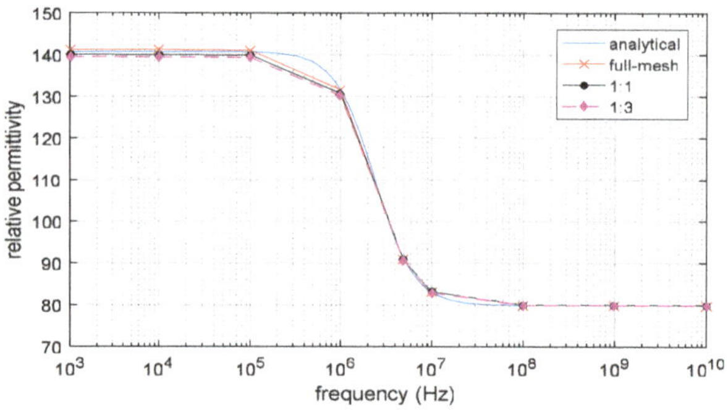

Figure 14. Calculated relative permittivity of the analytical solution and FEM simulation.

4. Conclusions

This paper proposed a method to accelerate FEM calculation with bio-cell models. The idea is to replace the thin cell membrane (full-mesh model) with an equivalent thicker cell membrane (reduce-mesh model). Then the number of meshing elements of the full-mesh model is reduced, and thus the computing time is reduced.

According to the simulation results, the reduce-mesh model can be used in both 2D and 3D FEM simulations. The amount of computing time is significantly reduced with an error no more than 0.5% in 2D simulation. The error on 3D simulation result is no more than 2%. All simulation results are validated by measurements and analytical results.

The proposed acceleration method is validated to be fast and accurate on cell models and the acceleration method has potential for all other thin shell FEM models.

Author Contributions: J.T. and W.Y. designed, planned and analysed the major acceleration method and prepared and reviewed the manuscript. M.L. helped in building the 3D FEM simulation server. Y.X. helped in building the experimental set-up for validation and reviewed the manuscript. All authors have read and agreed to the published version of the manuscript.

References

1. Gimsa, J.; Schnelle, T.; Zechel, G.; Glaser, R. Dielectric spectroscopy of human erythrocytes: Investigations under the influence of nystatin. *Biophys. J.* **1994**, *66*, 1244–1253. [CrossRef]
2. Awayda, M.S.; Driessche, W.; Helman, S.I. Frequency-dependent capacitance of the apical membrane of frog skin: Dielectric relaxation processes. *Biophys. J.* **1999**, *76*, 219–232. [CrossRef]
3. Mukhopadhyay, S.C.; Gooneratne, C.P. A novel planar-type biosensor for noninvasive meat inspection. *IEEE Sens. J.* **2007**, *7*, 1340–1346. [CrossRef]
4. Jaffrin, M.Y.; Morel, H. Body fluid volumes measurements by impedance: A review of bioimpedance spectroscopy (BIS) and bioimpedance analysis (BIA) methods. *Med. Eng. Phys.* **2008**, *30*, 1257–1269. [CrossRef] [PubMed]
5. Morimoto, T.; Kimura, S.; Konishi, Y.; Komaki, K.; Uyama, T.; Monden, Y.; Kinouchi, D.Y.; Iritani, D.T. A study of the electrical bio-impedance of tumors. *J. Investig. Surg.* **1993**, *6*, 25–32. [CrossRef] [PubMed]
6. Kerner, T.E.; Paulsen, K.D.; Hartov, A.; Soho, S.K.; Poplack, S.P. Electrical impedance spectroscopy of the breast: Clinical imaging results in 26 subjects. *IEEE Trans. Med. Imaging* **2002**, *21*, 638–645. [CrossRef] [PubMed]
7. Romsauerova, A.; McEwan, A.; Horesh, L.; Yerworth, R.; Bayford, R.H.; Holder, D.S. Multi-frequency electrical impedance tomography (EIT) of the adult human head: Initial findings in brain tumours, arteriovenous malformations and chronic stroke, development of an analysis method and calibration. *Physiol. Meas.* **2006**, *27*, S147. [CrossRef]

8. Schwan, A.; Herman, P. Electrical properties of tissue and cell suspensions. *Adv. Biol. Med. Phys.* **1957**, *5*, 147–209.

9. Schwan, A.; Herman, P. Electrical properties of tissues and cell suspensions: Mechanisms and models. In Proceedings of the 16th Annual International Conference of the IEEE Engineering in Medicine and Biology Society, Baltimore, MD, USA, 3–6 November 1994.

10. Damez, J.L.; Clerjon, S.; Abouelkaram, S.; Lepetit, J. Dielectric behavior of beef meat in the 1–1500 kHz range: Simulation with the Fricke/Cole–Cole model. *Meat Sci.* **2007**, *77*, 512–519. [CrossRef]

11. Stubbe, M.; Gimsa, J. Maxwell's Mixing Equation Revisited: Characteristic Impedance Equations for Ellipsoidal Cells. *Biophys. J.* **2015**, *109*, 194–208. [CrossRef]

12. Asami, K.; Tetsuya, H.; Naokazu, K. Dielectric approach to suspensions of ellipsoidal particles covered with a shell in particular reference to biological cells. *Jpn. J. Appl. Phys.* **1980**, *19*, 359. [CrossRef]

13. Pauly, H.; Schwan, H.P. Impedance of a suspension of ball-shaped particles with a shell; a model for the dielectric behavior of cell suspensions and protein solutions. *Z. Naturforsch.* **1959**, *14*, 125. [CrossRef]

14. Tuncer, E.; Stanisław, M.; Gubański, C.; Nettelblad, B. Dielectric relaxation in dielectric mixtures: Application of the finite element method and its comparison with dielectric mixture formulas. *J. Appl. Phys.* **2001**, *89*, 8092–8100. [CrossRef]

15. Asami, K. Dielectric dispersion in biological cells of complex geometry simulated by the three-dimensional finite difference method. *J. Phys. D Appl. Phys.* **2006**, *39*, 492. [CrossRef]

16. Mejdoubi, A.; Brosseau, C. Finite-element simulation of the depolarization factor of arbitrarily shaped inclusions. *Phys. Rev. E* **2006**, *74*, 031405. [CrossRef]

17. Takashima, S.; Asami, K.; Takahashi, Y. Frequency domain studies of impedance characteristics of biological cells using micropipet technique. *Biophys. J.* **1988**, *54*, 995. [CrossRef]

18. Fricke, H. The Maxwell-Wagner dispersion in a suspension of ellipsoids. *J. Phys. Chem.* **1953**, *57*, 934–937. [CrossRef]

19. Jin, J.M. *The Finite Element Method in Electromagnetics*; Wiley-IEEE Press; John Wiley & Sons: Hoboken, NJ, USA, 2015; pp. 1–876.

20. Bíró, O. Edge element formulations of eddy current problems. *Comput. Methods Appl. Mech. Eng.* **1999**, *169*, 391–405. [CrossRef]

21. O'Toole, M.D.; Marsh, L.A.; Davidson, J.L.; Tan, Y.M.; Armitage, D.W.; Peyton, A.J. Non-contact multi-frequency magnetic induction spectroscopy system for industrial-scale bio-impedance measurement. *Meas. Sci. Tech.* **2015**, *26*, 035102. [CrossRef]

22. Georgii, J.; Rudiger, W. A streaming approach for sparse matrix products and its application in Galerkin multigrid methods. *Electron. Trans. Numer. Anal.* **2010**, *37*, 263–275.

23. Fritschy, J.; Horesh, L.; Holder, D.S.; Bayford, R.H. Using the GRID to improve the computation speed of electrical impedance tomography (EIT) reconstruction algorithms. *Physiol. Meas.* **2005**, *26*, S209. [CrossRef]

24. Lu, M.Y.; Anthony, P.; Yin, W.L. Acceleration of Frequency Sweeping in Eddy-Current Computation. *IEEE Trans. Magn.* **2017**, *53*, 1–8. [CrossRef]

25. Gheorghiu, E. Measuring living cells using dielectric spectroscopy. *Bioelectrochem. Bioenerg.* **1996**, *40*, 133–139. [CrossRef]

26. Sekine, K. Application of boundary element method to calculation of the complex permittivity of suspensions of cells in shape of D∞ h symmetry. *Bioelectrochemistry* **2000**, *52*, 1–7. [CrossRef]

27. Beving, H.; Eriksson, L.E.G.; Davey, C.L.; Kell, D.B. Dielectric properties of human blood and erythrocytes at radio frequencies (0.2–10 MHz); dependence on cell volume fraction and medium composition. *Eur. Biophys. J.* **1994**, *23*, 207–215. [CrossRef] [PubMed]

28. Di Biasio, A.; Cametti, C. Effect of shape on the dielectric properties of biological cell suspensions. *Bioelectrochemistry* **2007**, *71*, 149–156. [CrossRef]

29. Saville, D.A.; Bellini, T.; Degiorgio, V.; Mantegazza, F. An extended Maxwell–Wagner theory for the electric birefringence of charged colloids. *J. Chem. Phys.* **2000**, *113*, 6974–6983. [CrossRef]

30. Davis, L.C. Polarization forces and conductivity effects in electrorheological fluids. *J. Appl. Phys.* **1992**, *72*, 1334–1340. [CrossRef]
31. Zhou, Y.Y.; Wang, A.P.; Zhou, P.; Wang, H.; Chai, T.Y. Dynamic performance enhancement for nonlinear stochastic systems using RBF driven nonlinear compensation with extended Kalman filter. *Automatica* **2020**, *112*, 108693. [CrossRef]
32. Tang, J.W.; Yin, W.L.; Lu, M.Y. Bio-impedance spectroscopy for frozen-thaw of bio-samples: Non-contact inductive measurement and finite element (FE) based cell modelling. *J. Food Eng.* **2020**, *272*, 109784. [CrossRef]

8

In Vivo Tumor Vascular Imaging with Light Emitting Diode-Based Photoacoustic Imaging System

Marvin Xavierselvan [1], Mithun Kuniyil Ajith Singh [2] and Srivalleesha Mallidi [1,3,*]

[1] Department of Biomedical Engineering, Tufts University, Medford, MA 02155, USA; marvin.xavierselvan@tufts.edu
[2] Research & Business Development Division, Cyberdyne INC, Cambridge Innovation Center, 3013 Rotterdam, The Netherlands; mithun_ajith@cyberdyne.jp
[3] Wellman Center for Photomedicine, Massachusetts General Hospital, Harvard Medical School, Boston, MA 02114, USA
* Correspondence: Srivalleesha.mallidi@tufts.edu

Abstract: Photoacoustic (PA) imaging has shown tremendous promise for imaging tumor vasculature and its function at deeper penetration depths without the use of exogenous contrast agents. Traditional PA imaging systems employ expensive and bulky class IV lasers with low pulse repetition rate, due to which its availability for preclinical cancer research is hampered. In this study, we evaluated the capability of a Light-Emitting Diode (LED)-based PA and ultrasound (US) imaging system for monitoring heterogeneous microvasculature in tumors (up to 10 mm in depth) and quantitatively compared the PA images with gold standard histology images. We used a combination of a 7 MHz linear array US transducer and 850 nm excitation wavelength LED arrays to image blood vessels in a subcutaneous tumor model. After imaging, the tumors were sectioned and stained for endothelial cells to correlate with PA images across similar cross-sections. Analysis of 30 regions of interest in tumors from different mice showed a statistically significant R-value of 0.84 where the areas with high blood vessel density had high PA response while low blood vessel density regions had low PA response. Our results confirm that LED-based PA and US imaging can provide 2D and 3D images of tumor vasculature and the potential it has as a valuable tool for preclinical cancer research.

Keywords: LED; photoacoustic imaging; ultrasound; tumor imaging

---

1. Introduction

The critical role of vasculature for tumor growth and metastasis is undisputed. Tumor aggressiveness and the extent of the aberrant tumor vascular structure and function are highly correlated. To meet the increasing needs for oxygen and nutrients, cancers induce neovascularization, one of the hallmarks of cancer [1]. The heterogeneity in tumor vasculature [2] affects drug distribution [3,4] and, as a result, impact treatment outcomes. Indeed, many anti-angiogenic agents or therapies that can prune these blood vessels and prevent nutrients from reaching the tumors have been developed [5]. Monitoring the dynamic changes in tumor vasculature post therapy is key for prognosis [6]. Several imaging modalities have been used to study changes in tumor vasculature both at structural and functional level. More recently, photoacoustic (PA) imaging has gained tremendous popularity for imaging tumor vasculature [7–10]. PA imaging involves detection of acoustic waves generated when the optical absorbers such as hemoglobin in the blood are irradiated with nanosecond pulsed light and undergo thermo-elastic expansion and contraction [11]. The acoustic waves are picked up by the ultrasound (US) transducer and processed to generate a PA image [11,12]. Notably, two features of PA imaging that make it highly suitable to image vasculature are: 1. ability to image blood vessels without exogenous contrast agents and 2. ability to complement US imaging that provides structural information of the tumor.

Traditionally PA imaging systems use lasers (typically Nd: YAG pumped optical parametric oscillator lasers) for exciting the optical absorbers and employ a US transducer (array or single element) to receive the generated acoustic wave. These lasers are expensive, bulky with large spatial occupancy, and often have low repetition rate which leads to low image frame rate and acquisition speed. These limitations hinder the wide adaption of PA imaging systems in both preclinical and clinical applications. Advances in semiconductor industry have led to the creation of powerful Light-Emitting Diodes (LED) which are compact, portable, affordable, and energy-efficient. AcousticX by Cyberdyne Inc. (Tsukuba, Japan) is a LED-based system that can perform PA and US imaging at high frame rates. These LEDs can be fired with a pulse repetition frequency (PRF) from 1 to 4 kHz. Despite generating low optical output (400 μJ/pulse when using two 850 nm arrays), the high PRF of LEDs offers the possibility of averaging several frames which results in generating real-time PA images with reasonable signal-to-noise ratio (SNR) [13–17]. Furthermore, the spatial resolution and SNR provided by LED-based PA imaging is very similar and comparable to laser-based PA systems [13]. Due to the inherent advantages of the LED-based PA system, several research groups have explored its ability for various potential applications [15,16,18–21]. None of these studies provide validation of the generated PA image with histology. In this study, for the first time to the best of our knowledge, we report the LED-based PA imaging system's ability to image microvasculature in subcutaneous murine tumor xenografts and validate the results using histology.

2. Materials and Methods

2.1. LED-Based PA Imaging System

An AcousticX system integrated with a 7 MHz US transducer (128 elements, −6 dB bandwidth is 80%) and two 850 nm LED arrays (for deeper light penetration) attached on either side of the transducer at a 30° angle was used for in vivo imaging (Figure 1A–C). The mean lateral and axial resolutions of AcousticX when using a 7 MHz transducer are 460 and 220 μm, respectively [14,19]. Each LED array had height, length and width dimensions of 12.4, 86.5, and 10.2 mm, respectively, and had 144 individual LEDs arranged in 4 rows (36 elements/row). The PRF of the LED array could be varied between 1, 2, 3, and 4 kHz. In this study, we operated the LED arrays at a PRF of 4 kHz to acquire and save PA images of the tumor vasculature at a frame rate of approximately 10 Hz i.e., 384 PA frames were continuously averaged to generate one display image. For offline MATLAB analysis, a higher number of frames (12,800) was averaged to enhance the PA image SNR. The SNR was defined as SNR = S/σ, where S is the mean of the image amplitude in a signal region, and σ is the standard deviation of the image amplitude in a noise region. The signal region was empirically chosen as a rectangular region (4 by 4 pixels) near a feeding blood vessel on the tumor surface where the PA signal was apparent; the noise region was manually chosen to correspond to a rectangular region outside the tumor region.

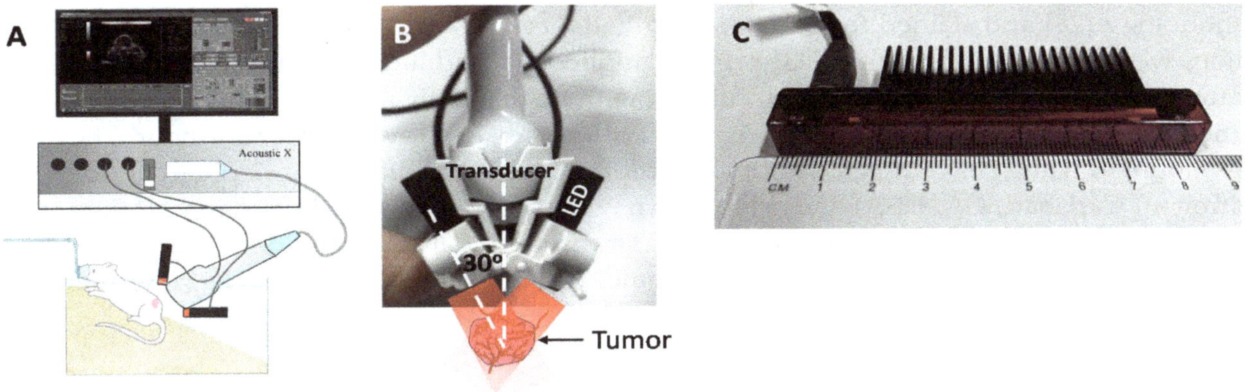

Figure 1. (**A**) Schematic of our experimental setup in which the Light-Emitting Diode (LED)-based photoacoustic (PA) system was utilized for imaging subcutaneous tumors in a mouse. (**B**,**C**) LED array used for illumination and the angle at which the LEDs are connected to the ultrasound transducer. (Scale bar = 2 mm).

2.2. *Animal Model*

All animal experiments were performed in compliance with the Institutional Animal Care and Use Committee (IACUC) of Massachusetts General Hospital (MGH). Swiss nu/nu female mice (aged 6–8 weeks, body weight 20–25 g) were raised in aseptic conditions in the institution's animal facility with a 12 h light and dark cycles. We used human hypopharyngeal squamous cell carcinoma (FaDu) xenograft model because these are highly vascularized tumors [22,23]. FaDu cells were cultured in Eagle's Minimum Essential Medium supplemented with 10% fetal bovine serum and 1% antibiotics (Penicillin and Streptomycin 1:1 *v*/*v*) in a T75 flask and maintained at 37 °C and 5% CO_2. At 80–90% confluency, cells were trypsinized and centrifuged to remove the supernatant. The cells were then suspended in a mixture of matrigel (BD Bioscience, CA) and phosphate buffered saline in 1:1 *v*/*v* at a density of 1 million cells per 100 μL and injected subcutaneously into mice.

2.3. *In-Vivo Photoacoustic Imaging*

A total of 3 mice were imaged using the AcousticX system when the tumors reached 6–8 mm in diameter as measured with a digital caliper (VWR 62379-531, Radnor, PA, USA). The mice were anesthetized using 2% isoflurane and placed in a warm water bath to achieve optical coupling with the US transducer as shown in Figure 1A. The LED arrays were positioned at a 30° angle (Figure 1B) to the US transducer to colocalize the light with the transducer focus. The US transducer was then vertically positioned such that the tumor was approximately at the focal region of the transducer (~20 mm depth). Radio frequency (RF) data and US/PA images for several cross-sections of the tumors were acquired and saved for further analysis. Motion artifacts in the tumor region due to mouse breathing were minimal as shown in Video S1 (captured at 10 Hz frame rate, see Supplementary materials). In the post-acquisition image analysis, frames with breathing motion were not included. The RF data was processed with previously reported algorithms [24–27] using custom written MATLAB code to obtain US/PA images of tumor vasculature. Three-dimensional imaging was performed by moving the US/PA transducer linearly across the XY plane with the aid of an in-built translation stage and the sequence was rendered in ImageJ.

2.4. *Histology*

Post imaging mice were sacrificed, and tumors were surgically removed without skin. The tumors were embedded and frozen in optical cutting temperature (OCT) compound in the same orientation as the US/PA image with the aid of fiducial markers placed prior to euthanasia. The frozen tumors were cryosectioned (5 μm) in the same plane as the US/PA images based on previously published methodology [28] and stained for platelet endothelial cell adhesion molecule-1 (or CD31). Tissue sections were incubated with anti-CD31 primary antibody (1:50 dilution; Rabbit polyclonal anti-CD31, Abcam) overnight at 4 °C, washed, and incubated with fluorescently tagged secondary antibody (1:100 dilution, Donkey Anti-Rabbit IgG NL637 Affinity Purified Ab, R&D systems) for one hour. The sections were mounted using slowfade gold antifade mountant with 4′,6-diamidino-2-phenylindole (DAPI, Invitrogen, Carlsbad, CA, USA) and sealed with coverslips. A whole-slide scanning fluorescence imaging system (Hamamatsu NanoZoomer 2.0-HT) was used to image the slides at 40 x magnification and images were saved in Hamamatsu Nanozoomer Digital Pathology Image (NDPI) format.

2.5. Image Processing

A 5x magnification of the fluorescence image was extracted from the NDPI file using ImageJ, rotated to match the PA image orientation and saved for further analysis in MATLAB (Figure 2). Several 1.25×1.85 mm^2 regions of interest (ROI) were chosen from the immunofluorescence (IF) and PA images for correlation analysis. This corresponds to 679×1005 and 5×50 pixels in IF and PA images, respectively. The background from a similar ROI area was calculated from a region outside the tumor area for both IF and PA images and subtracted from the tumor ROI values. The CD31 intensity from the ROI in IF images were summed and compared to the total PA signal intensity from the corresponding ROI in the PA image. Linear regression analysis was performed using GraphPad Prism software.

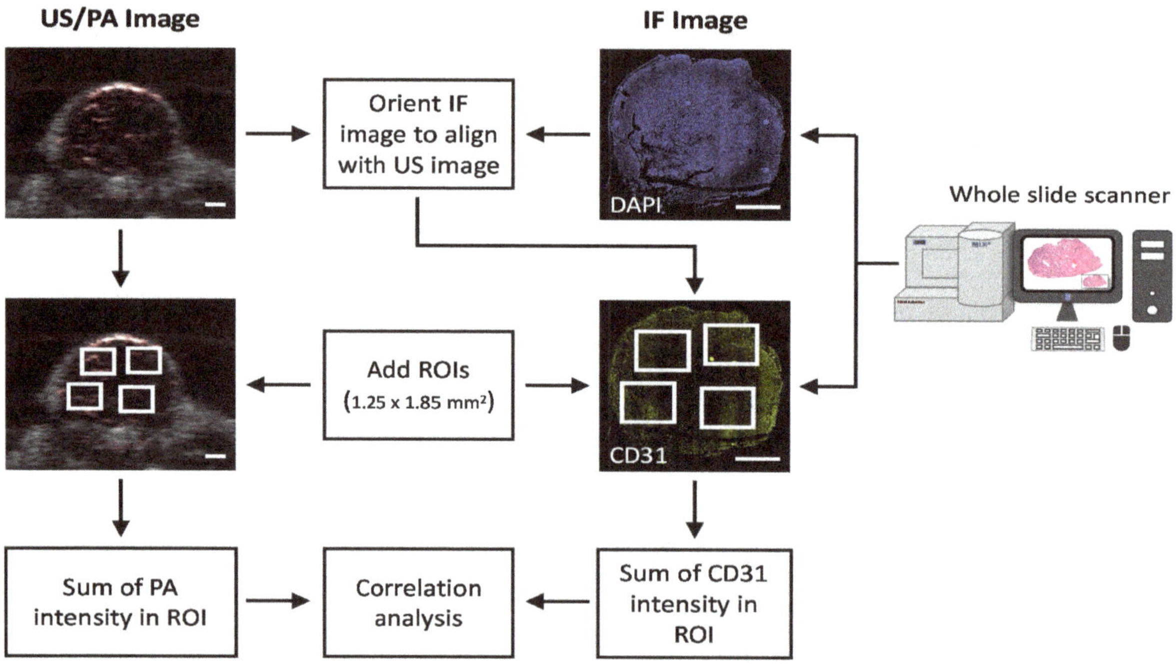

Figure 2. Flowchart describing the image processing methodology to correlate CD31 signal intensity with PA signals. (Scale bar = 2 mm).

3. Results

3.1. SNR Enhances with Frame Averaging

The PA image of a representative tumor acquired and processed at different frame rates (0.31–60 Hz) is shown in Figure 3A. To enhance the SNR and improve image quality, subsequent PA frames were averaged resulting in lower frame rate. This relationship between the frame rate and SNR of the PA image is displayed in Figure 3B, where low frame rate offers better SNR as expected. The low SNR of the image at higher frame rates may be attributed to the low output power of the LED, however, due to the high pulse repetition rate of LED excitation for PA data acquisition, more PA frames can be acquired and averaged to increase the SNR (Figure 3C). A frame rate of 10 Hz was chosen for data acquisition (2D and 3D acquisition) during the experiment as it provided the best possible SNR for near real-time combined US/PA imaging. To quantitatively compare the 2D images with IF images, the acquired PA images were further averaged to a final frame rate of 0.31 Hz to enhance the SNR by 20 dB, i.e., overall 12,800 frames were averaged to obtain an SNR of ~40 dB (Figure 3C). The enhanced SNR facilitated accurate comparison with histology images without the involvement of background noise.

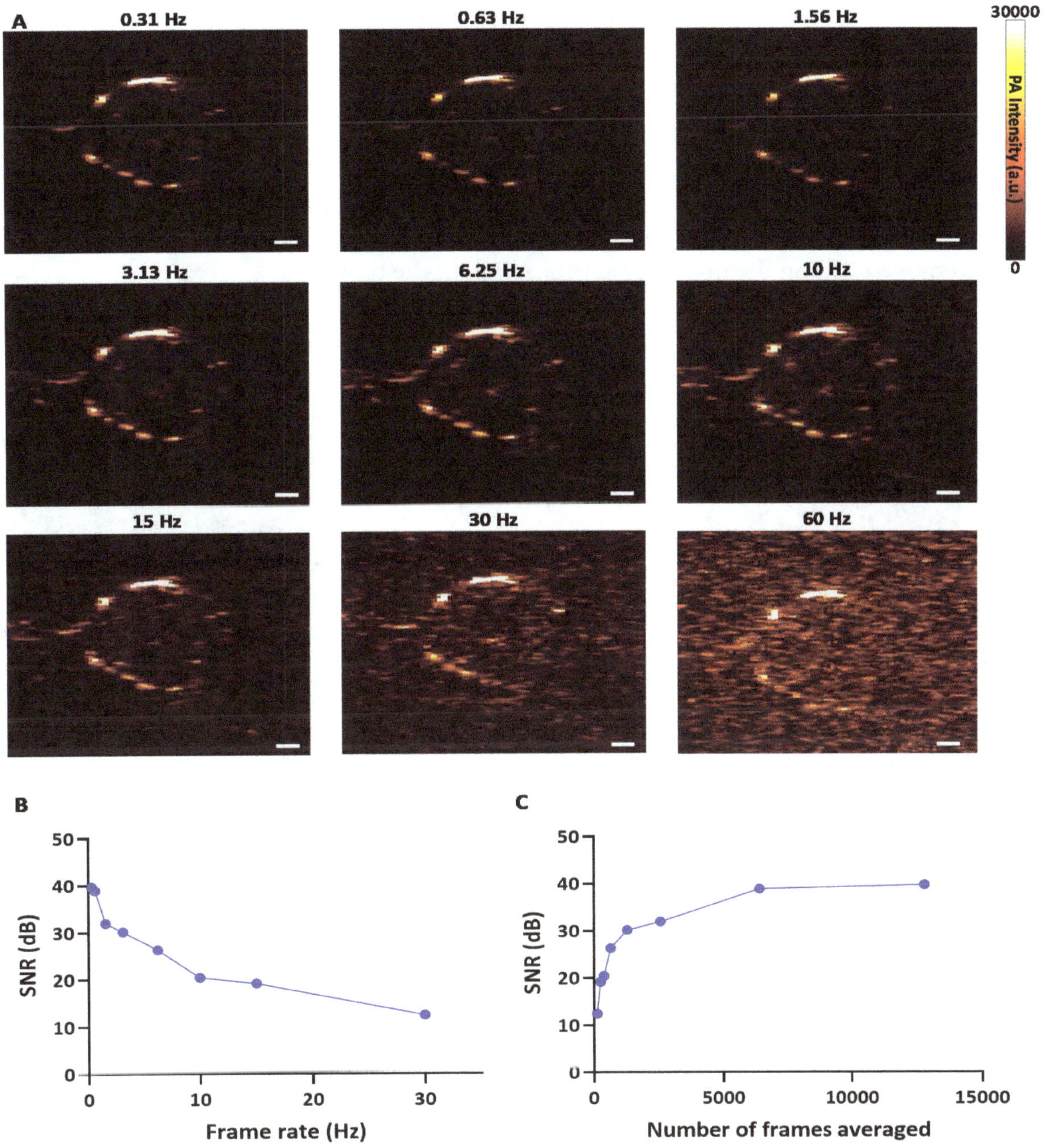

Figure 3. The signal-to-noise ratio (SNR) is enhanced by averaging several frames in the LED-based PA imaging system. (**A**) PA images of a tumor acquired and processed at different frame rates. (**B**) Relationship between the frame rate and SNR. (**C**) Plot detailing the SNR change with respect to the averaging of frames. (Scale bar = 2 mm).

3.2. Tumor Vascular Imaging with AcousticX

Figure 4A shows the overlay of the US image (in grayscale) with the PA image of two representative tumors (offline reconstructed). The B-mode US image depicts the shape and structure of the tumor (~6 to 10 mm in diameter and depth), and the PA image provides the blood vessels location inside and around the tumor. The PA image is displayed on a pseudo-colored hot map where low and high signals are represented by black and white, respectively. Subcutaneous tumors are fed by large blood vessels usually originating from the skin tissue above or the muscle tissue lying beneath the tumor, as visualized in Figure 4A. AcousticX can detect the PA signal not only from the surface of the tumor but also from the deep edge (~10 mm) of the tumor. The Hematoxylin and Eosin (H&E) stain is a standard histology stain to showcase tissue microanatomy. Figure 4B showcases the H&E image of the tumor at the same cross-section as the US/PA image where the tumor structure is analogous to the shape and size observed in the US image. Figure 4C shows the IF image of the tumor cross-section with CD31 stain for blood vessels (yellow) and DAPI for cell nuclei (blue). DAPI staining was performed to visualize the tumor structure and aided in selecting corresponding ROIs as the US/PA image. Qualitatively we noticed regions of the high PA signal have high vessel density on the IF images as displayed by the yellow arrows in Figure 4. The blood vessels on the top of the tumor (particularly Figure 4A top panel) are not strongly visualized in the IF image as these vessels were part of the skin above the tumors which was removed during the histological processing of the tissue.

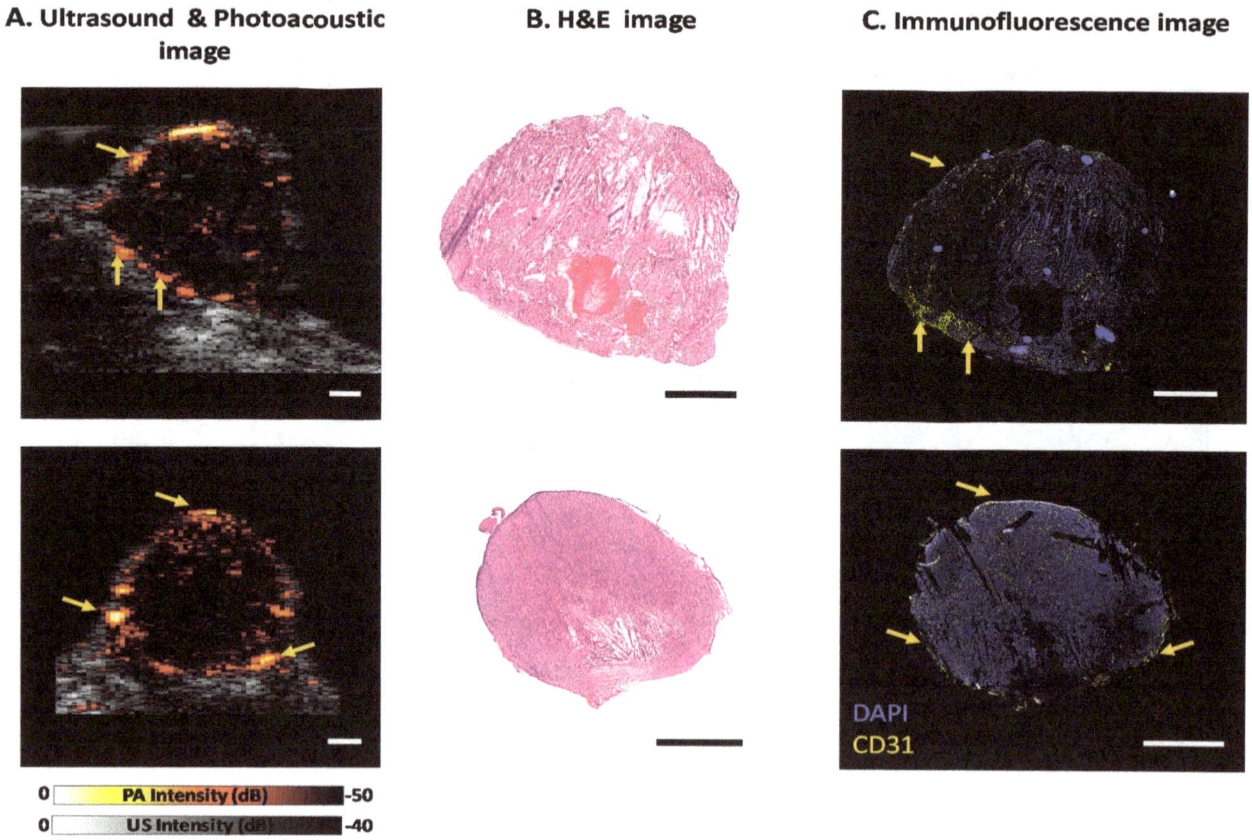

Figure 4. Evaluation of AcousticX on subcutaneous tumor xenografts in mice. (**A**) Ultrasound and photoacoustic image overlay of the tumor vasculature of two mice. Images of the Mouse 1 tumor acquired at a frame rate of 10 Hz are shown in Video 1. Motion due to breathing was minimal and only frames that did not have motion artifacts were used for image analysis. (**B**) H&E stain of the tumor cross-section. (**C**) Immunofluorescence stain for blood vessels in yellow and cell nuclei in blue. (Scale bar on all images = 2 mm, Video S1, MP4, 1.7 MB).

3.3. Correlation of PA Signal with Histology

The correlation plot between the PA signal from blood vessels and CD31 intensity from the IF image is displayed in Figure 5. As expected, we observed that larger blood vessels or areas with high blood vessel density had a high PA signal while the micro vessels or low blood vessel density regions had a low signal. The overall R-value for correlation was 0.84 and individual R-values for the three tumors used in the study were 0.65, 0.91 and 0.91. The differences in the R-values among the tumors were due to the inter-tumor heterogeneity in the vasculature and biological variations across different animals. The results obtained here with the LED-based PA imaging system are on par with reports using traditional laser-based PA imaging systems. For example, Mallidi et al. [28] and Bar-Zion et al. [29] qualitatively demonstrated good spatial co-registration between tumor vascular oxygenation maps obtained from PA imaging and hypoxia markers such as pimonidazole or carbonic anhydrase IX. Gerling et al. [30] observed an excellent R-value of 0.95 when quantitatively correlating oxygenation saturation measurements from PA imaging to the intensity of pimonidazole in the tumor, however, there were only six points in this correlation. Furthermore, the PA signals were averaged over the entire tumor underplaying the intra-tumor heterogeneity. In our study we divided the tumor region into several ROIs to consider both high and low vascular regions. In addition, these studies [28–30] utilized higher frequency transducers with limitations in imaging depth. It is obvious that some microvascular structures inside the tumors may be not within the detection limits of the 7 MHz transducer used in our study, which would have resulted in slightly lower correlation between PA signals and CD31 intensity in certain regions of the tumor. Nevertheless, we clearly demonstrate a good correlation between histology and PA images generated using an LED source with comparatively less optical output energy.

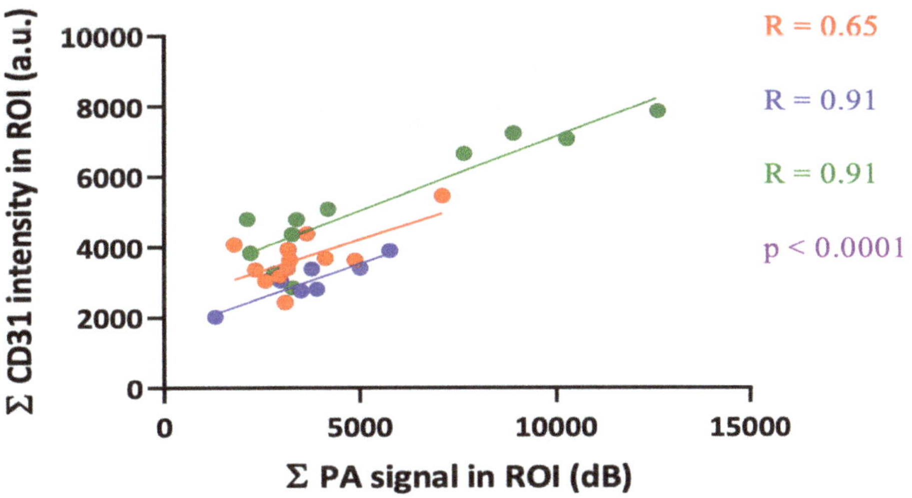

Figure 5. Correlation between background subtracted signal intensity from PA images and CD31 immunofluorescence (IF) image. Each color represents data from different mice. A total of 30 ROIs from three mice were used in our analysis. The R-value for correlation based on Pearson's coefficient was calculated between the CD31 intensity from the IF image and PA signals from blood vessels.

3.4. 3D Tumor Imaging with AcousticX

An LED-based photoacoustic imaging system can also be used to visualize vasculature in 3D. Figure 6 shows the overlay of a US/PA image of tumor acquired by AcousticX at a frame rate of 10 Hz and reconstructed in 3D using ImageJ. A corresponding video showcasing the 3D rendering of US/PA images of the tumor is shown in Video S2. Figure 6C shows the structure of the tumor in different cross-sectional planes. The measurements obtained from AcousticX images have good agreement with the caliper measurements for the tumor size (length, width, and depth). Two LED arrays on either side of the US transducer delivered a total optical energy output of 400 μJ/pulse on the skin surface. In the absence of optical scattering, the irradiation area at the US focus will be approximately 50 × 7 mm in the YX-plane, with a maximum radiant exposure of 0.11 mJ/cm^2, which is orders of magnitude lower than the ANSI safety limit and the radiant exposure in laser-based PA imaging systems. It is encouraging that the system used in this study could visualize tumor vasculature in vivo at an imaging depth of 10 mm, considering the low pulse energies provided by the LED arrays.

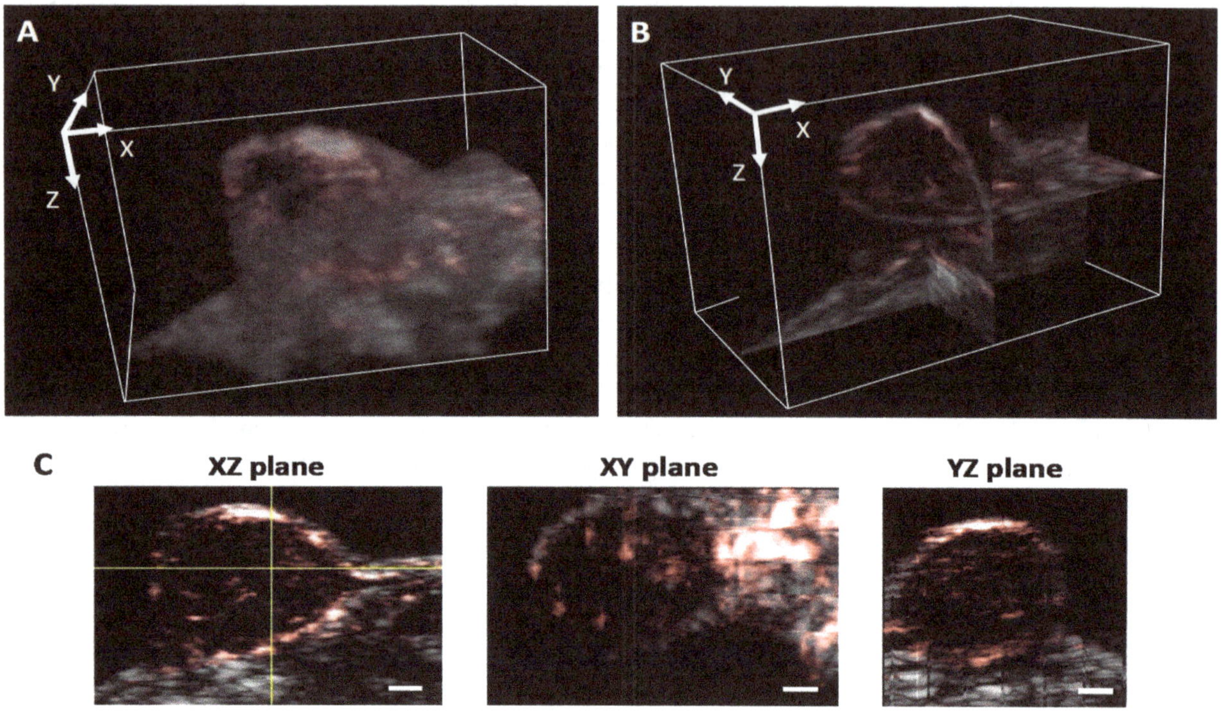

Figure 6. (**A**) Overlay of ultrasound and photoacoustic images of tumors reconstructed in 3D (Video 2) and (**B**) in orthoslice view. (**C**) Tumor images displayed in different 2D planes. (Scale bar = 2 mm, Video S2, MOV, 779 kB).

4. Discussion

In preclinical cancer research, rodent models are widely used to study the complex physiological process involved in tumor formation and therapy response. The tumor is grown either subcutaneously or orthotopically at the site of the origin of tumor cells. The maximum size for subcutaneous tumors is less than 1–2 cm in diameter, and orthotopic tumors depending on the organ can vary between 3 and 6 mm in diameter. The length of the LED array in AcousticX is 8.65 cm [14] and is significantly larger than that of the tumors generally seen in preclinical research. Hence most of the light from the LED arrays is delivered outside of the tumor. Considering this, the imaging depth of ~10 mm we achieved demonstrated the high sensitivity of the system, which is commendable. Better light delivery strategies to illuminate tumors efficiently may help in improving the imaging depth and SNR further.

Currently the AcousticX system is integrated with a 7 MHz ultrasound transducer that has limitations in spatial resolution. Higher frequency transducers offer better resolution and our future work involves integrating these transducers with LED arrays to enhance image resolution. In addition to improvements in spatial resolution, image SNR can be enhanced through novel beamforming algorithms. Traditional beamforming algorithms are based on "delay and sum" and "delay-multiply and sum" methodology. Although they are simple to implement in imaging systems, they generate low quality images with low contrast, especially when the data is noisy. Recent studies have shown that the "double stage delay-multiply and sum" algorithm improves lateral resolution and offers high contrast for an LED-based PA imaging system [31,32]. Moreover, in this study we used a single wavelength (850 nm) LED array that provides deeper light penetration to image tumor vasculature. The availability of high-power multi-wavelength LED arrays will enable imaging blood oxygen saturation levels in the tumor vasculature [33,34]. This information is key for monitoring treatment response and predicting recurrence. These multi-wavelength LED arrays can also enable the imaging of tumor via receptor targeted exogenous contrast agents [15,18,25,27], as previously demonstrated by us and others with traditional pulsed laser sources [9,35–41]. With the availability of low-cost multi-wavelength PA imaging systems, our future studies will aim at developing and monitoring various targeted therapies guided by multi-wavelength PA imaging that can provide vascular information with information on the localization of targeted contrast agents.

5. Conclusions

In summary, we demonstrate the capability of an LED-based PA imaging system for monitoring tumor vasculature in vivo. The PA images obtained are in good correlation with the gold standard IF images. With the widespread rise of PA imaging technology, new improved reconstruction algorithms, high frequency transducers, better illumination strategies, and multi-wavelength LED arrays, we can expect LED-based PA imaging to become a promising tool and play a highly significant role in both preclinical research and clinical applications.

Author Contributions: Conceptualization, M.X., M.K.A.S., and S.M.; methodology, M.X. and S.M.; software, M.X. and M.K.A.S.; validation, M.X. and S.M.; formal analysis, M.X.; investigation, M.X. and S.M.; resources, S.M.; data curation, M.X. and M.K.A.S.; writing—original draft preparation, M.X. and S.M.; writing—review and editing, M.X., M.K.A.S., and S.M.; visualization, M.X. and S.M.; supervision, S.M.; project administration, S.M.; funding acquisition, S.M. All authors have read and agreed to the published version of the manuscript.

Acknowledgments: The authors would like to thank the Pathology core at the Wellman Center for Photomedicine, MGH for sectioning the tissues and access to the NanoZoomer imaging system. We also would like to thank Annika Schaad at Tufts University for help with the Figure 1 schematic drawing.

References

1. Hanahan, D.; Weinberg, R.A. Hallmarks of cancer: The next generation. *Cell* **2011**, *144*, 646–674. [CrossRef] [PubMed]
2. Eberhard, A.; Kahlert, S.; Goede, V.; Hemmerlein, B.; Plate, K.H.; Augustin, H.G. Heterogeneity of angiogenesis and blood vessel maturation in human tumors: Implications for antiangiogenic tumor therapies. *Cancer Res.* **2000**, *60*, 1388–1393. [PubMed]
3. Garattini, S.; Fuso Nerini, I.; D'Incalci, M. Not only tumor but also therapy heterogeneity. *Ann. Oncol.* **2018**, *29*, 13–19. [CrossRef] [PubMed]
4. Stylianopoulos, T.; Munn, L.L.; Jain, R.K. Reengineering the Tumor Vasculature: Improving Drug Delivery and Efficacy. *Trends Cancer* **2018**, *4*, 258–259. [CrossRef] [PubMed]
5. Vasudev, N.S.; Reynolds, A.R. Anti-angiogenic therapy for cancer: Current progress, unresolved questions and future directions. *Angiogenesis* **2014**, *17*, 471–494. [CrossRef] [PubMed]
6. Cai, W.; Gambhir, S.S.; Chen, X. Methods in Enzymology. In *Angiogenesis: In Vivo Systems, Part B*; Academic Press: Cambridge, MA, USA, 2008; Volume 445, pp. 141–176.
7. Laufer, J.; Johnson, P.; Zhang, E.; Treeby, B.; Cox, B.; Pedley, B.; Beard, P. In vivo preclinical photoacoustic imaging of tumor vasculature development and therapy. *J. Biomed. Opt.* **2012**, *17*, 56016. [CrossRef]
8. Bohndiek, S.E.; Sasportas, L.S.; Machtaler, S.; Jokerst, J.V.; Hori, S.; Gambhir, S.S. Photoacoustic Tomography Detects Early Vessel Regression and Normalization During Ovarian Tumor Response to the Antiangiogenic Therapy Trebananib. *J. Nucl. Med.* **2015**, *56*, 1942–1947. [CrossRef]

9. Mallidi, S.; Luke, G.P.; Emelianov, S. Photoacoustic imaging in cancer detection, diagnosis, and treatment guidance. *Trends Biotechnol.* **2011**, *29*, 213–221. [CrossRef]
10. Brown, E.; Brunker, J.; Bohndiek, S.E. Photoacoustic imaging as a tool to probe the tumour microenvironment. *Dis. Model. Mech.* **2019**, *12*, 039636. [CrossRef]
11. Xu, M.; Wang, L.V. Photoacoustic imaging in biomedicine. *Rev. Sci. Instrum.* **2006**, *77*, 41101. [CrossRef]
12. Gigan, S. Optical microscopy aims deep. *Nat. Photonics* **2017**, *11*, 14–16. [CrossRef]
13. Agrawal, S.; Kuniyil Ajith Singh, M.; Yang, X.; Albahrani, H.; Dangi, A.; Kothapalli, S.-R. *Photoacoustic Imaging Capabilities of Light Emitting Diodes (LED) and Laser Sources: A Comparison Study*; Oraevsky, A.A., Wang, L.V., Eds.; Photons Plus Ultrasound: Imaging and Sensing: San Francisco, CA, USA, 2020.
14. Hariri, A.; Lemaster, J.; Wang, J.; Jeevarathinam, A.S.; Chao, D.L.; Jokerst, J.V. The characterization of an economic and portable LED-based photoacoustic imaging system to facilitate molecular imaging. *Photoacoustics* **2018**, *9*, 10–20. [CrossRef] [PubMed]
15. Zhu, Y.; Xu, G.; Yuan, J.; Jo, J.; Gandikota, G.; Demirci, H.; Agano, T.; Sato, N.; Shigeta, Y.; Wang, X. Light Emitting Diodes based Photoacoustic Imaging and Potential Clinical Applications. *Sci. Rep.* **2018**, *8*, 9885. [CrossRef] [PubMed]
16. Joseph Francis, K.; Boink, Y.E.; Dantuma, M.; Ajith Singh, M.K.; Manohar, S.; Steenbergen, W. Tomographic imaging with an ultrasound and LED-based photoacoustic system. *Biomed. Opt. Express* **2020**, *11*, 2152–2165. [CrossRef] [PubMed]
17. Agrawal, S.; Fadden, C.; Dangi, A.; Yang, X.; Albahrani, H.; Frings, N.; Heidari Zadi, S.; Kothapalli, S.R. Light-Emitting-Diode-Based Multispectral Photoacoustic Computed Tomography System. *Sensors* **2019**, *19*, 4861. [CrossRef] [PubMed]
18. Jo, J.; Xu, G.; Zhu, Y.; Burton, M.; Sarazin, J.; Schiopu, E.; Gandikota, G.; Wang, X. Detecting joint inflammation by an LED-based photoacoustic imaging system: A feasibility study. *J. Biomed. Opt.* **2018**, *23*, 1–4. [CrossRef]
19. Xia, W.; Kuniyil Ajith Singh, M.; Maneas, E.; Sato, N.; Shigeta, Y.; Agano, T.; Ourselin, S.; West, S.J. Handheld Real-Time LED-Based Photoacoustic and Ultrasound Imaging System for Accurate Visualization of Clinical Metal Needles and Superficial Vasculature to Guide Minimally Invasive Procedures. *Sensors* **2018**, *18*, 1394. [CrossRef]
20. Zhu, Y.; Lu, X.; Dong, X.; Yuan, J.; Fabiilli, M.L.; Wang, X. LED-Based Photoacoustic Imaging for Monitoring Angiogenesis in Fibrin Scaffolds. *Tissue Eng. Part C Methods* **2019**, *25*, 523–531. [CrossRef]
21. Hariri, A.; Zhao, E.; Jeevarathinam, A.S.; Lemaster, J.; Zhang, J.; Jokerst, J.V. Molecular imaging of oxidative stress using an LED-based photoacoustic imaging system. *Sci. Rep.* **2019**, *9*, 1–10.
22. Lauk, S.; Zietman, A.; Skates, S.; Fabian, R.; Suit, H.D. Comparative Morphometric Study of Tumor Vasculature in Human Squamous Cell Carcinomas and Their Xenotransplants in Athymic Nude Mice. *Cancer Res.* **1989**, *49*, 4557–4561.
23. Seshadri, M.; Mazurchuk, R.; Spernyak, J.A.; Bhattacharya, A.; Rustum, Y.M.; Bellnier, D.A. Activity of the vascular-disrupting agent 5,6-dimethylxanthenone-4-acetic acid against human head and neck carcinoma xenografts. *Neoplasia* **2006**, *8*, 534–542. [CrossRef] [PubMed]
24. Jaeger, M.; Schüpbach, S.; Gertsch, A.; Kitz, M.; Frenz, M. Fourier reconstruction in optoacoustic imaging using truncated regularized inversek-space interpolation. *Inverse Probl.* **2007**, *23*, S51–S63. [CrossRef]
25. Xia, W.; Maneas, E.; Trung Huynh, N.; Kuniyil Ajith Singh, M.; Montaña Brown, N.; Ourselin, S.; Gilbert-Kawai, E.; West, S.J.; Desjardins, A.E. *Imaging of Human Peripheral Blood Vessels during Cuff Occlusion with a Compact LED-Based Photoacoustic and Ultrasound System*; Oraevsky, A.A., Wang, L.V., Eds.; Photons Plus Ultrasound: Imaging and Sensing: San Francisco, CA, USA, 2019.
26. Hussain, A.; Petersen, W.; Staley, J.; Hondebrink, E.; Steenbergen, W. Quantitative blood oxygen saturation imaging using combined photoacoustics and acousto-optics. *Opt. Lett.* **2016**, *41*, 1720–1723. [CrossRef] [PubMed]
27. Kuniyil Ajith Singh, M.; Sato, N.; Ichihashi, F.; Sankai, Y. In Vivo Demonstration of Real-Time Oxygen Saturation Imaging Using a Portable and Affordable LED-Based Multispectral Photoacoustic and Ultrasound Imaging System. In Proceedings of the Photons Plus Ultrasound: Imaging and Sensing 2019, San Francisco, CA, USA, 27 February 2019.
28. Mallidi, S.; Watanabe, K.; Timerman, D.; Schoenfeld, D.; Hasan, T. Prediction of tumor recurrence and therapy monitoring using ultrasound-guided photoacoustic imaging. *Theranostics* **2015**, *5*, 289–301. [CrossRef]

29. Bar-Zion, A.; Yin, M.; Adam, D.; Foster, F.S. Functional Flow Patterns and Static Blood Pooling in Tumors Revealed by Combined Contrast-Enhanced Ultrasound and Photoacoustic Imaging. *Cancer Res.* **2016**, *76*, 4320–4331. [CrossRef]
30. Gerling, M.; Zhao, Y.; Nania, S.; Norberg, K.J.; Verbeke, C.S.; Englert, B.; Kuiper, R.V.; Bergstrom, A.; Hassan, M.; Neesse, A.; et al. Real-time assessment of tissue hypoxia in vivo with combined photoacoustics and high-frequency ultrasound. *Theranostics* **2014**, *4*, 604–613. [CrossRef]
31. Miri Rostami, S.R.; Mozaffarzadeh, M.; Ghaffari-Miab, M.; Hariri, A.; Jokerst, J. GPU-accelerated Double-stage Delay-multiply-and-sum Algorithm for Fast Photoacoustic Tomography Using LED Excitation and Linear Arrays. *Ultrason. Imaging* **2019**, *41*, 301–316. [CrossRef]
32. Mozaffarzadeh, M.; Hariri, A.; Moore, C.; Jokerst, J.V. The double-stage delay-multiply-and-sum image reconstruction method improves imaging quality in a LED-based photoacoustic array scanner. *Photoacoustics* **2018**, *12*, 22–29. [CrossRef]
33. Xavierselvan, M.; Mallidi, S. LED-Based Functional Photoacoustics—Portable and Affordable Solution for Preclinical Cancer Imaging. In *LED-Based Photoacoustic Imaging: From Bench to Bedside*; Kuniyil Ajith Singh, M., Ed.; Springer: Singapore, 2020; pp. 303–319.
34. Zhu, Y.; Feng, T.; Cheng, Q.; Wang, X.; Du, S.; Sato, N.; Kuniyil Ajith Singh, M.; Yuan, J. Towards Clinical Translation of LED-Based Photoacoustic Imaging: A Review. *Sensors* **2020**, *20*, 2484. [CrossRef]
35. Mallidi, S.; Larson, T.; Tam, J.; Joshi, P.P.; Karpiouk, A.; Sokolov, K.; Emelianov, S. Multiwavelength Photoacoustic Imaging and Plasmon Resonance Coupling of Gold Nanoparticles for Selective Detection of Cancer. *Nano Lett.* **2009**, *9*, 2825–2831. [CrossRef]
36. Obaid, G.; Bano, S.; Mallidi, S.; Broekgaarden, M.; Kuriakose, J.; Silber, Z.; Bulin, A.L.; Wang, Y.; Mai, Z.; Jin, W.; et al. Impacting Pancreatic Cancer Therapy in Heterotypic in Vitro Organoids and in Vivo Tumors with Specificity-Tuned, NIR-Activable Photoimmunonanoconjugates: Towards Conquering Desmoplasia? *Nano Lett.* **2019**, *19*, 7573–7587. [CrossRef] [PubMed]
37. Li, P.-C.; Wang, C.-R.C.; Shieh, D.-B.; Wei, C.-W.; Liao, C.-K.; Poe, C.; Jhan, S.; Ding, A.-A.; Wu, Y.-N. In vivo Photoacoustic Molecular Imaging with Simultaneous Multiple Selective Targeting Using Antibody-Conjugated Gold Nanorods. *Opt. Express* **2008**, *16*, 18605–18615. [CrossRef] [PubMed]
38. Yang, H.W.; Liu, H.L.; Li, M.L.; Hsi, I.W.; Fan, C.T.; Huang, C.Y.; Lu, Y.J.; Hua, M.Y.; Chou, H.Y.; Liaw, J.W.; et al. Magnetic gold-nanorod/ PNIPAAmMA nanoparticles for dual magnetic resonance and photoacoustic imaging and targeted photothermal therapy. *Biomaterials* **2013**, *34*, 5651–5660. [CrossRef] [PubMed]
39. Pan, D.; Pramanik, M.; Senpan, A.; Allen, J.S.; Zhang, H.; Wickline, S.A.; Wang, L.V.; Lanza, G.M. Molecular photoacoustic imaging of angiogenesis with integrin-targeted gold nanobeacons. *FASEB J.* **2011**, *25*, 875–882. [CrossRef] [PubMed]
40. Wu, D.; Huang, L.; Jiang, M.S.; Jiang, H. Contrast agents for photoacoustic and thermoacoustic imaging: A review. *Int. J. Mol. Sci.* **2014**, *15*, 23616–23639. [CrossRef] [PubMed]
41. Pan, D.; Kim, B.; Wang, L.V.; Lanza, G.M. A brief account of nanoparticle contrast agents for photoacoustic imaging. *WIREs Nanomed. Nanobiotechnol.* **2013**, *5*, 517–543. [CrossRef]

9

Portable and Affordable Light Source-Based Photoacoustic Tomography

Mithun Kuniyil Ajith Singh [1] and Wenfeng Xia [2,*]

1 Research and Business Development Division, CYBERDYNE INC., Stationsplein 45, A4.004, 3013 AK Rotterdam, The Netherlands; mithun_ajith@cyberdyne.jp
2 School of Biomedical Engineering & Imaging Sciences, King's College London, King's Health Partners, St Thomas' Hospital, London SE1 7EH, UK
* Correspondence: wenfeng.xia@kcl.ac.uk

Abstract: Photoacoustic imaging is a hybrid imaging modality that offers the advantages of optical (spectroscopic contrast) and ultrasound imaging (scalable spatial resolution and imaging depth). This promising modality has shown excellent potential in a wide range of preclinical and clinical imaging and sensing applications. Even though photoacoustic imaging technology has matured in research settings, its clinical translation is not happening at the expected pace. One of the main reasons for this is the requirement of bulky and expensive pulsed lasers for excitation. To accelerate the clinical translation of photoacoustic imaging and explore its potential in resource-limited settings, it is of paramount importance to develop portable and affordable light sources that can be used as the excitation light source. In this review, we focus on the following aspects: (1) the basic theory of photoacoustic imaging; (2) inexpensive light sources and different implementations; and (3) important preclinical and clinical applications, demonstrated using affordable light source-based photoacoustics. The main focus will be on laser diodes and light-emitting diodes as they have demonstrated promise in photoacoustic tomography—the key technological developments in these areas will be thoroughly reviewed. We believe that this review will be a useful opus for both the beginners and experts in the field of biomedical photoacoustic imaging.

Keywords: photoacoustic imaging; photoacoustic computed tomography; light-emitting diodes; laser diodes

---

1. Introduction

Photoacoustic imaging (PAI) is an emerging biomedical imaging modality that is based on the detection of ultrasound (US) waves generated from tissue in response to the absorption of temporally varying optical energy [1–5]. Typically, in PAI, short-pulsed or temporally modulated light is delivered to a tissue surface, and the light then propagates diffusively through the tissue during which a portion of the optical energy is selectively absorbed by various light absorbing structures, such as endogenous tissue chromophores and exogenous contrast agents [2]. These endogenous tissue chromophores include DNA/RNA, oxy- and deoxy-hemoglobin, lipid, and melanin; exogenous contrast agents include small molecular dyes, organic nanostructures, metal and carbon nanoparticles, and genetically encoded chromophores [3]. The absorption of the time-varying optical energies leads to rapid and subtle local temperature rises, and subsequently, the generation of broadband US waves in the MHz frequency range. These initial pressure waves propagate outwards and can be received by US detectors at the tissue surface to form images of the absorbing structures. Since optical absorption spectra of common tissue chromophores (hemoglobin, melanin, lipid, etc.) are well known, it is possible to tune the light excitation wavelength and functionally characterize the tissue using multispectral PAI [1]. For example, one can quantitatively detect oxygen saturation inside a blood vessel with high spatial and temporal resolution at depths up to a few centimeters, which is unachievable using any other imaging modalities. PAI involves US detection and it is straight forward to implement this technique in conventional US imaging equipment, offering structural, functional, and molecular imaging details in a single image acquisition [6]. PAI is undoubtedly one of the fastest growing research-based medical imaging modalities in recent times. However, one of the key factors hindering the clinical translation of this promising technique is the requirement of bulky and expensive solid-state lasers for tissue illumination [7]. In this review, after covering the principles of PAI, we will focus on affordable light sources (light-emitting diodes and laser diodes) that are being explored as alternative excitation sources for photoacoustic (PA) tomography, demonstrate its applications, and also discuss the advantages and disadvantages of different illumination sources in PAI. To focus more on PA tomography (PAT) using light-emitting diodes (LEDs) and laser diodes (LDs), we exclude developments and applications demonstrating PA microscopy and endoscopy.

2. Principles of Photoacoustic Imaging

Optical tissue imaging utilizes spectroscopic features of light–tissue interactions, such as scattering, absorption, and polarization. Since many tissue molecules possess signature optical properties (especially absorption), this interaction is quite powerful in characterizing tissue at functional and molecular levels. Figure 1 shows the optical absorption spectra of prominent tissue chromophores, such as hemoglobin, melanin, lipid, and water. The rich spectroscopic contrast of these molecules and their relations to a spectrum of diseases make optical imaging very useful [1–3]. However, purely light-based imaging techniques suffer from poor resolution at depths larger than a few mm, due to high scattering in the tissue [1]. While in US imaging, the tissue is insonified using sound waves and echoes are used to generate acoustic reflectivity maps [8]. This is one of the most popular medical imaging modalities with several advantages, including a high portability, affordability, accessibility, and spatial and temporal resolution. Even though US imaging offers tissue anatomical information in real time, it can provide insufficient contrast for soft tissues, and insufficient sensitivity for differentiating malignant and benign abnormalities in deep tissue [6,9].

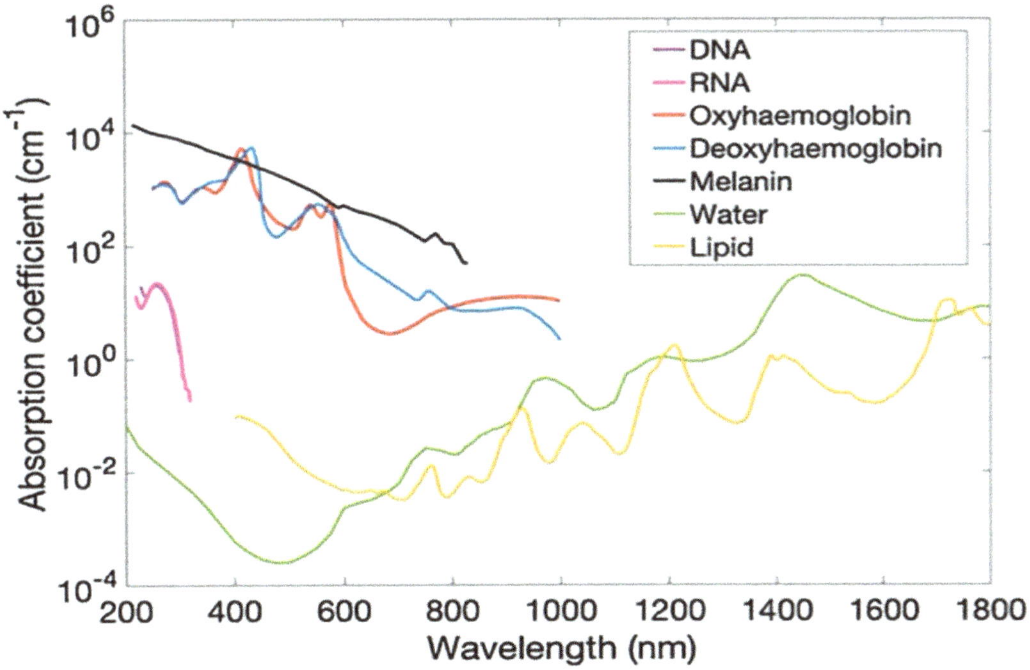

Figure 1. Absorption coefficient spectra (μa) of endogenous tissue chromophores, including DNA, RNA, oxyhemoglobin, deoxyhemoglobin (150 g L^{-1}), melanin, water, and lipid. Adapted with permission from T. Zhao, A. E. Desjardins, S. Ourselin, T. Vercauteren, W. Xia, Photoacoustics, Vol.16, Article ID100146, 2019.

2.1. Generation of Photoacoustic Signals

The basic idea of the photoacoustic effect was described by Alexander Graham Bell long back in 1880 [10]. When pulsed light is shone on a sample that absorbs a fraction of the incident energy, the optical absorption will result in a temperature rise, leading to thermoelastic expansion of the absorbing object. This sudden pressure rise propagates as a sound wave, which then can be detected using conventional US transducers. By detecting the pressure waves, one can localize their sources (i.e., where the light was absorbed) and obtain important functional and molecular information about the studied sample [1]. The basic idea of PA imaging is schematized in Figure 2.

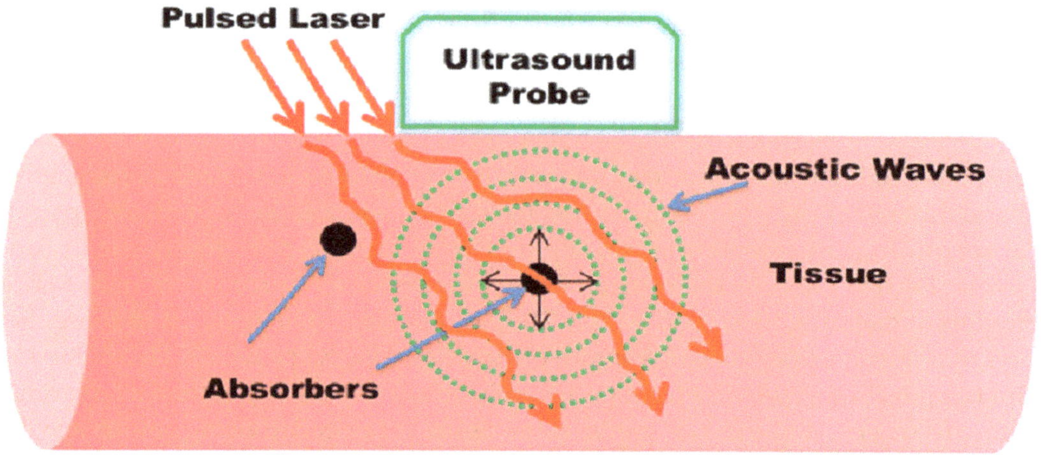

Figure 2. Basic principle of biomedical photoacoustic imaging. Reproduced with permission from Handheld Probe-Based Dual Mode Ultrasound/Photoacoustics for Biomedical Imaging. In: Olivo M., Dinish U. (eds) Frontiers in Biophotonics for Translational Medicine.

To generate broadband PA signals (sound waves) in the sample efficiently and obtain high-resolution images, the light pulse must be shorter than both the thermal relaxation time τ_{th} (thermal confinement) and the stress relaxation time τ_s (stress confinement), respectively, defined by Equations (1) and (2) [1,11].

$$\tau_{th} = \frac{d_c^2}{\alpha_{th}} \tag{1}$$

where d_c is the characteristic dimension of the structure of interest and α_{th} is the thermal diffusivity.

$$\tau_s = \frac{d_c}{v_s} \tag{2}$$

where v_s is the speed of sound in the tissue (~1540 m/s).

Let us consider a 15 μm optically absorbing structure inside the tissue. In this case, τ_{th} and τ_s will be 1.4×10^{-3} s and 1×10^{-8} s, respectively. Thus, it is clear that the pulse width of the tissue illumination source must be shorter than 10 ns to spatially resolve this 15 μm structure in a PA image. It is also important to note that the detection bandwidth of the US probe also must be high to achieve such high-resolution images, which will be discussed in greater detail later in Section 2.4. The optically induced initial pressure distribution p_0 can be estimated as

$$p_0(r) = \Gamma\, \mu_a\,(r) F(r) \tag{3}$$

where r refers to a spatial location within the heated volume, μ_a is the optical absorption distribution of the absorbing structure, F is the local fluence, Γ is the Grüneisen coefficient, and a the dimensionless thermodynamic constant that defines the conversion efficiency of heat energy to pressure, and can be expressed as

$$\Gamma = \beta v_s^2 / C_p \tag{4}$$

where β is the isobaric volume expansion coefficient and C_p is the specific heat at a constant pressure. It can be seen that p_0 depends on a number of parameters. Although several studies have shown that Γ can be a source of PA contrast in tissue [12], PA image contrast is generally assumed to be dominated by the local optical absorption μ_a and the local fluence F, which is a product of optical absorption and scattering. Considering the strong light attenuation in the tissue, F decreases exponentially with tissue depth; however, optical fluence variations at a given depth in the tissue are usually much smaller compared to those of μ_a. As such, PA imaging is often considered as an imaging modality that is based on optical absorption of the tissue; however, it is important to note that the PA image signal is not directly proportional to μ_a.

2.2. Illumination Sources

The characteristics of the illumination sources mainly define the quality of the PA images and contribute to the high cost of the whole PAI system. PAI systems conventionally use solid-state lasers, such as Q-switched Nd: YAG lasers coupled with optical parametric oscillators (OPO). These lasers usually offer pulse widths in the range of 5–20 ns, which is very much suitable for high-resolution PAI. However, these bulky laser sources are very expensive and are not suitable for use in a clinical setting (for example in an operating room or an outpatient clinic) [13–17]. Recently, there has been significant research in the area of affordable light sources for PAI. Laser diodes (LDs) and light-emitting diodes (LEDs) are the most common PAI illumination sources, which offer high portability, affordability, and energy efficiency [13–17]. Solid-state lasers, LDs, and LEDs have completely different characteristics (pulse width, pulse repetition rate (PRR), optical output, and cost) and have their own advantages and disadvantages. Table 1 shows a comparison of the light sources used in PAI.

Table 1. Comparison of different light sources used in photoacoustic imaging. * Cost includes the driving electronics and may vary based on different features, number of wavelengths, etc. Integration to a US probe may also involve extra development cost. LD, Laser diode; LED: Light-emitting diode; DPSS: Diode-pumped solid-state; PRR, pulse repetition rate. Adapted with permission from Y. Zhu, T. Feng, Q. Cheng, X. Wang, S. Du, N. Sato, J. Yuan and M. Kuniyil Ajith Singh, Sensors, Vol.20, Article ID2484, 2020.

	Energy (mJ)	PRR (Hz)	Pulse Width (ns)	Cost *	Advantages	Disadvantages
Solid-state lasers	5–120	10–200	<10	$70–200 K	Powerful, ~5 cm penetration depth, tunable wavelength	Bulky size, eye protection and laser safe rooms needed
LD	0.5–2.5	~1 K–6 K	30–200	~$10–25 K	Integration in a handheld probe feasible, high PRR	Limited penetration depth, eye protection and laser safe rooms needed, wavelength tuning not possible
LED	0.2	~200–16 K	30–100	$10–15 K	Integration in a handheld probe feasible, high PRR, wide wavelength range, no need of laser-safe rooms and eye-safety goggles	Limited penetration depth, wavelength tuning not possible
Q-switched DPSS laser	1	100 K	2–10	-	High PRR, low pulse width, Reasonably high optical energy per pulse	Less number of wavelengths (266 nm, 355 nm, 532 nm, 1064 nm) available and spectral tuning may be cumbersome
High-energy DPSS laser	200	200	10–30	-	High optical output per pulse, reasonably high PRR	Less number of wavelengths (266 nm, 355 nm, 532 nm, 1064 nm) available and spectral tuning may be cumbersome

2.3. Optical Absorption

As shown in Figure 1, intrinsic optical absorbers in the tissue possess the signature absorption characteristics and the spatial distributions of these absorbers can be quantified in PAI with a high spatial resolution and large imaging depths [1]. For example, PAI offers excellent contrast for blood. Since oxyhemoglobin and deoxyhemoglobin have different optical absorption spectra, careful selection of the excitation wavelengths (even two wavelengths with good absorption difference would suffice) can help in obtaining oxygen saturation maps of the tissue with an unprecedented resolution (micro-vasculature level) [16]. Apart from intrinsic absorbers, it is feasible to image exogenous contrast agents by selecting the light wavelengths based on the absorption peak of them [17]. Considering the low absorption of water and high absorption of blood, near infrared (NIR) wavelengths are most commonly used in PAI for achieving higher imaging depths.

2.4. Ultrasound Propogation and Detection

The velocity of the US waves in tissue is considered constant at 1540 m/s in general. Variations are typically less than 10%, and are usually not accounted for, unless the sample is highly heterogenous. Acoustic scattering in tissue is roughly three orders of magnitude lower than optical scattering and this is the key reason for a higher imaging depth in PAI compared to other optical imaging modalities that rely on optical focusing [1–5]. One important factor to consider acoustically is the attenuation in the tissue, which can be modelled as below.

$$\alpha = af^{b}\ [\mathrm{dB/cm}] \tag{5}$$

where a is a tissue dependent constant, b is a power law factor whose value is usually ranged between 1 and 2 in the soft tissue, and f is the frequency expressed in MHz. In general, for soft tissue, α is considered as 1 dB cm^{-1} MHz^{-1} on average; it can reach as high as 20 dB cm^{-1} MHz^{-1} for bone (assuming $b = 1$ in both cases). As such, the characteristics of the frequency-dependent acoustic attenuation are similar to those of a low pass filter so that higher frequency signals are attenuated more in tissue. Although the PA signals can be extremely broadband with frequency contents ranging from several tens of kHz to several tens of MHz, depending on the size of the object, frequency-dependent acoustic attenuation in tissue has limited the maximum frequency content that can arrive at the detector side and thus fundamentally limits the achievable spatial resolution. The spatial resolution of a PA tomography system also depends on other factors, including the frequency bandwidth of the US detector, the active surface area of the detector element, number of detector elements, detector aperture, and image reconstruction algorithms. Moreover, as the acoustic sensitivity of an US detector decreases with the increase in frequency (which largely determines the spatial resolution), there is a trade-off between the imaging depth and spatial resolution. For example, according to a recent study by Xia et al. [18], the measured axial resolution using resolution targets immersed in water for a PAI system with a linear array US probe (central frequency: 9 MHz; −6 dB bandwidth: 77%; active surface area: 5 mm × 0.3 mm; number of element: 128; and detector aperture: 38.4 mm) was 0.22 mm and remained consistent over a depth range of 13 to 36 mm; the lateral resolution depended on the spatial location, ranging from 0.35 mm to 0.76 mm over the same depth range.

Linear array piezoelectric probes are commonly used as US detectors for PAI similar to those used for conventional US imaging. As such, real-time interleaved US and PA imaging can be performed with the same US detector and DAQ electronics [6]. US detection in PAI mode is the same as that in the US mode, except that in this case no US transmissions are performed. This dual modality approach offers many advantages involving complementary contrast and easiness in clinical translation. US imaging is a well-accepted imaging modality and it would be easier for clinicians to accept PAI as an additional technique along with conventional US imaging [7]. Typical frequencies for US imaging are in the range of 1–25 MHz. For utilizing the full benefits of PA imaging, it is important to develop new US probes with a higher bandwidth and sensitivity as the PA signals are usually broadband

and their amplitudes are much lower than the pulse echo signals in US imaging. There have been significant developments in this area recently [6]. Acoustic waves can be detected using single-element transducers (and employing scanning) or using an array of elements as in conventional US probes (planar, cylindrical, or spherical) to enable 2D or 3D imaging.

2.5. Image Reconstruction

PAI involves the detection of acoustic signals generated by optical absorption, and image reconstruction strategies are thus stemmed from both optical and US imaging. Basic PA image reconstruction aims to retrieve the spatial distribution of the initial PA pressure or locations of the absorbed optical energy [11]. This is usually termed the acoustic inversion problem and uses various algorithms that originate from the US and sonar world. From the distribution of the initial PA pressure, it is desired to reconstruct a distribution of the optical absorption coefficient, especially when multiple wavelengths are used for PA excitation; however, this is a non-linear problem due to the wavelength-depended optical attenuation of the tissue, which is termed the optical inversion problem. Reconstruction of the optical absorption coefficient is usually termed quantitative PA imaging [11].

There has been extensive research in the area of PA image reconstruction and different methods have been reported. Time reversal, Fourier domain analysis, analytic back-projection, radon transfer, and model-based algorithms are some of the most commonly applied methods. Kuchment et al. reported a detailed review about the different PA-based image reconstruction methods [19]. Based on the type of acoustic detection probes (linear arrays, curved arrays, etc.) and the computational capability, one can choose the right image reconstruction algorithm. Considering the ease in implementation and speed offered, back-projection is the most commonly used image reconstruction technique for processing PA data [1]. Figure 3 illustrates the concept of back-projection algorithms when the PA detection geometry is linear/planar. In this case, each detector element at a specific location records the PA data using the speed of sound (c) and time of flight (t), and then the recorded time-resolved signals are back-projected over a spherical surface of radius R = ct into the imaging volume [1].

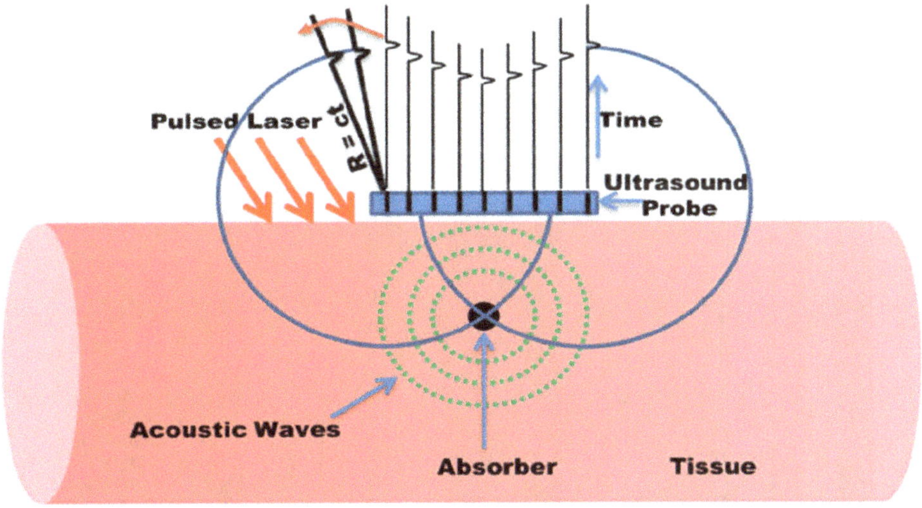

Figure 3. Back-projection PAI reconstruction for a planar detection geometry. Reproduced with permission from Handheld Probe-Based Dual Mode Ultrasound/Photoacoustics for Biomedical Imaging. In: Olivo M., Dinish U. (Eds) Frontiers in Biophotonics for Translational Medicine.

This method is comparable to the conventional delay-and-sum beamformer, which is the most common algorithm employed in US imaging using phased arrays. It is important to note that a US-based delay-and-sum reconstruction algorithm can be used for PAT data by reducing the time-of-flight to half (PA data traverse half the time in tissue when compared to US signals). This offers the possibility to switch between these two image reconstruction modes at a high speed, which is a key requirement in handheld dual-mode PA/US imaging systems. However, the image quality offered by such an approach is not up to the mark. To solve this issue, there have been tremendous developments in the area of frequency domain algorithms, offering superior image quality with computing speeds suitable for systems suitable for real-time imaging [20,21].

3. LED-Based Photoacoustic Tomography

In recent years, there have been significant developments in the use of high-power LEDs in biomedical PAI, especially for superficial imaging applications [13,22]. In this section, we review the developments in this area after discussing briefly the characteristics of the LEDs and its advantages and disadvantages.

3.1. High-Power LEDs Suitable for Photoacoustic Tomography

An LED is a semiconductor device (P–N junction) that emits light when an electrical current passes through it. Free electrons are the majority charge carriers in N-type semiconductors. On the other hand, holes are the main charge carriers in P-type semiconductors. A P–N junction is formed when the N-type and P-type semiconductors are joined together. When a voltage is applied across the P–N junction diode (forward bias), holes (from P-substrate) and electrons (from N-substrate) move towards the junction, resulting in plenty of electrons and holes in the junction region. This fosters a strong electron–hole radiative recombination and consequent emission of photons. In case of LEDs, the radiative recombination process is dependent on spontaneous emission in which electrons in a high energy state (E_2) move down to a lower energy state (E_1) and combine with the available holes. The difference in energy between these two states ($E_g = E_2 - E_1$) results in spontaneous emission of photons in random directions [23].

3.2. High-Power LEDs—Technical Aspects

3.2.1. Emission Wavelength

When considering the biomedical imaging applications, a key advantage of LEDs over LDs is the availability of a wide range of wavelengths. As shown in Figure 4, LEDs are available even in the visible wavelengths in which the optical absorption of hemoglobin is quite high [23].

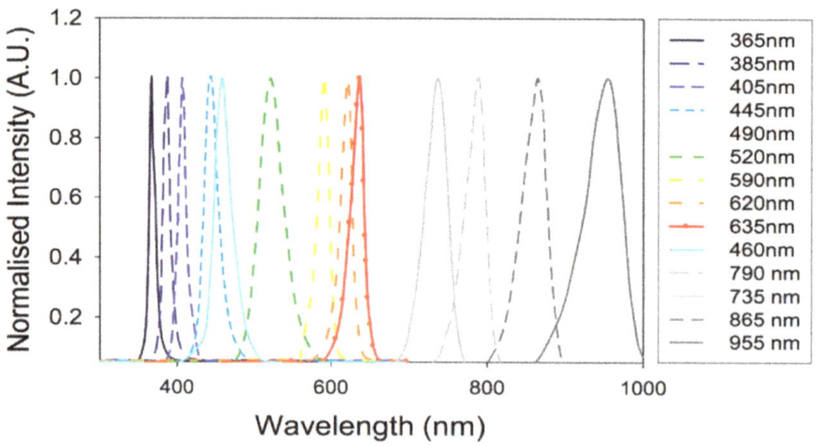

Figure 4. Optical spectra for a range of commercially available LEDs. Reproduced with permission from T. J. Allen and P. C. Beard, Biomedical Optics Express, Vol.7, Article ID1260, 2016.

Materials used for designing the semiconductor (P–N junction) and its energy bandgap (E_g) are the factors that define the emission wavelength of the LEDs. Thus, one can tune the emission wavelength (visible to NIR range suitable for PAI) of LEDs by carefully selecting the semiconductor material [23]. For example, NIR wavelengths, the most suitable wavelengths for deep-tissue PAI can be developed by using aluminum gallium arsenide (AlxGa1-xAs). By changing the mole fraction (x) of the aluminum (Al) in AlxGa1-xAs, it is straightforward to tune the wavelength range from 624 nm to 920 nm. For obtaining wavelengths in the visible range (570–650 nm), aluminum gallium indium phosphide ((AlxGa1-x)0.5In0.5P) is the right candidate for the semiconductor material. In this case, by increasing the mole fraction (x) of the aluminum (Al), one can reduce the emission wavelength. For even shorter wavelengths (440–550 nm), it is recommended to use indium gallium nitride (InGaN) as the semiconductor material. An increase in indium (In) will result in shifts of emission from shorter to longer wavelengths. The materials used to design LEDs with different wavelengths are summarized in Table 2. With the availability in a wide range of wavelengths, LED illumination is very well suited for multispectral PAI [22].

Table 2. Summary of the materials used to design LEDs with different wavelengths.

Wavelength (nm)	440–550	570–650	624–920
Material	InGaN	AlGaInP	AlGaAs

3.2.2. Overdriving LEDs

LEDs are designed to be used for continuous wave (CW) operation and its rated current is valid in this mode. However, it is possible to operate LEDs in the pulsed mode by driving it with higher current pulses of lower duty cycles (less than <0.1%). This way, one can safely increase the optical output and use these affordable devices for PAI [22,24]. Even though LED manufacturers do not provide specifications for pulsed operation, recent studies have demonstrated that it is safe to drive LEDs using a higher current (ten times their rated current) at a duty cycle lower than 0.1% without any noticeable damage [24].

To operate LEDs in the pulsed mode, special electronic drivers are required. Pulsed LED drivers are most commonly composed of a capacitor, which is used as a storage element that discharges through the LED when a fast-switching device (metal oxide semiconductor field-effect transistors (MOSFETs) are used commonly) is activated. Figure 5 shows a schematic of a typical LED driver.

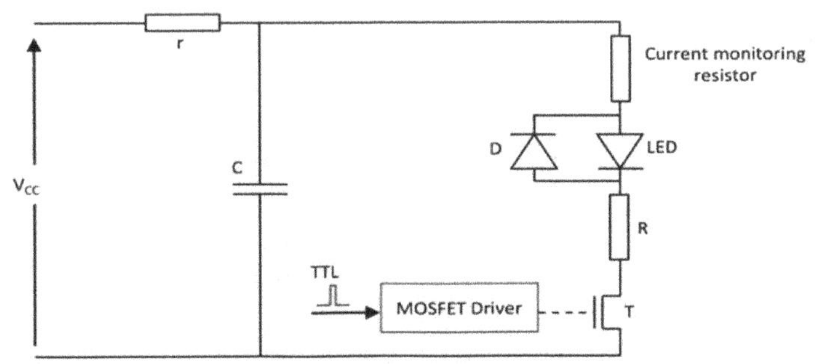

Figure 5. Schematic of a typical LED driver for the pulse operation mode. Vcc is the voltage provided by the power supply, T is the transistor used to switch the LED on and off, C is the storage capacitor, R is the limiting resistor, r is the charging resistor, D is a diode, and MOSFET is a metal oxide semiconductor field-effect transistor. Reprinted with permission from High-Power Light Emitting Diodes; An Alternative Excitation Source for Photoacoustic Tomography. In: Kuniyil Ajith Singh M. (eds) LED-Based Photoacoustic Imaging.

3.2.3. Optical Output Power

In its default continuous wave mode, typical high-power LEDs can provide optical output up to a few watts, which is dependent on the wavelength and also the size of the elements [24]. It is essential to use the LED elements within its allowed current rating (usually around 1 A). For avoiding heating issues, high power LED elements are usually mounted on heatsinks. However, it is critical to consider the amount of heat generated, especially when the goal is to integrate a light source and US probe in a single housing for handheld PA and US imaging. Photographs of two representative high-power LEDs are shown in Figure 6, where Figure 6a shows a device with a large emitting area (9 mm^2) and Figure 6b shows a multi-wavelength device composed of 4 LED elements, each with a smaller emitting area (1 mm^2) and at a different wavelength and mounted on a metal-core printed circuit (MCPC) board for efficient heat removal.

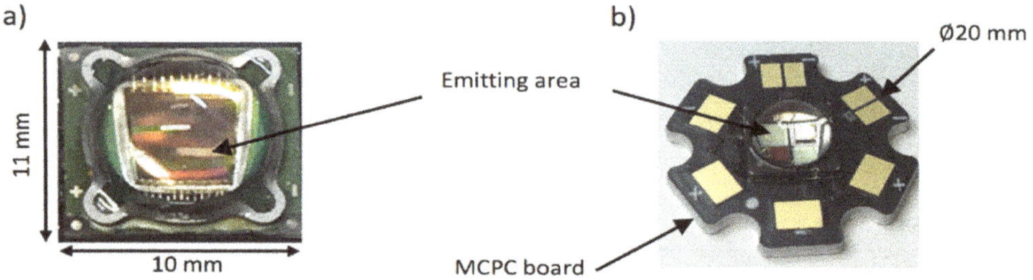

Figure 6. Photographs of high-power LEDs: (**a**) high-power LED (SST-90) with an emitting area of 9 mm^2; (**b**) high-power multi-wavelength LED (LZ4-00MC00, LedEngin, Inc., California, USA), composed of 4 LEDs emitting at 452, 520, 520, and 618 nm, each with a 1 mm^2 emitting area and mounted on a metal-core printed circuit (MCPC) board. These devices are encapsulated in spherical glass lenses. Reprinted with permission from High-Power Light Emitting Diodes; An Alternative Excitation Source for Photoacoustic Tomography. In: Kuniyil Ajith Singh M. (Eds) LED-Based Photoacoustic Imaging. Progress in Optical Science and Photonics, vol 7.

In recent years, the possibility of using multiple LED elements as an array have also been explored to generate a higher optical output required for PAT. Figure 7 shows a photograph of an LED array with 750 nm and 850 nm LED elements arranged in an interleaved manner (left panel, 36 elements per row, 4 rows in total) and also the integrated PA and US probe in which the LED arrays are fixed on a conventional linear array US probe (right panel). These high-power LED arrays are commercialized by CYBERDYNE INC (Tsukuba, Japan) for research use [25].

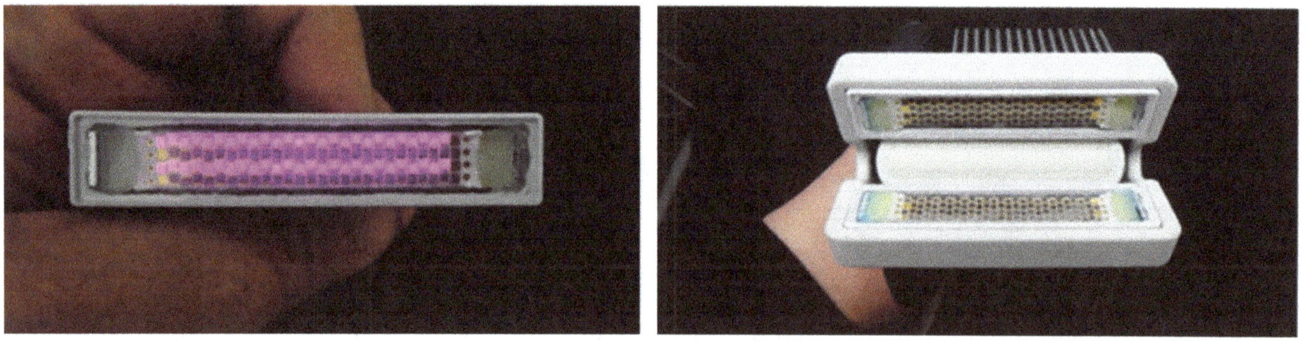

Figure 7. Photograph of an LED array developed by CYBERDYNE INC with four rows of LED elements, in which Rows 1 and 3 are 850 nm elements, and Rows 2 and 4 are 750 nm elements (**left**). In this picture, the 850 nm elements are activated and captured using an IR camera. Photograph of a LED-based PA/US probe developed by CYBERDYNE INC, in which two LED arrays (750/850 nm) are placed on both sides of a linear array US probe (7 MHz) (**right**).

3.2.4. Pulse Repetition Rate (PRR)

The typical PRR of conventional solid-state lasers are in the range of 10–200 Hz. For obtaining good signal-to-noise ratios (SNRs) in deep tissue PAI, it is usually required to perform signal averaging over multiple imaging frames, leading to low frame rates in a solid-state laser-based PAI system. On the other hand, PRRs of LEDs are in the KHz range and this will help to average more frames to improve SNR, without compromising the temporal resolution. Moreover, the large PRR makes high-speed PAT a possibility. LED arrays at 850 nm with a PRR of 16 KHz have been reported by Zhu et al. recently and they demonstrated dynamic PAI using commercially available LED arrays and conventional linear array US probes [26].

3.2.5. Pulse Width

The pulse width of LEDs are tens of nanoseconds (30–100 ns), whereas that of the solid-state lasers is usually less than ten nanoseconds. The temporal pulse width imposes a limit on the spatial resolution of the PAI systems [1]. For example, if an LED element with a 70 ns pulse width is used as the excitation source, the finest spatial resolution that is potentially achievable can be roughly estimated as 105 μm (= 70 ns × 1500 μm/μs). However, conventional US probes (5–7 MHz probes) have reception bandwidth limits and thus further limits its axial resolution to approximately 200–300 μm. One may generate broad bandwidth PA signals when the excitation pulse width is low (for example, 5 ns as in a solid-state laser), but detection sensitivity beyond the US bandwidth is usually very low and the spatial resolution is thus limited by the bandwidth of the US probe. It has been demonstrated that the pulse widths of LEDs are suitable for deep tissue imaging using conventional US probes [13]. A recent study also has shown that tuning the pulse width of the LEDs is feasible and this would be helpful if transducers with different center frequencies and bandwidths are used for the detection [27].

3.2.6. Spatial Divergence of LEDs

Conventional high-power LEDs have larger emission angles when compared to other sources. The spatial divergence of commercially available high-power LED arrays (CYBERDYNE INC, Tsukuba, Japan) is approximately +/−60° [28,29], which is acceptable in PAT where a relatively large illumination area is usually required. However, because of the large divergence and larger emission area (~1 mm^2), it is difficult to collimate the light and couple it to optical fibers for applications like minimally invasive PA imaging [9,30–32]. In terms of eye/skin safety, high spatial divergence in combination with a low optical output makes LEDs a safer alternative to solid-state lasers for non-invasive PAI [20].

3.3. *Technical Developments in LED-Based Photoacoustic Tomography*

The first report on the use of LEDs as an illumination source in PAI was from Jansen in 2011 [33]. In this work, a 627 nm LED element was used (Luxeon LXHL_PD09), which has been measured to yield approximately 250 mW of light output when supplied with 1 A DC current. Using a special electronic driver, the LED was supplied with 60-ns current pulses with a peak value of 40 A, resulting in a pulse energy of 400 nJ per pulse with a pulse width of 60 ns and a PRR of 200 Hz. Light focusing was performed to generate the fluence required for generating a PA response. To obtain PA signals from a non-realistic gelatin-based phantom, 50,000 A-lines were averaged. Owing to significant developments in the field of solid-state technology, there have been significant developments in LED technology (optical output, PRR, and pulse width), which resulted in the step-by-step development of LED-based PAI technology after 2011.

In 2013, Allen and Beard worked on this further and demonstrated that LEDs can be used as illumination sources in biomedical PA imaging [34]. In this work, they demonstrated the potential of using LEDs as an alternative excitation source in multispectral PA imaging. Recently, the same group achieved an imaging depth of 1.5 cm in tissue mimicking phantoms when using LEDs as an illumination source in PA imaging [24]. In this work, they obtained an LED output power of 10 μJ/pulse by overdriving 620 nm elements and averaging thousands of frames to improve the SNR. Figure 8a shows a schematic of the experimental setup used by them. Figure 8b shows a raw RF signal obtained and 8c shows a reconstructed image. With the same PRR of 200 Hz, as in the previous study, they achieved a frame rate that is 1000 times better, thanks to the higher optical output achieved using a MOSFET-based electronic driver.

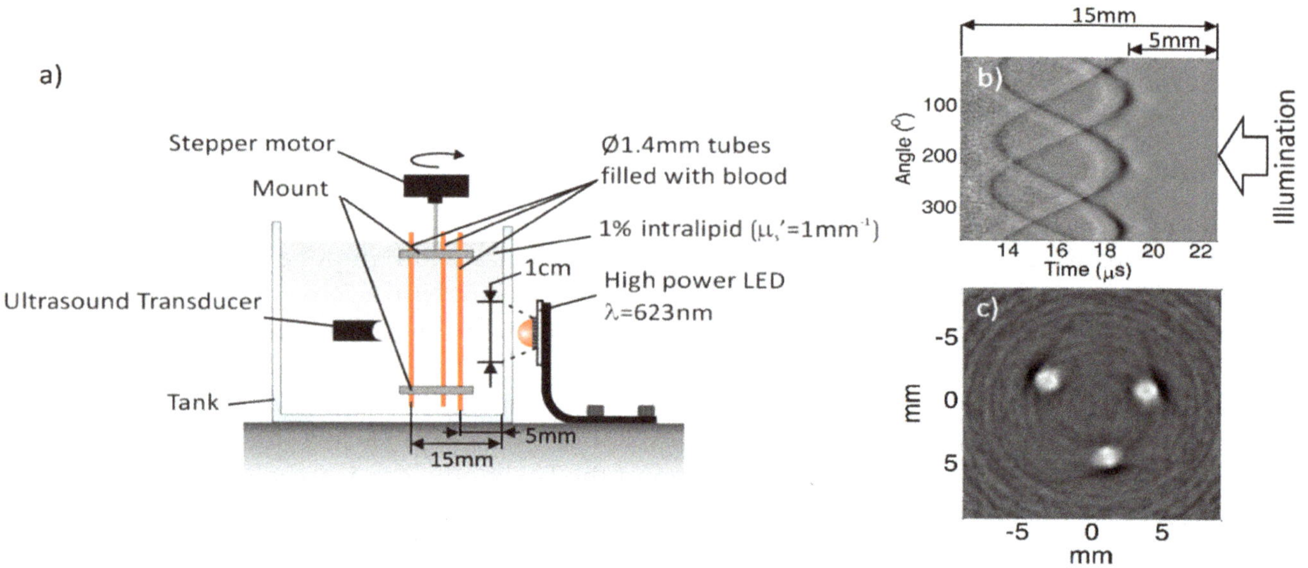

Figure 8. (**a**) Experimental setup; (**b**) RF PA signals of three 1.4 mm tubes filled with human blood immersed in water mixed with intralipid; (**c**) final reconstructed PA image. Optical output energy attained = 9 μJ. Number of frames averaged: 5000.

Although these pioneering works demonstrated the feasibility of using LEDs as illumination sources in PAI, no in vivo results have been reported. The main reason behind this is the optical energy of the LEDs, which is magnitudes lower than that of a solid-state laser or even some LDs. In 2015, Agano et al. demonstrated that it was feasible to combine hundreds of high-power LED elements in a rectangular package and could be pulsed simultaneously to perform biomedical PAI [35–37]. Using this novel technology, a high-power LED-array-based PA imaging system (AcousticX) was commercialized by a Japanese company (PreXion Corporation, later the technology was acquired by CYBERDYNE, INC, Japan).

With AcousticX, a single LED element provided an output energy of 0.024 μJ per pulse, with a pulse duration of 70 ns and 1 A DC current. By developing LED elements with a double stack structure, arranging them in an array, and applying 20 times the rated current, a light output of 200 μJ per pulse at a wavelength of 850 nm was achieved. Two of these arrays were kept on both sides of a linear array US probe for performing real-time PA and US imaging. The repetition rate of this first commercial LED-based PAI system was 4 KHz.

The system was thoroughly characterized by several research groups for its spatial resolution and imaging depth, and subsequently its capability for functional, structural, and molecular imaging was demonstrated [26,38–42]. Figure 9 shows a photograph of the system and the PA and US images of a human volunteer's wrist, which was acquired in a real-time handheld operation, demonstrating the capability of obtaining a complementary contrast (structural details from the US image and vasculature details from PA image) in a single measurement [18].

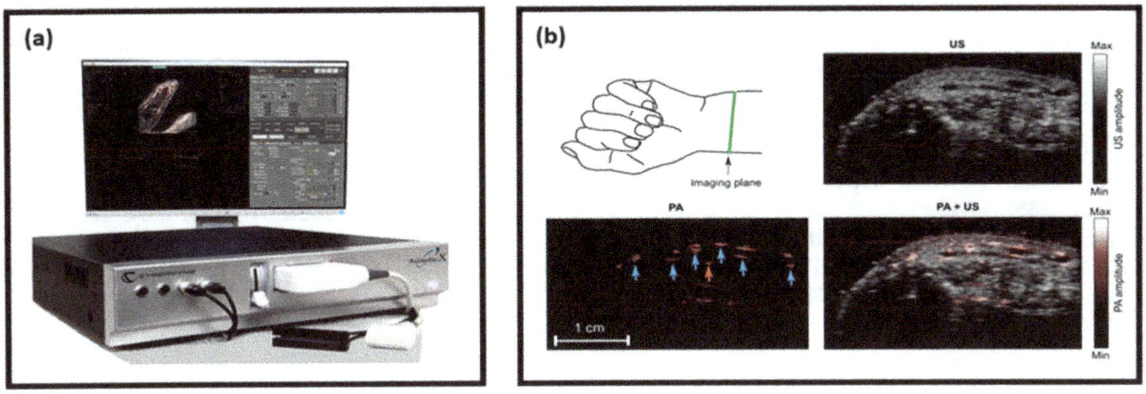

Figure 9. (**a**) Photograph of the LED-based PA and US imaging system—AcousticX; (**b**) US (gray colormap), PA (hot colormap), and US/PA overlay cross-section images of a human volunteer's wrist acquired at a frame rate of 10 Hz. Blood vessels are marked using blue arrows in the PA image.

In another study [7], utilizing the high temporal resolution of LED-based PAI, it was also possible to scan through an area of interest to generate 3D maps of the vasculature on a human volunteer's foot dorsum, as shown in Figure 10. The total time required to generate such a high-resolution 3D PA image with a large field-of-view was less than 15 s, including scanning and image reconstruction and rendering [7].

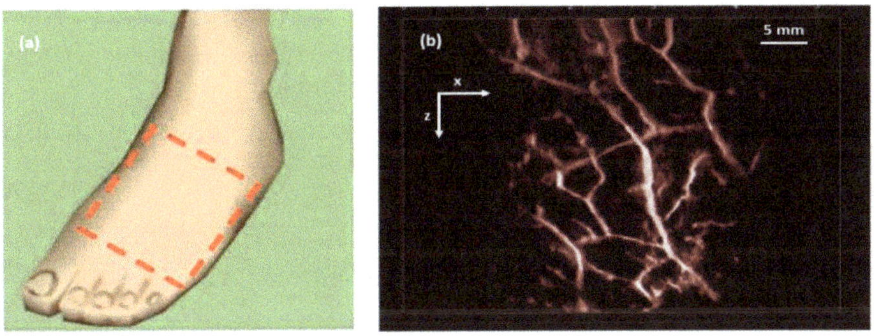

Figure 10. (**a**) Dashed box showing the imaging area on a human volunteer's foot dorsum; (**b**) 3D maximum intensity projection PA image of the area marked in (**a**), clearly visualizing the vasculature network. Adapted with permission from. Reprinted with permission from Clinical Translation of Photoacoustic Imaging—Opportunities and Challenges from an Industry Perspective. In: Kuniyil Ajith Singh M. (Eds) LED-Based Photoacoustic Imaging.

The system has been recently used extensively by several research groups in a number of studies to explore its potential preclinical and clinical applications [43–51], which are summarized in Table 3. All these reports clearly demonstrated the potential of LED-based PAI in structural, functional, and molecular imaging applications in a preclinical and a clinical setting. Even though the optical output power of the LEDs or LED arrays are not comparable to a solid-state laser, it is encouraging that LED-based PAI is able to consistently achieve an imaging depth of around 5–10 mm. The main reason for this is the high PRR (~16 KHz), which allows averaging over a large number of image frames while maintaining a good temporal resolution; one can easily achieve video rates even after averaging hundreds of frames. Considering the portability, affordability, safety, and ease-of-use, LED-based PAI holds strong potential in clinical translation of PA imaging as an additional modality along with conventional pulse-echo US imaging.

Table 3. Summary of the preclinical and clinical applications of LED-based PAI. Adapted with permission from Y. Zhu, T. Feng, Q. Cheng, X. Wang, S. Du, N. Sato, J. Yuan and M. Kuniyil Ajith Singh, Sensors, Vol.20, Article ID2484, 2020.

Target	Application		Depth (mm)	Contrast Agent	Wavelength (nm)
Medical needles, Vasculature	Guidance of minimally invasive procedures with peripheral tissue targets [18]	Phantom and ex vivo studies	38	N/A	850
Vasculature	Imaging of human placental vasculature [48]		7	N/A	850
Tumor	Imaging of intraocular tumors [26]		10	N/A	850
Vasculature	Non-invasive monitoring of angiogenesis [51]	Animal in vivo	10	N/A	850
Ulcer	Noninvasive imaging of pressure ulcers [47]		10	N/A	690
Oxygen saturation	Oxygen saturation imaging in rheumatoid arthritis [39]		5	N/A	750/850
Molecular	Detection and monitoring of reactive oxygen and nitrogen species [49]		10	CyBA	850
Tumor/Contrast agents	Imaging of tumor using contrast enhancement [44]		10	NC	850
Cells/Contrast agents	Imaging of molecular-labelled cells [38]		10	DiR	850
Vasculature	Imaging of peripheral microvasculature and function [26]	Healthy human	10	N/A	690/850
Vasculature	Simultaneous imaging of veins and lymphatic vessels [40]		10	ICG	940/820
Finger joints	Full view tomography of finger joints [28]		5	N/A	850
Finger joints	Imaging of inflammatory arthritis [42]	Patient	5	N/A	850
Skin	Imaging of port wine stain [43]		10	N/A	850

4. Laser Diode-Based Photoacoustic Tomography

Just like LEDs, LDs are also used as an excitation source in PAT, as an alternative to bulky and expensive lasers [52]. With high optical energy (when compared to LEDs) and compactness, pulsed LDs are suitable for performing deep-tissue PAT. In this section, after discussing some of the technical details, specifications, and development of LD-based PAT, we shortly introduce the applications that demonstrate the use of this technique. For the technical aspects, we will focus on the key differences when compared to LEDs.

4.1. High-Power Pulsed Laser Diodes

LD is a semiconductor laser device in which the laser beam is produced at the interface region in a P–I–N (positive–interface–negative) diode region. They are electrically pumped semiconductor laser sources. They convert the input electric energy into light energy, in comparison with conventional lasers in which the input light energy from a flash lamp is converted into laser output [14]. The energy efficiency of these bulky lasers is not high, and this results in an enormous amount of heat generation (water cooling, etc., is thus required, which increases the footprint of the device). On the other hand, the energy efficiency of an LD is very high and thus a minimal amount of heat will be generated.

In recent years, there have been multiple studies about the development and use of pulsed LDs in PAT [14,15,53].

4.2. *Pulsed Laser Diodes—Technical Aspects*

4.2.1. Emission Wavelengths

Conventionally, continuous wave laser diodes are available in a wide range of wavelengths (visible to NIR range). However, pulsed LDs are available only in the NIR range, most probably because of the lower optical energy generated when overdriven with the short pulses required in PAI. In the NIR range, pulsed LDs offer a far higher optical energy when compared to LEDs and thus are ideal sources of illumination in multispectral PAI of deep tissue.

Even though the fundamental process of light generation of LEDs and LDs are the same, LDs generate stimulated emissions and are considered as laser sources with a high spatial coherence. Just as in LEDs, semiconductor materials and their energy band gaps are the deciding factors for the emission wavelengths in LDs. Interestingly, there are some semiconductor compounds in which the bandgap energy can be altered by varying the details of the composition. For example, to achieve shorter wavelengths, one can increase the bandgap energy by increasing the aluminum content (increased x) in AlxGa1-xAs. Table 4 gives a summary of the semiconductor compounds used for developing LDs with different wavelengths. Even though the visible wavelength range is listed here, these are not commonly available in the pulsed mode.

Table 4. Summary of the materials used to design LDs with different wavelengths.

Wavelength (nm)	630–670	720–850	900–1100
Material	AlGaInP/GaAs	AlGaAs/GaAs	InGaAs/GaAs

4.2.2. Pulsed Laser Diode Drivers

Even though continuous wave modulations have also been explored to drive LDs, the most common way is to pulse modulate to generate the short light pulses required for PAI [15,54]. A typical LD driver circuit is shown in Figure 11 and the basic idea of driving is similar to that of an LED driver detailed in Section 3.2.2 (charging and discharging of a capacitor).

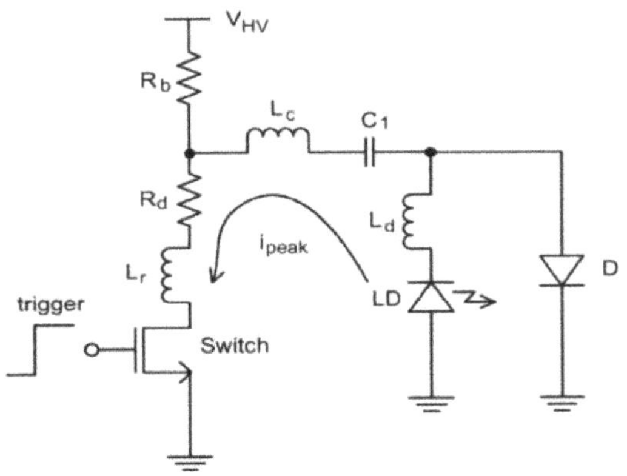

Figure 11. Typical laser driver circuit. Reproduced with permission from H. Zhong, T. Duan, H. Lan, M. Zhou, F. Gao, Sensors, Vol.18, Article ID2264, 2018.

The pulse current flows from the LD to the switching device, as illustrated by the arrow in Figure 11. In order to attain the lower pulse width and boost the peak current, the parasitic inductance (L_r, L_c and L_d) should be as small as possible [15,55]. Usually the time constant for these circuits are fixed and tuning of the pulse width is not an option. It is worth mentioning that LEDs on the other hand has already proven to generate light pulses of different pulse widths (30–100 ns). To the best of our knowledge, the most efficient LD driver in the literature so far was reported in 2016, with a size of 40×50 mm^2, a PRR up to 10 kHz, and a pulse energy of 1.7 mJ per pulse with a pulse width of 40 ns [56]. In this work, Canal et al. reported the possibility of integrating a high power LD in its own driver electronic board to save space (Figure 12) and thus opening up the possibility to develop handheld PA probes.

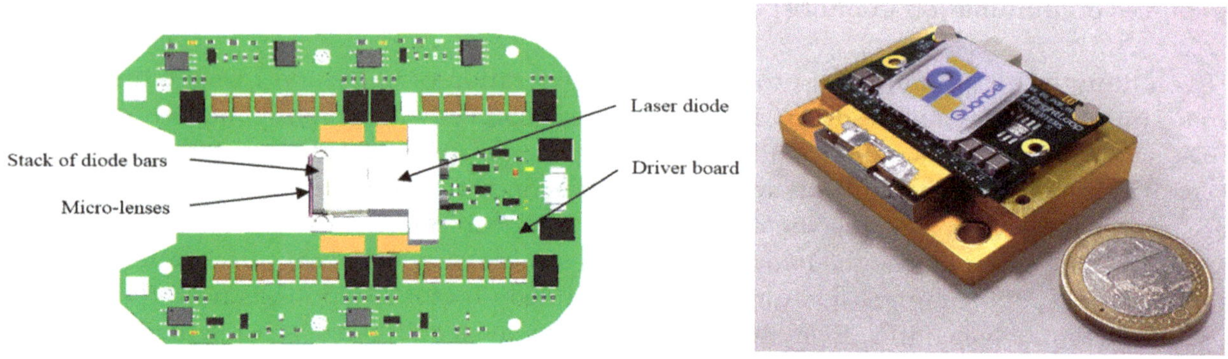

Figure 12. Schematic diagram of the diode laser source showing implementation of the laser diode within the driver board (**left**). An ultra-short pulse laser source integrating a mini-laser diode providing 1.7 mJ in pulses as short as 40 ns from Quantel, France (**right**). Adapted with permission from Proc. SPIE 9887, Biophotonics: Photonic Solutions for Better Health Care V, 98872B (2016).

4.2.3. Optical Output Power

Conventional pulsed LDs generate laser pulses of relatively low energies over a range of few hundreds of nanojoules to a few microjoules per pulse. However, similar to LEDs, with high PRR LDs (~10 KHz), one can average multiple frames and improve the SNR and imaging depth without much impact on the temporal resolution. Recent developments in semiconductor technology also had positive impacts on the field of LDs. Using diode-stacking technology and ultracompact drivers, a maximum output energy of 1.7 mJ per pulse was reported in 2016 [56]. Combined with a PRR of 10 KHz and a pulse width of 40 ns, these powerful LDs hold strong potential in deep-tissue high-resolution PAI. Figure 13 shows a schematic comparing diode bars with single and multiple active regions.

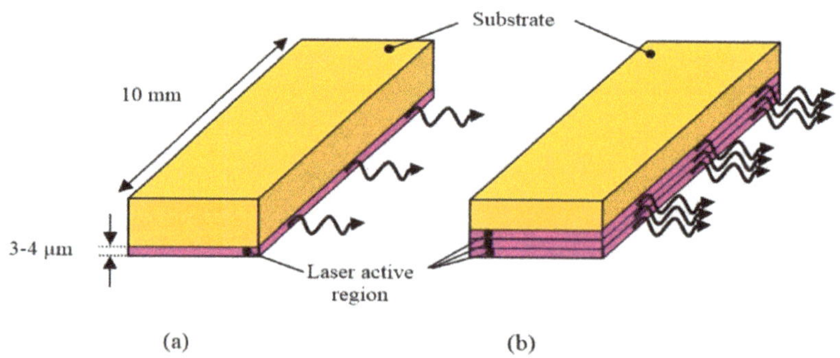

Figure 13. Schematic diagram of (**a**) a standard diode bar and (**b**) a multiple active region diode bar. Adapted with permission from Proc. SPIE 9887, Biophotonics: Photonic Solutions for Better Health Care V, 98872B (2016).

4.2.4. Pulse Repetition Rate

Typically, pulsed LDs can be driven at repetition rates of 1–10 KHz, which is far higher than the PRR of conventional lasers. To the best of our knowledge, the highest PRR reported for an LD is 10 KHz, which is high enough to be useful for compensating for a low output pulse energy [56]. In this regard, there is flexibility to average multiple frames, maintaining the real-time imaging capability just as in the case of LEDs. Since LDs are coherent light sources as lasers, it is also important to consider the maximum permissible exposure when using higher PRR to ensure light safety, especially in a clinical setting [53].

4.2.5. Pulse Width

Pulse widths of commercially available pulsed LDs are in the range of 30–200 ns [53]. This range is higher than that of a conventional solid-state laser, which is capable of delivering 5–10 ns pulses. However, as discussed before, if stress and thermal confinement can be met, such a low pulse width is not a necessity for deep-tissue PAT. For example, when using 100 ns LDs as an illumination source, the maximum PA signal frequency expected will be around 10 MHz, which is well within the detection bandwidths of US transducers suitable for imaging deep-tissue structures. However, for high-resolution imaging of shallow structures using high-frequency US probes, the pulse widths of the LDs may not be sufficient; also, it is important to mention that the pulse energy of the LD-generated light pulses will drop when the pulse width is reduced. Pulse width-tunable LDs are yet to be reported, which may be because of the technical difficulties in the driver circuit.

4.2.6. Spatial Divergence of LD

The spatial divergence of LDs is larger than that of solid-state lasers but smaller than that of LEDs in general, with angles of up to 40 degrees in the axis perpendicular to the diode arrays ("fast axis") and 10 degrees in the parallel axis ("slow axis") [57]. It has been shown that one can efficiently reshape the divergent beam from LDs to be used in an integrated PA and US probe [57]. However, tight optical focusing with these high-power LDs is not feasible due to their multimode nature, which limits their application in optical-resolution PA microscopy.

4.3. *Technical Developments in LD-Based Photoacoustic Tomography*

To the best of our knowledge, the first report on using LDs as a PA illumination source was from Allen and Beard back in 2005 [58]. In this work, they used a pulsed LD (P GAF5S24 from EG&G; wavelength: 905 nm; and pulse duration: 200 ns) driven by a commercially available electronic driver (PCO–7120 from DEI). In this proof-of-concept work, they used a non-realistic phantom (ink-filled cell) and the light was delivered to it using a multimode fiber coupled to the diode. Apart from showing the feasibility of generating PA signals using an LD, they also studied the impact of pulse duration in PAI. In another work immediately after this, Kolkman et al. demonstrated that it was feasible to generate PA signals from superficial blood vessels in a human volunteer [59]. They used a commercially available pulsed laser diode module (iRLS, Laser Components GmbH, Germany) and compared its PAI efficiency with a conventional solid-state laser. The LD used was of 905 nm wavelength with a pulse duration of 112 ns and a PRR of 5 kHz, and offered a maximum optical energy of 23 μJ per pulse. Acoustic detection was performed using a double-ring sensor that can generate 1D depth images (A-scans), which then can be used to generate 2D images by rendering multiple A-lines together. Using this setup, for the first time they demonstrated that LDs could image blood vessels in vivo. However, in this encouraging study, the time for one scan (above 3 min) and the imaging depth (1 mm) was not optimal.

In late 2016, Allen and Beard improved their 905 nm LD-based PAT system and showed that it was feasible to image a tissue-mimicking blood vessel phantom effectively [60]. This work confirmed that LDs can very well be an alternative to solid-state lasers for superficial PA imaging applications. In this system, the maximum PRR was 5 kHz and the pulse width was tunable from 50–500 ns. Pulse width settings of 65 ns (pulse energy: 24 μJ) and 500 ns (pulse energy: 184 μJ) were used to demonstrate how pulse width affects PA image quality because of stress confinement requirements. A 3.5 MHz single-element PZT focused transducer was used for acoustic detection and 5000 PA frames were averaged to generate one image. Even though slightly slow because of limitations in electronics and data transfer, this work was a solid demonstration of LD-based PAT. Key issues to resolve for using LD-based PAT for in vivo applications were pulse energy and time of acquisition and processing.

After these pioneering works on the use of LDs in PAI, there have been significant developments in the field of combining PAI with conventional pulse-echo US imaging. In this regard, by 2014, Daoudi et al. reported an integrated US and PA imaging probe with a high-power LD (Quantel, France) and all optical components integrated inside one housing along with a commercially available 7 MHz linear array US probe (ESAOTE Europe) [57]. The wavelength of the LD was 805 nm, which emitted 130 ns pulses with an optical energy of 0.56 mJ per pulse. The PRR was 10 kHz, opening up the possibility to average multiple frames to improve the SNR without sacrificing the frame rate. Figure 14 shows a photograph of this dual-modality PA and US system. As one can see, the probe is quite portable and well suited for a real-time handheld operation in a clinical setting.

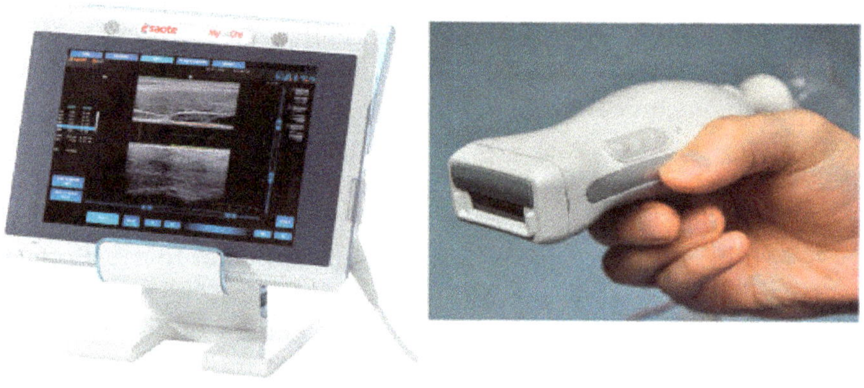

Figure 14. Portable imaging scanner combining photoacoustics and ultrasound. Left is the ultrasound scanner system and right is the picture of the probe integrating the laser module and ultrasound transducer array. Reprinted with permission from K. Daoudi, P.J. van den Berg, O. Rabot, A. Kohl, S. Tisserand, P. Brands, and W. Steenbergen, Optics Express, Vol.22, pp. 26365–26374, 2014.

A key feature of this probe design is that all optical components, including the deflecting prism, diffractive optical elements, diode stack, micro-cylindrical lenses, and aluminum cooling rim, were packaged inside a single casing along with a 128-element US probe (Figure 15a). Along with reporting the design of the probe, they performed a detailed characterization of the system and demonstrated the feasibility of in vivo real-time imaging on a human finger. An imaging depth of 4 mm was achieved in the human finger measurement at a frame rate of 20 Hz (Figure 15b,c). Higher imaging depths (10–15 mm) were achieved in phantom studies, but at a higher PRF, which cannot be used in human experiments because of laser safety regulations. Radiant exposure of 1.3 mJ/cm^2 on the skin with an illumination spot size of 18.2 × 2.3 mm^2 was achieved in this prototype, resulting in the possibility of imaging micro-vasculature with unprecedented contrast and resolution. The same system was later used for multiple preclinical applications and early clinical pilot studies [61–66]. Adding multiple diode stacks with different wavelengths can make this system a power tool with excellent structural, functional, and molecular imaging capability.

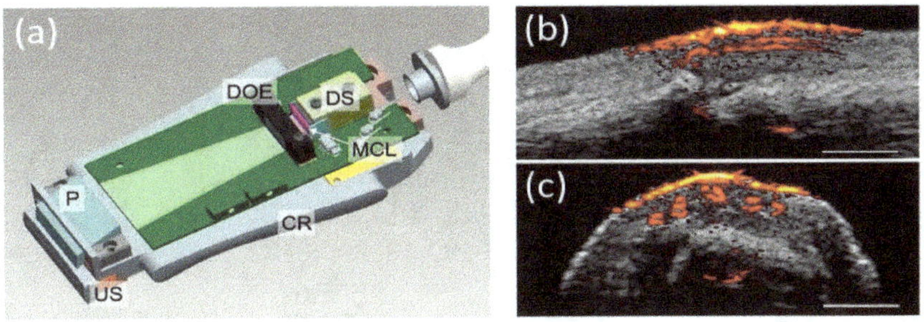

Figure 15. (**a**) A schematic of the handheld PA and US probe. US: ultrasound array transducer; P: deflecting prism; DOE: diffractive optical elements; DS: diode stack; MCL: micro-cylindrical lenses; CR: aluminum cooling rim. Photoacoustic/ultrasound images of a human proximal interphalangeal joint in the (**b**) sagittal and (**c**) transverse planes. Adapted with permission from K. Daoudi, P.J. van den Berg, O. Rabot, A. Kohl, S. Tisserand, P. Brands, and W. Steenbergen, Optics Express, Vol.22, pp. 26365–26374, 2014.

In late 2015, Upputuri et al. demonstrated the possibility of PAT using LD excitation and scanning of a single-element US transducer [67]. Using a powerful LD from Quantel (wavelength: 803 nm; pulse energy: 1.4 mJ; and PRR: 7 KHz) and a conventional single-element US transducer rotating around the object, they achieved to obtain an image every 3 s and they also demonstrated an imaging depth of 2 cm in phantom studies, which is commendable. They also compared the results with an OPO-based laser system in similar settings. This system was upgraded by them with multiple single-element transducers and used in multiple preclinical applications recently [68–70]. Figure 16 shows a schematic of the PLD-PAT system designed for in vivo small animal brain imaging and Figure 17 shows images of brain vasculature in a 95 g female rat acquired non-invasively with PAT at different scan times.

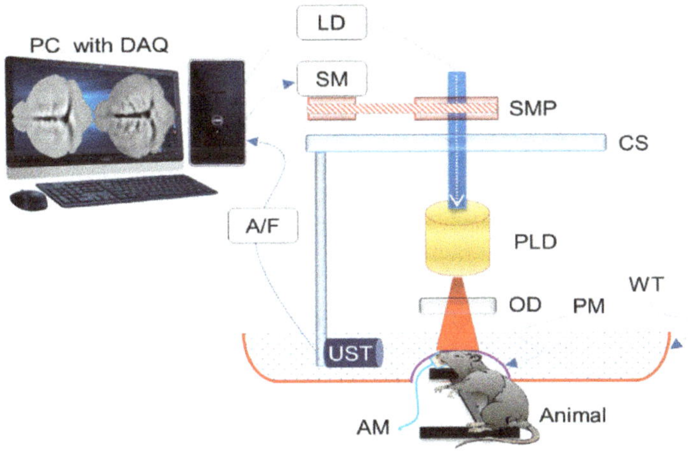

Figure 16. Schematic of the PLD-PAT system for in vivo small animal brain imaging: PLD, pulsed laser diode; OD, optical diffuser; CS, circular scanning plate; SMP, stepper motor pulley unit; UST, ultrasound transducer; A/F, amplifier/filter unit; LD, laser driver unit; SM, stepper motor; PC, personal computer; WT, water tank; DAQ, data acquisition card; AM, anesthesia machine; PM, transparent polythene membrane. Reproduced with permission from P. K. Upputuri and M. Pramanik, Journal of Biomedical Optics, Vol.22, Article ID090501, 2017.

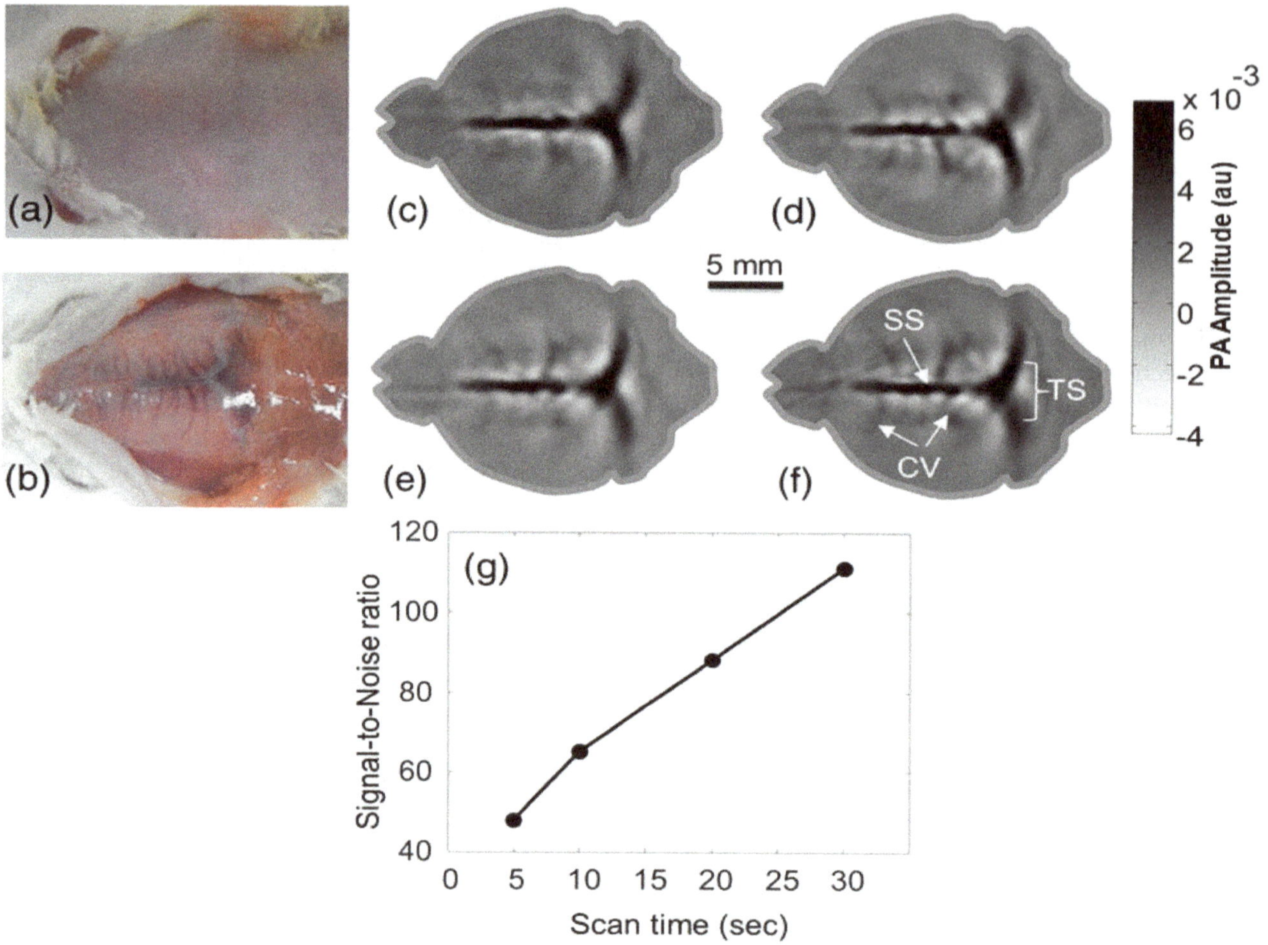

Figure 17. Images of brain vasculature in a 95 g female rat acquired non-invasively with a laser diode-based photoacoustic tomography system at different scan times: photograph of rat brain before (**a**) and after (**b**) removing the scalp. In vivo brain images at a (**c**) 5-s, (**d**) 10-s, (**e**) 20-s, and (**f**) 30-s scan time. (**g**) SNR of the in vivo images as a function of scan time. SS, sagittal sinus; TS, transverse sinus; CV, cerebral veins. Adapted with permission from P. K. Upputuri and M. Pramanik, Journal of Biomedical Optics, Vol.22, Article ID090501, 2017.

Out of these PLD-PAT works, a recent study from Rajendran et al. [69] is commendable. In this work, the authors used their LD-PAT setup for detecting changes in the sagittal sinus due to intra-cranial hypotension in a rat model. A key advantage of this LD-PAT setup is the cost reduction because of (1) not using US probes with multiple elements; (2) not using multichannel DAQ systems; and (3) replacement of bulky and expensive lasers with LDs. In another recent work from the same group, Upputuri et al. [71] demonstrated a pulsed LD-based PA temperature sensing system for monitoring tissue temperature in real time. The system takes advantages of a laser diode with a high repetition rate (7000 Hz), a near-infrared wavelength (803 nm), and a relatively high energy (1.42 mJ/pulse). Results gave a direct confirmation that this LD-based PAI system is capable of providing local temperature information at a high temporal resolution of 1 ms and high sensitivity of 0.31 °C.

Even though no LD-based PAT system is available commercially, several research studies (Table 5) have validated the potential of LD-based PAT in multiple preclinical and clinical applications, in which encouraging imaging depths were achieved despite low pulse energies when compared with lasers. Pulsed LDs are powerful, portable, and cost-effective, and it is believed that LD-based PAT could be a complementary modality to conventional clinical US imaging [72].

Table 5. Summary of the preclinical and clinical applications of LD-based PAI. ICG, indocyanine green.

Target	Application		Depth (mm)	Contrast Agent	Wavelength (nm)
Vasculature	Detection of intraplaque hemorrhage in carotid artery [62]	Phantom and ex vivo studies	20	N/A	808
Vasculature	Dynamic imaging studies (for example in cardiovascular medicine) [73]		20	N/A	803
Red blood cells	Non-invasive blood flow imaging [66]		7	N/A	805
Vasculature	Detection of liver fibrosis [64]	Animal in vivo	5	N/A	808
Cortical vasculature	Brain imaging [68]		5	ICG	803
Cerebro-spinal fluid volume level	Detection of venous sinus distension by measuring intra-cranial hypertension [69]		5	N/A	803
Vasculature and perfusion	Vascular/dermal pathologies [63]	Healthy human	5	N/A	805
Vasculature	Detection of intraplaque hemorrhage in carotid artery [65]		15	N/A	808
Finger joints	Imaging of rheumatoid arthritis [57]		5	N/A	808
Finger joints	Imaging of rheumatoid arthritis [61]	Patient	5	N/A	808

5. Discussion

In this review, we focused on the basics of PAI and the use of affordable light sources (LEDs and LDs) as illumination sources in PAT. After a short introduction to the physical phenomenon behind biomedical PAI, we elaborated on the key specifications and technological developments in the area of high-power LEDs and LDs and detailed their use as illumination sources in PAT. It is encouraging that even with low optical energies, LED and LD-based PAT systems have already demonstrated their potential in a wide range of functional (oxygen saturation imaging, blood flow imaging, etc.) and molecular imaging applications (tracking contrast agents, pharmacokinetic studies, etc.), thanks to the high PRR (maximum reported PRR for LED: 16 KHz; LD: 10 KHz) and possibility to average over a large number of frames to improve the SNR [13–15]. With these affordable light source-based PAT systems, several in vivo preclinical and clinical pilot studies have reported imaging depths of above 8–10 mm, at frame rates unachievable for conventional laser-based systems [13–15]. Apart from the technical aspects in developing an LED and LD-based PAT system, we also shortly introduced the wide variety of preclinical applications and clinical pilot studies reported using these. Divergence of the LEDs and their large beam size when using an array of LDs make these semiconductors not the optimum choice for PA microscopy applications where a tight light focus is an important requirement [23]. However, there are some reports on the use of LEDs and LDs for microscopic and shallow-depth imaging applications, too [74–79]. We did not include these details in this review as our main focus was on tomographic setups and applications.

PAI is already matured in the research setting and has demonstrated its unprecedented potential in a wide range of biomedical imaging applications. However, the clinical translation of this promising technology is not happening at the expected pace. One of the important reasons for this is the requirement of bulky, slow, and expensive pulsed lasers. In the last decade, there have been significant developments in the semiconductor device technology and use of portable and affordable devices like LEDs and LDs became popular as pulsed light sources in PAT. Q-switched solid-state lasers with water-cooling are indeed not an optimal choice for use in a clinical setting because of their sizes, power consumption, costs, and also skin/eye safety aspects (users and patients must wear eye safety glasses and systems must be installed in a laser-safe room). The PRRs of these lasers are also slow and real-time imaging can be challenging, especially when frame averaging is a requirement for improving SNR. Considering the portability, affordability, and dynamic imaging capability aspects, both LEDs and LDs hold strong potential in replacing solid-state lasers, especially for superficial and sub-surface imaging applications, such as in rheumatology, dermatology, and cardiovascular medicine. Handheld US imaging is one of the most popular medical imaging modalities and it is seamless to implement PAT in conventional clinical pulse-echo US equipment. In such handheld systems, integration of LEDs and LDs in a single housing along with a US probe will be a straightforward development and an important aspect to consider in these integrated probes is the mechanism for absorbing the heat generated because of high-speed pulsing. In terms of eye and skin safety, LDs with its coherent nature is similar to that of a conventional laser and the requirements of eye-safety goggles and laser-safe rooms remain important. Even though the fundamental light generation processes for LEDs and LDs are similar, LEDs do not generate stimulated emissions and they possess a broad optical bandwidth and their spatial coherence is low. Considering these factors, LEDs are not practically considered as laser sources and thus could be potentially used as an eye/skin-safe light sources for PAI given the low optical fluence, and the system could be installed in non-laser safe rooms, too, making it an ideal choice for using in a resource-limited clinical setting [13].

Even though LEDs and LDs have shown their potential in biomedical PAT, the pulse energy of these diodes is still a bottleneck when compared to a solid-state laser, and this limits their use only to superficial imaging applications. The maximum pulse energy reported by an LED source (when used in an array form) is 200 μJ at an 850 nm wavelength. When two such arrays are used on both sides of an US probe, the total light output will be 400 μJ per pulse. In such a setting, the maximum imaging depth achieved in vivo was reported to be around 10 mm, with a combined US and PA frame rate above 10 Hz. On the other hand, LDs are more powerful and a pulse energy above 2 mJ is achievable. However, in an animal/human in vivo situation, so far no LD-based PAI studies has reported an imaging depth above 5–6 mm. An exception is the study from Jaeger et al., in which a carotid artery at a depth of 15 mm was visualized using an integrated probe with an 808 nm LD and a 7 MHz linear array probe. This was achieved by applying an algorithm called DCA (deformation compensated averaging) to reduce the clutter and thereby improving the SNR. It is not straightforward to use a clinical US system for PA detection as highly sensitive and broadband detection with high amplification is very important to achieve high imaging depths. In a nutshell, the maximum imaging depth currently achievable using LED and LED-based PAI systems is less than 2 cm, making it difficult to target deep-tissue imaging applications. Imaging depth in PAI is dependent on several factors, including illumination (type of illumination source, optical output power, wavelength, illumination area, etc.), acoustic detection strategies (sensitivity, directionality, spatial distributions of the US detectors, and noise performance of DAQ, etc.), and image processing and reconstruction algorithms. The conventional solid-state laser-based PAT has already achieved an excellent imaging depth above 6 cm in phantom studies and 3–4 cm in in vivo clinical pilot studies [80]. It is worth mentioning that a higher imaging depth (4 cm) was achieved using curved US probes in a computed tomographic setup [81,82]. Using clinical linear array US probes, to the best of our knowledge, an imaging depth above 2 cm has not been demonstrated in vivo even when using bulky and powerful solid-state lasers as illumination sources. We believe that further advancements in semiconductor device technology and lighting industry in general will improve the pulse energy offered by LDs and LEDs in the near future, thus making these devices well-suited for PAT applications. Theoretically, it is feasible to improve the SNR and thereby imaging depth by increasing the PRR and thus offering more room to increase frame averaging. However, heat generation (especially in fully integrated US/PA probes) and also laser safety will be serious concerns when the PRR is extremely high. It is also well known that when the N frames are averaged, the SNR will be improved only by $\sqrt{N}$. Several US-received side strategies and AI-based methods have also been reported for improving the image quality [65,83–91]. We foresee that developments in the area of semiconductor devices and low noise electronics, combined with advanced image reconstruction and enhancement algorithms, will accelerate the clinical translation of affordable light sources based PAI. Since SNR is a key problem to solve, use of novel coded excitation schemes [24,92] and implementation of clutter and reflection artifact reduction algorithms [65,93] also will have a significant impact in clinical translation of LED and LD-based PAT. When compared to OPO-based lasers, one of the key disadvantages of LEDs and LDs is the difficulty in obtaining multiple illumination wavelengths for multispectral PAI [13]. When multiple diode elements with different wavelengths are embedded in an arrayed form, the pulse energy will be further reduced, which then has a serious impact on the imaging depth. Dual-wavelength LED-based PAT for applications like oxygen saturation imaging and differentiation of veins and lymphatic vessels are already reported [25,40]. However, in a complex situation with more than two optical absorbers in the tissue, OPO-based laser systems are still preferred because of the wide range of wavelengths available and fast tuning capability.

The pulse duration of the excitation light source is one of the key factors that has an impact on PA signal generation and image quality. It is well known that a short pulse width is important for satisfying the stress confinement criteria and generating broadband PA signals suitable for high-resolution images. Typical pulsed lasers offer a pulse width in the range of 3–10 ns, which then can generate broadband PA signals from the optically absorbing objects. For example, a 3.5 ns light pulse can generate PA signals with frequencies up to 300 MHz, depending on the size of the targets. Such high frequencies from deep tissue will be heavily attenuated and will not reach the US probe. If one has to detect such signals from superficial tissue, it is important to use high frequency US probes with a super-high reception bandwidth. Even though this is feasible technically, applications will be limited to PA microscopy. When using a conventional mid-frequency US probe suitable for deep tissue imaging, the US detection efficiency with frequencies above 12–14 MHz is extremely low [13]. Considering these factors, we believe that such a low pulse width is not an absolute necessity, provided that the stress confinement is met. As discussed before, a very low pulse widths will be only interesting for PA microscopy imaging applications with imaging depth less than 1–2 mm.

In this review, we mainly focused on LEDs and LDs as these are the most common and well-explored affordable PAT light source, especially in the NIR wavelength range, which is the most suitable range of light wavelengths for deep tissue imaging applications [14,15,53]. However, in recent years there have been several other reports too on affordable illumination strategies in PAT. In 2016, Wong et al. reported on the use of a single Xenon flash lamp as a light source in PAT [94]. In this promising work, the PRR of the Xenon lamp could be controlled between 10–100 Hz and 3 mJ of energy was carried in pulses with a 1 μs pulse width. Using a 0.5 MHz ring-shape detector, the authors demonstrated the feasibility of the imaging tissue, mimicking phantoms (imaging depth: 3.5 cm) and a whole mouse body in vivo. Recently, there have been promising reports on the use of diode-pumped solid-state lasers (DPSSLs) as a light source in PAT. PDSSLs are portable and energy efficient, and thus a promising light source for PAI in a resource-limited setting. Wang et al. used a compact high-power DPSSL (Montfort Laser GmbH Inc., Germany) for deep tissue single wavelength in vivo PAT imaging [95]. This laser source has a miniature size of $13.2 \times 14.0 \times 6.5$ cm^3, a weight of 1.6 kg, and an average power output of 4 W, with a high pulse energy of up to 80 mJ at the wavelength 1064 nm with a PRR up to 50 Hz. Using this DPSSL-based system, the authors successfully imaged murine whole-body vascular structures and cardiac functions in vivo, and mapped the arm, palm, and breast vasculatures of living human subjects. One of the key advantages of these DPSSLs are the possibility of fiber coupling and consequent focusing, which is very much important for PA microscopy imaging applications (this is not possible using LED and LEDs). Recently, Jeng et al. reported on the use of a compact 700–900 nm tunable DPSSL with a pulse energy of around 1 mJ over the range of wavelengths and a PRR of 1 KHz [96]. In this work, the authors demonstrated automatic laser-fluence compensation in spectroscopic PAT and inter-wavelength motion correction using US speckle tracking, which has never been shown before in real-time systems. The 50-Hz video rate PAUS system was demonstrated in vivo using a murine model of drug delivery monitoring. As an energy-efficient and portable illumination source, pulsed fiber lasers were also explored as a PAT illumination source. Using a fiber laser emitting at 1060 nm, with a maximum pulse energy of 0.8 mJ and a Fabry Perot ultrasound scanner, Allen et al. demonstrated the potential of 3D PAT with a realistic blood vessel phantom and the palm vasculature of a human volunteer [97]. Frequency domain PAI systems using continuous-wave modulated laser diodes and LEDs have also been developed recently for several biomedical applications [98,99].

Since short-pulsed light can have a serious impact on the eyes/skin, it is very important to keep the optical pulse energy within the maximum permissible exposure (MPE) limit by following, e.g., the American National Standards Institute (ANSI). Even though the LEDs used in PAI generate pulsed light, they are not considered as laser sources and at present there are no safety standards defined in this regard, to the best of our knowledge. Light from LEDs is optically broad and non-coherent, making it considerably safer to use in a clinical setting as compared to lasers in general (divergence of LEDs is also high, and no safety issues are expected unless the light source is kept very close to the eyes). As a high PRR pulsed laser source, it is very important to consider the MPE limits of the LDs. One may get an initial impression that portable devices like LDs with a low optical power will be completely safe for the eyes and skin. Unfortunately, this is not the case because the light density on the skin will be high when the repetition rate is very high (a large number of light pulses over a period of time). ANSI has clear definitions for this and the safety limits for the skin depend on the light wavelength, pulse width, duration of the exposure, and illumination area [51]. For example, let us consider the case of 800-nm wavelength (λ), the MPE limit for the skin over an exposure time (t) of 0.5 s (assumption) is given by $1.1 \times 10^{(2(\lambda-700)/1000)} \times t^{0.25}$ J/cm^2 = ~1.47 J/cm^2. For an LD with a PRR of 2 KHz, the MPE per pulse becomes ~0.735 mJ/cm^2 (1.47/2000). If the LD can deliver optical energy of 1 mJ per pulse, the light beam must be expanded in such a way that the total area of illumination is about 1.36 cm^2 (1/0.735). From this, it is clear that for increasing the PRR for the same exposure time of 0.5 s, the MPE per pulse must be lower than 0.735 mJ/cm^2. In a nutshell, the total pulse energy density will be lower when one increases the PRR, subsequently reducing the possibility of averaging and thus SNR reduction. In clinical PAI, it is of paramount importance to carefully select the pulse energy, PRR, illumination area, and time of exposure for keeping up with the MPE safety limits [52].

6. Conclusions

Compact, fast, affordable, and energy-efficient light sources are important requirements for accelerating the clinical translation of PAI. LEDs and LDs fit very well into this category and have been explored extensively in recent years as an illumination source in PAI. This review, which is focused on affordable light source-based PAI, is timely considering the fact that this promising technology is facing an exciting transition from bench to bedside.

In this paper, we first covered the basic theory of PAI, clearly conveying the key advantages of the technique, including optical contrast and acoustic resolution/imaging depth. In the first section, we also shortly introduced the different light sources used in PAI with its specifications, including pulse energy, PRR, pulse width, and cost. After this, the principles of light generation and basic performance characteristics of both LEDs and LDs were discussed with a focus on the advantages and disadvantages when they are used as a light source in PAI. The historical developments (from single-point measurements to in vivo imaging and to commercialization) of both LED- and LD-based PAI systems were also discussed, listing out the key preclinical and clinical application demonstrations.

Even though LEDs and LDs possess some disadvantages, such as low optical energy, lack of spectral tuning capability, and long pulse widths, they are portable, affordable, and energy-efficient light sources. Apart from point-of-care biomedical imaging, LEDs and LDs would be an ideal choice for wearable PA equipment and may find a plethora of applications in the field of therapeutic drug monitoring. Integration of LED- or LD-based PAI to a clinical US scanner will have an easier clinical acceptance when compared to laser-based PAI. We expect that dual-mode US and PA equipment utilizing affordable light sources will have a significant impact on bedside diagnostic imaging, accelerating the translation of this technology from research labs to clinics.

Author Contributions: Conceptualization, M.K.A.S. and W.X.; writing—original draft preparation, M.K.A.S.; writing—review and editing, W.X.; supervision, W.X.; project administration, W.X.; funding acquisition, W.X. All authors have read and agreed to the published version of the manuscript.

References

1. Beard, P. Biomedical photoacoustic imaging. *Interface Focus* **2011**, *1*, 602–631. [CrossRef] [PubMed]
2. Manohar, S.; Razansky, D. Photoacoustics: A historical review. *Adv. Opt. Photonics* **2016**, *8*, 586–617. [CrossRef]
3. Wang, L.V. Multiscale photoacoustic microscopy and computed tomography. *Nat. Photonics* **2009**, *3*, 503–509. [CrossRef]
4. Omar, M.; Aguirre, J.; Ntziachristos, V. Optoacoustic mesoscopy for biomedicine. *Nat. Biomed. Eng.* **2019**, *3*, 354–370. [CrossRef]
5. Wang, L.V.; Yao, L.V.W.J. A practical guide to photoacoustic tomography in the life sciences. *Nat. Methods* **2016**, *13*, 627–638. [CrossRef]
6. Singh, M.K.A.; Steenbergen, W.; Manohar, S. Handheld Probe-Based Dual Mode Ultrasound/Photoacoustics for Biomedical Imaging. In *Frontiers in Biophotonics for Translational Medicine*; Progress in Optical Science and Photonics; Springer: Singapore, 2015; Volume 3, pp. 209–247. [CrossRef]
7. Singh, M.K.A.; Sato, N.; Ichihashi, F.; Sankai, Y. Clinical Translation of Photoacoustic Imaging—Opportunities and Challenges from an Industry Perspective. In *LED-Based Photoacoustic Imaging*; Progress in Optical Science and Photonics; Springer: Singapore, 2020; Volume 7, pp. 379–393. [CrossRef]
8. Szabo, T.L. *Diagnostic Ultrasound Imaging: Inside Out*; Elsevier BV: Amsterdam, The Netherlands, 2014.
9. Zhao, T.; Desjardins, A.E.; Ourselin, S.; Vercauteren, T.; Xia, W. Minimally invasive photoacoustic imaging: Current status and future perspectives. *Photoacoustics* **2019**, *16*, 100146. [CrossRef]
10. Bell, A.G. On the production and reproduction of sound by light. *Am. J. Sci.* **1880**, *118*, 305–324. [CrossRef]
11. Lutzweiler, C.; Razansky, D. Optoacoustic Imaging and Tomography: Reconstruction Approaches and Outstanding Challenges in Image Performance and Quantification. *Sensors* **2013**, *13*, 7345–7384. [CrossRef]
12. Tian, C.; Xie, Z.; Fabiilli, M.L.; Wang, X. Imaging and sensing based on dual-pulse nonlinear photoacoustic contrast: A preliminary study on fatty liver. *Opt. Lett.* **2015**, *40*, 2253–2256. [CrossRef]
13. Zhu, Y.; Feng, T.; Cheng, Q.; Wang, X.; Du, S.; Sato, N.; Yuan, J.; Singh, M.K.A. Towards Clinical Translation of LED-Based Photoacoustic Imaging: A Review. *Sensors* **2020**, *20*, 2484. [CrossRef]
14. Erfanzadeh, M.; Zhu, Q. Photoacoustic imaging with low-cost sources; A review. *Photoacoustics* **2019**, *14*, 1–11. [CrossRef] [PubMed]
15. Zhong, H.; Duan, T.; Lan, H.; Zhou, M.; Gao, F. Review of Low-Cost Photoacoustic Sensing and Imaging Based on Laser Diode and Light-Emitting Diode. *Sensors* **2018**, *18*, 2264. [CrossRef] [PubMed]
16. Li, M.; Tang, Y.; Yao, J. Photoacoustic tomography of blood oxygenation: A mini review. *Photoacoustics* **2018**, *10*, 65–73. [CrossRef]
17. Mallidi, S.; Luke, G.P.; Emelianov, S. Photoacoustic imaging in cancer detection, diagnosis, and treatment guidance. *Trends Biotechnol.* **2011**, *29*, 213–221. [CrossRef]
18. Xia, W.; Singh, M.K.A.; Maneas, E.; Sato, N.; Shigeta, Y.; Agano, T.; Ourselin, S.; West, S.J.; Desjardins, A.E. Handheld Real-Time LED-Based Photoacoustic and Ultrasound Imaging System for Accurate Visualization of Clinical Metal Needles and Superficial Vasculature to Guide Minimally Invasive Procedures. *Sensors* **2018**, *18*, 1394. [CrossRef]
19. Kuchment, P.; Kunyansky, L. Mathematics of thermoacoustic tomography. *Eur. J. Appl. Math.* **2008**, *19*, 191–224. [CrossRef]

20. Jaeger, M.; Schüpbach, S.; Gertsch, A.; Kitz, M.; Frenz, M. Fourier reconstruction in optoacoustic imaging using truncated regularized inverse k -space interpolation. *Inverse Probl.* **2007**, *23*, S51–S63. [CrossRef]
21. Niederhauser, J.J.; Jaeger, M.; Lemor, R.; Weber, P.; Frenz, M. Combined ultrasound and optoacoustic system for real-time high-contrast vascular imaging in vivo. *IEEE Trans. Med. Imaging* **2005**, *24*, 436–440. [CrossRef]
22. Singh, M.K.A. *LED-Based Photoacoustic Imaging*; Springer Nature Singapore Pte Ltd.: Singapore, 2020.
23. Allen, T.J. High-Power Light Emitting Diodes; An Alternative Excitation Source for Photoacoustic Tomography. In *LED-Based Photoacoustic Imaging*; Progress in Optical Science and Photonics; Springer: Singapore, 2020; Volume 7, pp. 23–43. [CrossRef]
24. Allen, T.J.; Beard, P.C. High power visible light emitting diodes as pulsed excitation sources for biomedical photoacoustics. *Biomed. Opt. Express* **2016**, *7*, 1260–1270. [CrossRef]
25. Singh, M.K.A.; Sato, N.; Sankai, Y.; Ichihashi, F. In vivo demonstration of real-time oxygen saturation imaging using a portable and affordable LED-based multispectral photoacoustic and ultrasound imaging system. *Photons Plus Ultrasound: Imaging Sens. 2019* **2019**, *10878*, 108785N. [CrossRef]
26. Zhu, Y.; Xu, G.; Yuan, J.; Jo, J.; Gandikota, G.; Demirci, H.; Agano, T.; Sato, N.; Shigeta, Y.; Wang, X. Light Emitting Diodes based Photoacoustic Imaging and Potential Clinical Applications. *Sci. Rep.* **2018**, *8*, 1–12. [CrossRef]
27. Singh, M.K.A. Effect of light pulse width on frequency characteristics of photoacoustic signal—An experimental study using a pulse-width tunable LED-based photoacoustic imaging system. *Int. J. Eng. Technol.* **2018**, *7*, 4300–4303.
28. Francis, K.J.; Boink, Y.E.; Dantuma, M.; Singh, M.K.A.; Manohar, S.; Steenbergen, W.; Joseph, F.K. Tomographic imaging with an ultrasound and LED-based photoacoustic system. *Biomed. Opt. Express* **2020**, *11*, 2152–2165. [CrossRef]
29. Francis, K.J.; Boink, Y.E.; Dantuma, M.; Singh, M.K.A.; Manohar, S.; Steenbergen, W. Light Emitting Diodes Based Photoacoustic and Ultrasound Tomography: Imaging Aspects and Applications. In *LED-Based Photoacoustic Imaging*; Progress in Optical Science and Photonics; Springer: Singapore, 2020; Volume 7, pp. 245–266. [CrossRef]
30. Xia, W.; Nikitichev, D.I.; Mari, J.M.; West, S.J.; Pratt, R.; David, A.L.; Ourselin, S.; Beard, P.C.; Desjardins, A.E. Performance characteristics of an interventional multispectral photoacoustic imaging system for guiding minimally invasive procedures. *J. Biomed. Opt.* **2015**, *20*, 086005. [CrossRef]
31. Mari, J.M.; Xia, W.; West, S.J.; Desjardins, A.E. Interventional multispectral photoacoustic imaging with a clinical ultrasound probe for discriminating nerves and tendons: An ex vivo pilot study. *J. Biomed. Opt.* **2015**, *20*, 110503. [CrossRef] [PubMed]
32. Singh, M.K.A.; Parameshwarappa, V.; Hendriksen, E.; Steenbergen, W.; Manohar, S. Photoacoustic-guided focused ultrasound for accurate visualization of brachytherapy seeds with the photoacoustic needle. *J. Biomed. Opt.* **2016**, *21*, 120501. [CrossRef] [PubMed]
33. Hansen, R.S. Using high-power light emitting diodes for photoacoustic imaging. *SPIE Med. Imaging* **2011**, *7968*, 79680. [CrossRef]
34. Allen, T.J.; Beard, P.C. Light emitting diodes as an excitation source for biomedical photoacoustics. In Proceedings of the Photons Plus Ultrasound: Imaging and Sensing 2013, San Francisco, CA, USA, 4 March 2013; p. 85811F. [CrossRef]
35. Agano, T.; Sato, N.; Nakatsuka, H.; Kitagawa, K.; Hanaoka, T.; Morisono, K.; Shigeta, Y. Comparative experiments of photoacoustic system using laser light source and LED array light source. In Proceedings of the Photons Plus Ultrasound: Imaging and Sensing 2015, San Francisco, CA, USA, 11 March 2015; p. 93233X. [CrossRef]
36. Agano, T.; Sato, N.; Nakatsuka, H.; Kitagawa, K.; Hanaoka, T.; Morisono, K.; Shigeta, Y. Attempts to increase penetration of photoacoustic system using LED array light souce. In Proceedings of the Photons Plus Ultrasound: Imaging and Sensing 2015, San Francisco, CA, USA, 11 March 2015; p. 93233Z. [CrossRef]
37. Agano, T.; Sato, N. Photoacoustic Imaging System using LED light source. In Proceedings of the 2016 Conference on Lasers and Electro-Optics (CLEO), San Jose, CA, USA, 5–10 June 2016; The Optical Society: Washington, DC, USA, 2016; p. ATh3N.5.
38. Hariri, A.; LeMaster, J.; Wang, J.; Jeevarathinam, A.S.; Chao, D.L.; Jokerst, J.V. The characterization of an economic and portable LED-based photoacoustic imaging system to facilitate molecular imaging. *Photoacoustics* **2018**, *9*, 10–20. [CrossRef]

39. Joseph, F.K.; Xavierselvan, M.; Singh, M.K.A.; Mallidi, S.; Van Der Laken, C.; Van De Loo, F.; Steenbergen, W. LED-based photoacoustic imaging for early detection of joint inflammation in rodents: Towards achieving 3Rs in rheumatoid arthritis research. In Proceedings of the Photons Plus Ultrasound: Imaging and Sensing 2020, San Francisco, CA, USA, 17 February 2020; p. 112400M. [CrossRef]
40. Singh, M.K.A.; Agano, T.; Sato, N.; Shigeta, Y.; Uemura, T. Real-time in vivo imaging of human lymphatic system using an LED-based photoacoustic/ultrasound imaging system. In Proceedings of the Photons Plus Ultrasound: Imaging and Sensing 2018, San Francisco, CA, USA, 19 February 2018; p. 1049404. [CrossRef]
41. Singh, M.K.A.; Shigeta, Y.; Hanaoka, T.; Agano, T.; Sato, N. High-speed photoacoustic imaging using an LED-based photoacoustic imaging system. In Proceedings of the Photons Plus Ultrasound: Imaging and Sensing 2018, San Francisco, CA, USA, 19 February 2018; p. 104943N. [CrossRef]
42. Jo, J.; Xu, G.; Zhu, Y.; Burton, M.; Sarazin, J.; Schiopu, E.; Gandikota, G.; Wang, X. Detecting joint inflammation by an LED-based photoacoustic imaging system: A feasibility study. *J. Biomed. Opt.* **2018**, *23*, 110501–110504. [CrossRef]
43. Cheng, Q.; Qian, M.; Wang, X.; Zhang, H.; Wang, P.; Wen, L.; Pan, J.; Gao, Y.; Wu, S.; Zhang, M.; et al. Diagnosis and Treatment Monitoring of Port-Wine Stain Using LED-Based Photoacoustics: Theoretical Aspects and First In-Human Clinical Pilot Study. In *LED-Based Photoacoustic Imaging*; Progress in Optical Science and Photonics; Springer Nature Singapore Pte Ltd.: Singapore, 2020; pp. 351–377.
44. Xavierselvan, M.; Mallidi, S. LED-Based Functional Photoacoustics—Portable and Affordable Solution for Preclinical Cancer Imaging. In *LED-Based Photoacoustic Imaging*; Progress in Optical Science and Photonics; Springer: Singapore, 2020; Volume 7, pp. 303–319. [CrossRef]
45. Agrawal, S.; Fadden, C.; Dangi, A.; Yang, X.; AlBahrani, H.; Frings, N.; Zadi, S.H.; Kothapalli, S.-R. Light-Emitting-Diode-Based Multispectral Photoacoustic Computed Tomography System. *Sensors* **2019**, *19*, 4861. [CrossRef]
46. Francis, K.J.; Booijink, R.; Bansal, R.; Steenbergen, W. Tomographic Ultrasound and LED-Based Photoacoustic System for Preclinical Imaging. *Sensors* **2020**, *20*, 2793. [CrossRef]
47. Hariri, A.; Chen, F.; Moore, C.; Jokerst, J.V. Noninvasive staging of pressure ulcers using photoacoustic imaging. *Wound Repair Regen.* **2019**, *27*, 488–496. [CrossRef]
48. Maneas, E.; Aughwane, R.; Huynh, N.; Xia, W.; Ansari, R.; Singh, M.K.A.; Hutchinson, J.C.; Sebire, N.J.; Arthurs, O.J.; Deprest, J.; et al. Photoacoustic imaging of the human placental vasculature. *J. Biophotonics* **2019**, *13*, e201900167. [CrossRef]
49. Hariri, A.; Zhao, E.; Jeevarathinam, A.S.; LeMaster, J.; Zhang, J.; Jokerst, J.V. Molecular imaging of oxidative stress using an LED-based photoacoustic imaging system. *Sci. Rep.* **2019**, *9*, 11378. [CrossRef]
50. Xia, W.; Maneas, E.; Huynh, N.T.; Singh, M.K.A.; Brown, N.M.; Ourselin, S.; Gilbert-Kawai, E.; West, S.J.; Desjardins, A.E. Imaging of human peripheral blood vessels during cuff occlusion with a compact LED-based photoacoustic and ultrasound system. In Proceedings of the Photons Plus Ultrasound: Imaging and Sensing 2019, San Francisco, CA, USA, 27 February 2019; p. 1087804. [CrossRef]
51. Zhu, Y.; Lu, X.; Dong, X.; Yuan, J.; Fabiilli, M.L.; Wang, X. LED-Based Photoacoustic Imaging for Monitoring Angiogenesis in Fibrin Scaffolds. *Tissue Eng. Part C Methods* **2019**, *25*, 523–531. [CrossRef]
52. Kalva, S.K.; Pramanik, M. *Photoacoustic Tomography with High-Energy Pulsed Laser Diodes*; SPIE Spotlight Series Book; SPIE-Intl Soc Optical Eng: Bellingham, WA, USA, 2020; Volume SL56, ISBN 9781510636620. Available online: https://spie.org/Publications/Book/2566566?SSO=1 (accessed on 28 October 2020).
53. Fatima, A.; Kratkiewicz, K.; Manwar, R.; Zafar, M.; Zhang, R.; Huang, B.; Dadashzadeh, N.; Xia, J.; Avanaki, K. (Mohammad) Review of cost reduction methods in photoacoustic computed tomography. *Photoacoustics* **2019**, *15*, 100137. [CrossRef]
54. Choi, S.S.S.; Mandelis, A. Review of the state of the art in cardiovascular endoscopy imaging of atherosclerosis using photoacoustic techniques with pulsed and continuous-wave optical excitations. *J. Biomed. Opt.* **2019**, *24*, 1–15. [CrossRef]
55. Nissinen, J.; Kostamovaara, J. A 4 a peak current and 2 ns pulse width CMOS laser diode driver for high measurement rate applications. In Proceedings of the 2013 ESSCIRC (ESSCIRC), Bucharest, Romania, 16–20 September 2013; Institute of Electrical and Electronics Engineers (IEEE): Bucharest, Romania, 2013; pp. 355–358.
56. Canal, C.; Laugustin, A.; Kohl, A.; Rabot, O. Portable multiwavelength laser diode source for handheld photoacoustic devices. *Biophotonics: Photonic Solutions for Better Health Care V* **2016**, *9887*, 98872. [CrossRef]

57. Daoudi, K.; Berg, P.V.D.; Rabot, O.; Kohl, A.; Tisserand, S.; Brands, P.; Steenbergen, W. Handheld probe integrating laser diode and ultrasound transducer array for ultrasound/photoacoustic dual modality imaging. *Opt. Express* **2014**, *22*, 26365–26374. [CrossRef]
58. Allen, T.J.; Cox, B.T.; Beard, P.C. Generating photoacoustic signals using high-peak power pulsed laser diodes. In Proceedings of the Photons Plus Ultrasound: Imaging and Sensing 2005: The Sixth Conference on Biomedical Thermoacoustics, Optoacoustics, and Acousto-optics, San Jose, CA, USA, 25 April 2005; SPIE-Intl Soc Optical Eng: Bellingham, WA, USA, 2005; Volume 5697, pp. 233–243.
59. Kolkman, R.G.M.; Steenbergen, W.; Van Leeuwen, T.G. In vivo photoacoustic imaging of blood vessels with a pulsed laser diode. *Lasers Med Sci.* **2006**, *21*, 134–139. [CrossRef] [PubMed]
60. Allen, T.J.; Beard, P.C. Pulsed near-infrared laser diode excitation system for biomedical photoacoustic imaging. *Opt. Lett.* **2006**, *31*, 3462–3464. [CrossRef]
61. Berg, P.J.V.D.; Daoudi, K.; Moens, H.J.B.; Steenbergen, W. Feasibility of photoacoustic/ultrasound imaging of synovitis in finger joints using a point-of-care system. *Photoacoustics* **2017**, *8*, 8–14. [CrossRef]
62. Arabul, M.U.; Heres, M.; Rutten, M.C.M.; Van Sambeek, M.R.; Van De Vosse, F.N.; Lopata, R.G.P. Toward the detection of intraplaque hemorrhage in carotid artery lesions using photoacoustic imaging. *J. Biomed. Opt.* **2016**, *22*, 41010. [CrossRef]
63. Heres, H.M.; Arabul, M.U.; Rutten, M.C.M.; Van De Vosse, F.N.; Lopata, R.G.P. Visualization of vasculature using a hand-held photoacoustic probe: Phantom and in vivo validation. *J. Biomed. Opt.* **2017**, *22*, 41013. [CrossRef]
64. Berg, P.J.V.D.; Bansal, R.; Daoudi, K.; Steenbergen, W.; Prakash, J. Preclinical detection of liver fibrosis using dual-modality photoacoustic/ultrasound system. *Biomed. Opt. Express* **2016**, *7*, 5081–5091. [CrossRef]
65. Jaeger, M.; Schwab, H.-M.; Almallouhi, Y.; Canal, C.; Song, M.; Sauget, V.; Sontrop, D.; Mulder, T.; Roumen, P.; Humblet, A.; et al. Deformation-Compensated Averaging for Deep-Tissue LED and Laser Diode-Based Photoacoustic Imaging Integrated with Handheld Echo Ultrasound. In *LED-Based Photoacoustic Imaging*; Progress in Optical Science and Photonics; Springer: Singapore, 2020; Volume 7, pp. 47–78. [CrossRef]
66. Berg, P.J.V.D.; Daoudi, K.; Steenbergen, W. Pulsed photoacoustic flow imaging with a handheld system. *J. Biomed. Opt.* **2016**, *21*, 026004. [CrossRef]
67. Upputuri, P.K.; Pramanik, M. Performance characterization of low-cost, high-speed, portable pulsed laser diode photoacoustic tomography (PLD-PAT) system. *Biomed. Opt. Express* **2015**, *6*, 4118–4129. [CrossRef]
68. Kalva, S.K.; Upputuri, P.K.; Pramanik, M. High-speed, low-cost, pulsed-laser-diode-based second-generation desktop photoacoustic tomography system. *Opt. Lett.* **2018**, *44*, 81–84. [CrossRef]
69. Rajendran, P.; Sahu, S.; Dienzo, R.A.; Pramanik, M. In vivo detection of venous sinus distension due to intracranial hypotension in small animal using pulsed-laser-diode photoacoustic tomography. *J. Biophotonics* **2020**, *13*, e201960162. [CrossRef]
70. Upputuri, P.K.; Pramanik, M. Dynamic in vivo imaging of small animal brain using pulsed laser diode-based photoacoustic tomography system. *J. Biomed. Opt.* **2017**, *22*, 1. [CrossRef]
71. Upputuri, P.K.; Das, D.; Maheshwari, M.; Yaowen, Y.; Pramanik, M. Real-time monitoring of temperature using a pulsed laser-diode-based photoacoustic system. *Opt. Lett.* **2020**, *45*, 718–721. [CrossRef]
72. Upputuri, P.K.; Pramanik, M. Fast photoacoustic imaging systems using pulsed laser diodes: A review. *Biomed. Eng. Lett.* **2018**, *8*, 167–181. [CrossRef]
73. Sivasubramanian, K.; Pramanik, M. High frame rate photoacoustic imaging at 7000 frames per second using clinical ultrasound system. *Biomed. Opt. Express* **2016**, *7*, 312–323. [CrossRef]
74. Hariri, A.; Fatima, A.; Mohammadian, N.; Mahmoodkalayeh, S.; Ansari, M.; Bely, N.; Nasiriavanaki, M. Development of low-cost photoacoustic imaging systems using very low-energy pulsed laser diodes. *J. Biomed. Opt.* **2017**, *22*, 75001. [CrossRef]
75. Zeng, L.; Piao, Z.; Huang, S.; Jia, W.; Chen, Z. Label-free optical-resolution photoacoustic microscopy of superficial microvasculature using a compact visible laser diode excitation. *Opt. Express* **2015**, *23*, 31026–31033. [CrossRef]
76. Wang, T.; Nandy, S.; Salehi, H.S.; Kumavor, P.D.; Zhu, Q. A low-cost photoacoustic microscopy system with a laser diode excitation. *Biomed. Opt. Express* **2014**, *5*, 3053–3058. [CrossRef]
77. Zeng, L.; Liu, G.; Yang, D.; Ji, X. Portable optical-resolution photoacoustic microscopy with a pulsed laser diode excitation. *Appl. Phys. Lett.* **2013**, *102*, 053704. [CrossRef]

78. Erfanzadeh, M.; Kumavor, P.D.; Zhu, Q. Laser scanning laser diode photoacoustic microscopy system. *Photoacoustics* **2018**, *9*, 1–9. [CrossRef]
79. Dai, X.; Yang, H.; Jiang, H. In vivo photoacoustic imaging of vasculature with a low-cost miniature light emitting diode excitation. *Opt. Lett.* **2017**, *42*, 1456–1459. [CrossRef]
80. Steinberg, I.; Huland, D.M.; Vermesh, O.; Frostig, H.E.; Tummers, W.S.; Gambhir, S.S. Photoacoustic clinical imaging. *Photoacoustics* **2019**, *14*, 77–98. [CrossRef]
81. Kruger, R.A.; Kuzmiak, C.M.; Lam, R.B.; Reinecke, D.R.; Del Rio, S.P.; Steed, D. Dedicated 3D photoacoustic breast imaging. *Med Phys.* **2013**, *40*, 113301. [CrossRef]
82. Lin, L.; Hu, P.; Shi, J.; Appleton, C.M.; Maslov, K.; Li, L.; Zhang, R.; Wang, L.V. Single-breath-hold photoacoustic computed tomography of the breast. *Nat. Commun.* **2018**, *9*, 1–9. [CrossRef]
83. Abu Anas, E.M.; Zhang, H.K.; Kang, J.; Boctor, E. Enabling fast and high quality LED photoacoustic imaging: A recurrent neural networks based approach. *Biomed. Opt. Express* **2018**, *9*, 3852–3866. [CrossRef]
84. Mozaffarzadeh, M.; Hariri, A.; Moore, C.; Jokerst, J.V. The double-stage delay-multiply-and-sum image reconstruction method improves imaging quality in a LED-based photoacoustic array scanner. *Photoacoustics* **2018**, *12*, 22–29. [CrossRef]
85. Singh, M.K.A.; Sivasubramanian, K.; Sato, N.; Ichihashi, F.; Sankai, Y.; Xing, L. Deep learning-enhanced LED-based photoacoustic imaging. In Proceedings of the Photons Plus Ultrasound: Imaging and Sensing 2020, San Francisco, CA, USA, 17 February 2020; p. 1124038. [CrossRef]
86. Farnia, P.; Najafzadeh, E.; Hariri, A.; Lavasani, S.N.; Makkiabadi, B.; Ahmadian, A.; Jokerst, J.V. Dictionary learning technique enhances signal in LED-based photoacoustic imaging. *Biomed. Opt. Express* **2020**, *11*, 2533–2547. [CrossRef]
87. Manwar, R.; Hosseinzadeh, M.; Hariri, A.; Kratkiewicz, K.; Noei, S.; Avanaki, K. Photoacoustic Signal Enhancement: Towards Utilization of Low Energy Laser Diodes in Real-Time Photoacoustic Imaging. *Sensors* **2018**, *18*, 3498. [CrossRef]
88. Chandramoorthi, S.; Thittai, A.K. Ultrasound Receive-Side Strategies for Image Quality Enhancement in Low-Energy Illumination Based Photoacoustic Imaging. In *LED-Based Photoacoustic Imaging*; Progress in Optical Science and Photonics; Springer: Singapore, 2020; Volume 7, pp. 79–112. [CrossRef]
89. Chandramoorthi, S.; Thittai, A.K. Enhancing Image Quality of Photoacoustic Tomography Using Sub-Pitch Array Translation Approach: Simulation and Experimental Validation. *IEEE Trans. Biomed. Eng.* **2019**, *66*, 3543–3552. [CrossRef]
90. Sowmiya, C.; Thittai, A.K. Noise Reduction in Inherently low-SNR PLD-based PAT images. In Proceedings of the TENCON 2019—2019 IEEE Region 10 Conference (TENCON), Kochi, India, 17–20 October 2019; Institute of Electrical and Electronics Engineers (IEEE): Kochi, India, 2019; pp. 106–108.
91. Zhang, H.K. Democratizing LED-Based Photoacoustic Imaging with Adaptive Beamforming and Deep Convolutional Neural Network. In *LED-Based Photoacoustic Imaging*; Progress in Optical Science and Photonics; Springer: Singapore, 2020; Volume 7, pp. 183–202. [CrossRef]
92. Xia, W.; Ginsberg, Y.; West, S.J.; Nikitichev, D.I.; Ourselin, S.; David, A.L.; Desjardins, A.E. Coded excitation ultrasonic needle tracking: An in vivo study. *Med Phys.* **2016**, *43*, 4065. [CrossRef]
93. Singh, M.K.A.; Jaeger, M.; Frenz, M.; Steenbergen, W. In vivo demonstration of reflection artifact reduction in photoacoustic imaging using synthetic aperture photoacoustic-guided focused ultrasound (PAFUSion). *Biomed. Opt. Express* **2016**, *7*, 2955–2972. [CrossRef]
94. Wong, T.T.W.; Zhou, Y.; Garcia-Uribe, A.; Li, L.; Maslov, K.; Lin, L.; Wang, L.V. Use of a single xenon flash lamp for photoacoustic computed tomography of multiple-centimeter-thick biological tissue ex vivo and a whole mouse body in vivo. *J. Biomed. Opt.* **2016**, 22, 041003. [CrossRef]
95. Wang, D.; Wang, Y.; Wang, W.; Luo, D.; Chitgupi, U.; Geng, J.; Zhou, Y.; Wang, L.; Lovell, J.F.; Xia, J. Deep tissue photoacoustic computed tomography with a fast and compact laser system. *Biomed. Opt. Express* **2016**, *8*, 112–123. [CrossRef] [PubMed]
96. Jeng, G.-S.; Li, M.-L.; Kim, M.W.; Yoon, S.J.; Pitre, J.J.; Li, D.S.; Pelivanov, I.; O'Donnell, M. *Real-Time Spectroscopic Photoacoustic/Ultrasound (PAUS) Scanning with Simultaneous Fluence Compensation and Motion Correction for Quantitative Molecular Imaging*; bioRxiv: New York, NY, USA, 2019.
97. Allen, T.J.; Alam, S.; Zhang, E.; Laufer, J.; Richardson, D.J.; Beard, P.C. Use of a pulsed fibre laser as an excitation source for photoacoustic tomography. In Proceedings of the Photons Plus Ultrasound: Imaging and Sensing 2011, San Francisco, CA, USA, 28 February 2011; p. 78991V. [CrossRef]

98. Lashkari, B.; Choi, S.S.S.; Dovlo, E.; Dhody, S.; Mandelis, A. Frequency-Domain Photoacoustic Phase Spectroscopy: A Fluence-Independent Approach for Quantitative Probing of Hemoglobin Oxygen Saturation. *IEEE J. Sel. Top. Quantum Electron.* **2015**, *22*, 127–136. [CrossRef]
99. Lashkari, B.; Mandelis, A. Comparison between pulsed laser and frequency-domain photoacoustic modalities: Signal-to-noise ratio, contrast, resolution, and maximum depth detectivity. *Rev. Sci. Instrum.* **2011**, *82*, 094903. [CrossRef] [PubMed]

10

EMG-Centered Multisensory Based Technologies for Pattern Recognition in Rehabilitation: State of the Art and Challenges

Chaoming Fang [1,†], Bowei He [2,†], Yixuan Wang [1], Jin Cao [3] and Shuo Gao [1,4,*]

1 School of Instrumentation and Optoelectronic Engineering, Beihang University, Beijing 100083, China; timefliesfang@buaa.edu.cn (C.F.); wangyixuan@buaa.edu.cn (Y.W.)

2 School of Automation Science and Electrical Engineering, Beihang University, Beijing 100083, China; 17374556@buaa.edu.cn

3 Department of Psychiatry, Massachusetts General Hospital, Harvard Medical School, Boston, MA 02138, USA; jcao9@mgh.harvard.edu

4 Beijing Advanced Innovation Center for Big Data-Based Precision Medicine, Beihang University, Beijing 100083, China

* Correspondence: shuo_gao@buaa.edu.cn

† These authors contribute equally to this work.

Abstract: In the field of rehabilitation, the electromyography (EMG) signal plays an important role in interpreting patients' intentions and physical conditions. Nevertheless, utilizing merely the EMG signal suffers from difficulty in recognizing slight body movements, and the detection accuracy is strongly influenced by environmental factors. To address the above issues, multisensory integration-based EMG pattern recognition (PR) techniques have been developed in recent years, and fruitful results have been demonstrated in diverse rehabilitation scenarios, such as achieving high locomotion detection and prosthesis control accuracy. Owing to the importance and rapid development of the EMG centered multisensory fusion technologies in rehabilitation, this paper reviews both theories and applications in this emerging field. The principle of EMG signal generation and the current pattern recognition process are explained in detail, including signal preprocessing, feature extraction, classification algorithms, etc. Mechanisms of collaborations between two important multisensory fusion strategies (kinetic and kinematics) and EMG information are thoroughly explained; corresponding applications are studied, and the pros and cons are discussed. Finally, the main challenges in EMG centered multisensory pattern recognition are discussed, and a future research direction of this area is prospected.

Keywords: multisensory; electromyography; pattern recognition; rehabilitation

---

1. Introduction

Monitoring and analyzing the patient's physiological information are of significance in the process of physical rehabilitation in order to evaluate the rehabilitation effect [1,2] and control auxiliary devices during the physical rehabilitation process. Conventionally, the physiological information is divided into physical and psychological information, e.g., muscle force information and the intention of the patient. To detect these two categories of information, various types of sensors, including electromechanical sensors (such as accelerometers [3,4], gyroscopes [5,6] and force sensors [7,8]), and biosensors (such as electromyography (EMG) [9–11] magnetoencephalography (MEG) and electroencephalogram (EEG)) have been utilized. Electromechanical sensors are capable of detecting the physical information effectively. For example, in [12], flex sensors and force sensitive sensors (FSRs) are utilized to detect the bending angle of the finger and the grasp force, respectively. The sensing information is then used for the control of robotic fingers in performing ten different tasks. In [13], the integrated use of accelerometer sensors, pulse sensors, and ambient sensors is reported for recognizing sedentary behavior with an accuracy of 95%. Nevertheless, biosensors are not only proven to reflect physical information, but convert the bioelectric signal, which is broadly treated as a direct link to human psychological information, into interpretable voltage amplitudes, and therefore have unique advantages in psychological detection over the electromechanical sensors [11,14]. Note that in the rehabilitation area, human psychological information normally refers to human intention information, which can be used to examine the synchronization level between human movements and human thinking. Hence, in this article, the detection of human intention, instead of human psychology, is focused.

Among all biosensor-captured information, EEG, MEG, and EMG are the three most relevant signals to human intention [15–17]. Among them, the EEG signal is of weak robustness due to the shortage of noninvasive electrodes in collecting a surface EEG signal, failing to provide high signal quality. MEG techniques, e.g., MRI, can offer accurate and rich information, but the time-consuming issue and huge machine volume block its use in rehabilitation. In contrast, EMG techniques enjoy relatively higher signal-noise ratio (SNR) and robustness than EEG means (especially during movements), and process information much faster than MEG techniques. Therefore, EMG is a more preferred choice for intention detection in the rehabilitation field.

Two widely used techniques to interpret the EMG signal are signal intensity registration and pattern recognition [18,19]. The former approach is based on the correlation between EMG signal intensity and quantified muscle force level [20,21]. However, the EMG amplitude of a muscle is usually determined by many uncontrollable factors, e.g., EMG crosstalk [22] and variation in muscle force [23], which will not only generate misinterpretations of the muscle activities, but also result in potential safety risks when such information is directly utilized in the exoskeleton for the motion functions impaired patients [18]. Alternatively, the latter approach offers higher accuracy in decoding EMG signals owing to the higher level of information, e.g., a set of motions or the movement intention can be extracted via raw data to provide deep insights in examining user's body condition. EMG PR was not popularized for its high computational cost compared to its counterpart, until being promoted by the rapid development of electronics and information technology in recent years. Now EMG PR has been broadly applied to disease diagnosis [24], intelligent prosthesis control [19], and gains continuing attentions from relevant researchers.

Generally, the recognition scenarios can be divided into upper limb PR and lower limb PR. In early years, research on EMG PR mainly focused on the recognition of the upper limb movements with great differences, e.g., largely changed arm movements [25]. This is because the EMG patterns of such movements are significantly different and therefore is easier to be recognized. Nevertheless, fine upper movements and lower limb movements are also important in many neuromuscular disease analysis, such as Parkinson's disease and myasthenia. Therefore, it is also important to create a reliable relationship between EMG signal and patients' intentions and physical conditions for these two kinds of movements.

However, using the EMG signal to interpret fine upper limb and lower limb motions is challenging. In terms of the former, small movements in the upper limbs like the finger or wrist only result in slight differences in EMG signals, giving rise to difficulties in effectively distinguishing the EMG signal of one pattern from others. For example, a hand movement recognition method using single-channel sEMG is presented in [26]. This work reached an accuracy of 86.7% in classifying nine finger movements, and the recognition accuracy and the pattern types are all lower than the multisensory approach [27]. As to the latter, interactions between lower limbs and unpredictable environments during movements can generate unexpected EMG patterns. For example, the muscle activity of lower limbs is often related to the flatness of terrains [28], or the different locomotion modes such as obstacle crossing [29] and stairs ascending/descending [30]. Therefore, utilizing only the EMG signal cannot satisfy the demand for reaching robust recognition performances at these complicated scenarios without learning environmental knowledge. A possible solution is to concurrently acquire the external information of the environment as well as the EMG signals, so that information from different dimensions can be integrated for further analysis and complementing each other.

In light of this, EMG-centered multisensory-based technologies emerge in recent years, and increasing demonstrations and attempts in three main rehabilitation scenarios have been reported globally. First, multisensory fusion EMG PR plays an important role in accurate and early diagnosis for neuromuscular diseases so that the patients could start the rehabilitation process before the diseases further develop. For example, in [31], the acceleration information of the muscles and forearm of the biceps brachii of the Parkinson's patient are collected simultaneously, 12 kinds of signal features were extracted for cluster analysis, and successfully achieved a diagnostic accuracy rate of more than 90%. Second, multi-sensor fusion can evaluate the rehabilitation process of patients and the effectiveness of the treatment in more dimensions. For example, in [32], the fusion analysis of the plantar force information of the Parkinson's patient and the myoelectric information of the anterior tibial muscle. The effect of a plantar sensory stimulation therapy on improving gait and motor output in Parkinson's patients were evaluated. Third, multisensory EMG PR is used as the control strategy for assistive devices such as intelligent prosthesis and exoskeleton [33–36], these auxiliary devices can effectively help patients in physical rehabilitation, and to a certain extent reduce the burden of the physical therapy. In addition, multi-sensor fusion also allows these devices to obtain higher security and a more comfortable user experience. For example, in [37], an exoskeleton hand is designed to help paralyzed people in rehabilitation training. It uses myoelectricity as an input to represent the patient's intention and uses angle information and gripping force information as feedback to provide reference and correction for EMG signals in real-time, ensuring that the rehabilitation action can be completed accurately. The above three application scenarios are conceptually depicted in Figure 1.

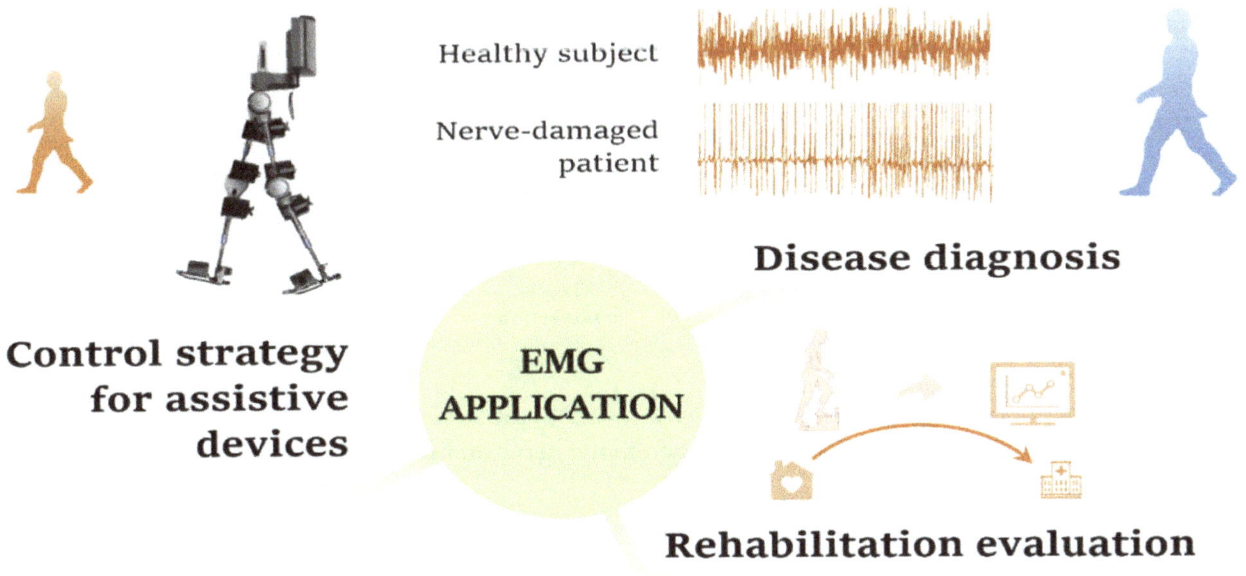

Figure 1. The conceptual depiction of the application scenarios of the electromyography (EMG) pattern recognition technique.

To provide a timely and systematic overview of the EMG based pattern recognition techniques using multisensory fusion strategies in the context of rehabilitation, this review article is composed. The paper is structured as follows: we first introduce the basic physiology knowledge relevant to EMG-based PR in Section 2. Then, in Section 3, a detailed explanation of the processing procedure and comparison of the state-of-the-art EMG PR is presented. Afterward, Section 4 explains the collaborations between EMG and multi-sensory information and presents diverse multisensory strategies successfully applied in different rehabilitation scenarios. Finally, the challenges faced by EMG PR and the prospect in resolving these challenges are summarized in Section 5.

2. Physiology Background

For reader convenience in understanding the working principle for EMG pattern recognition, some relevant physiological backgrounds, including the mechanism of EMG generation and the target patterns, are essential prior knowledge. This chapter will explain these physiological backgrounds, which helps readers to understand the characteristics of EMG signals and the design of recognition systems for the target patterns.

2.1. EMG Signal Overview

EMG is a type of technique used to evaluate and record a series of electrical signals that emanate from body muscles [38]. The principle of the generation of the EMG signal can be described as follows. Motor nerve cells produce electrical pulses under the control of the central nervous system in the cerebral cortex. These neural signals are transmitted to muscle fibers through axons and cause pulse sequences, which activate them to contract and produce muscle tension. Meanwhile, a current is generated in the human body that brings about transmembrane potential [39]. The transmembrane potential is the difference between the internal and external potentials of muscle cell membranes. When muscle cells are in a quiet state, the cell membrane potential is polarized. The potential difference between the inside and outside of the cell membrane under the polarization state is called resetting potential. Depolarization occurs when the cell is excited, and this trend will spread to around [40]. The corresponding action potential is defined as an electromyography signal. The above procedure is demonstrated in Figure 2.

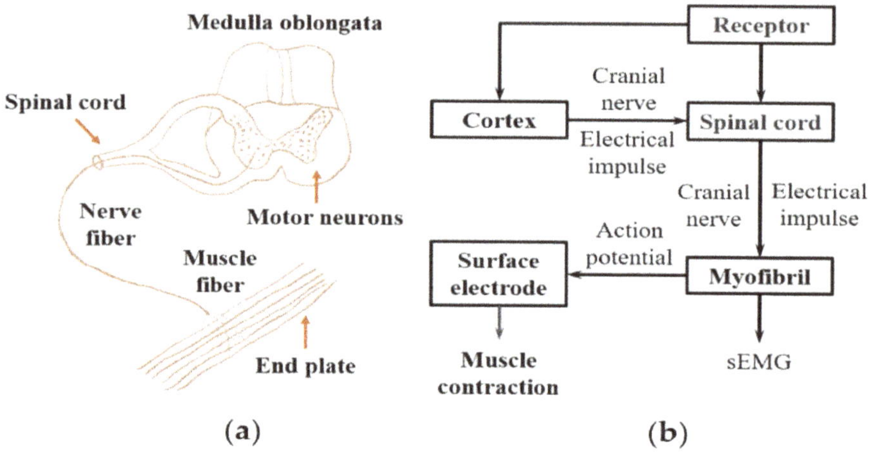

Figure 2. The principle of generation of the EMG signal. (**a**) the structure of the neuro-muscular system. (**b**) the schematic of the EMG signal transduction in the nerve and muscle system.

2.2. Human Movement Patterns

As the EMG signal is a bioelectrical signal controlled by the mutual effect of the receptors and nerve system of human beings, the pattern of the EMG signal relies on both the user's subjective intention and the interactive environment conditions while performing specific actions. In this section, we will introduce some frequently studied upper and lower limb patterns in relevant studies.

The upper limbs of the human body include a forearm, elbow, rear arm, wrist, and hand. The muscle mass of the upper limb is generally small and slender, and the movement range of the upper limb is not extensive. Compared with the lower limbs, the muscle strength of the upper limbs is generally weaker because the body does not need to be supported.

The main functions of the upper limbs are grasping, stretching, and expressing information with hand gestures. Therefore, the patterns in the upper limb can be divided into two categories: limb position and hand gestures. The classification of Limb positions has been elaborated comprehensively in [25], including P1: arm hanging at the side, elbow bent at 90 degrees; P2: straight arm reaching up (45 degrees from vertical); P3: straight arm hanging at side; P4: straight arm reaching forward. Hand gestures account for the dexterous movements of the hand, including wrist and finger movements. Wrist gestures are the hand movements that rotate the whole hand around the wrist joint, but finger gestures only involve the movements of the fingers. Reference [27] proposed a challenging set of 15 gestures in which 5 (thumb, index, middle, ring, pinky) are finger gestures, 6 are wrist gestures. The above patterns are demonstrated in Figure 3.

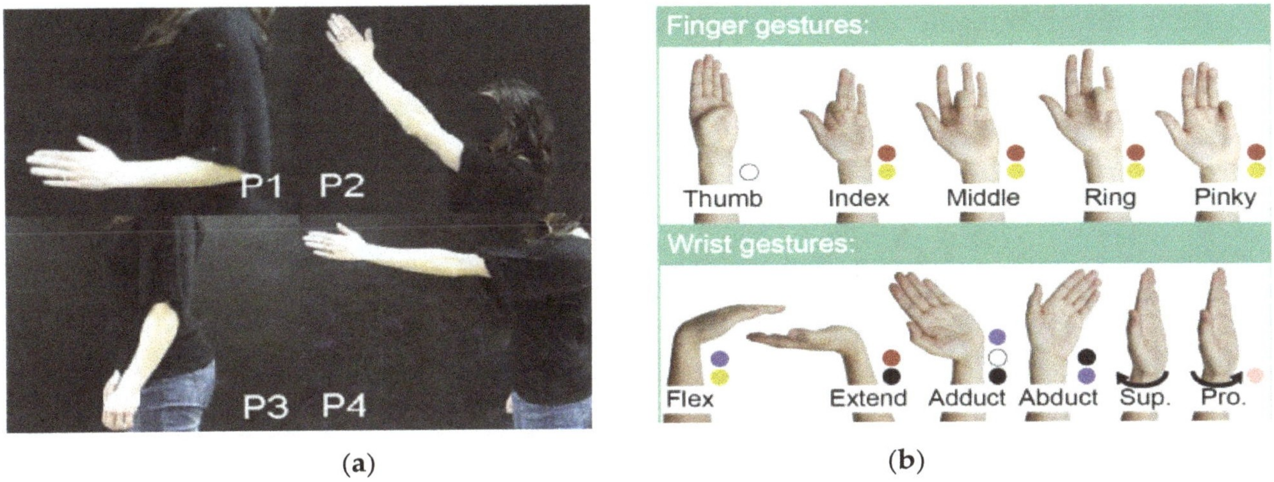

Figure 3. Two types of upper limb patterns. (**a**) the limb position, adopted from [25]. (**b**) hand gestures, adopted from [27].

The lower limbs of the human body include the hip, thigh, calf, foot, hip, knee, ankle, and other joint parts. The lower limb has the characteristics of larger muscle tissue and a larger joint movement angle [41]. Its function is mainly to support the human body and change the position of the human body. Depending on these physiological functions of the lower limbs, the activities most closely related to the lower limbs are often activities with the core of walking behavior, so the activity recognition based on the lower limbs can be roughly summarized in two aspects, namely, the locomotion mode and the gait phase.

The first one is locomotion mode, which aims at the process that the brain actively coordinates the limbs to make different actions when the human body is facing different environments in the real world. Specifically, up and downslope, walking on flat ground, up and downstairs are the most widely studied in the relevant research [35,42,43]. This is not only because these five sports modes are the most common and widespread scenes in life, but also because these modes have the process of overcoming the influence of gravity and changing the center of gravity of the body, so auxiliary equipment is needed to adjust the lower limbs [44,45]. In addition to these five kinds of sports modes, some work has also been done to study such sports modes as crossing obstacles [29,46], turning [29], standing, and sitting transition [47]. These locomotion modes are a more in-depth interpretation than simple actions, such as leg swinging, touchdown, etc., which is conducive to the auxiliary equipment to have a better understanding of the user's environment and generate adaptive control based on this.

Gait phase is another widely concerned lower limb mode, which is a scientific decomposition and utilization of human periodic walking movement. There are different ways to define the gait phases according to different usage scenarios. The simplest one is to divide the gait into two phases: namely, the stance phase and swing phase [3]. Generally, the heel strike (HC) and toe-off (TO) are used as the starting point of the stance phase and the swing phase, respectively [48]. However, this division is not accurate enough and is not applicable in scenes that require high continuity. In [42], a definition of the gait phase consisting of four phases is proposed and used for real-time recognition. In the most precise definitions, the gait cycle can be divided into eight phases [49].

The function of the gait phase is to provide auxiliary equipment to refine the human walking process and provide different auxiliary control in different gait segments [42,50]. The characteristics of the gait phase, such as continuity, duration, and so on, to describe the whole walking cycle of the human body, is a standard method in gait analysis and has been proved to be related to the diagnosis of some diseases [51]. Figure 4 shows the five most commonly studied locomotion modes, as well as a detailed definition of the gait phases.

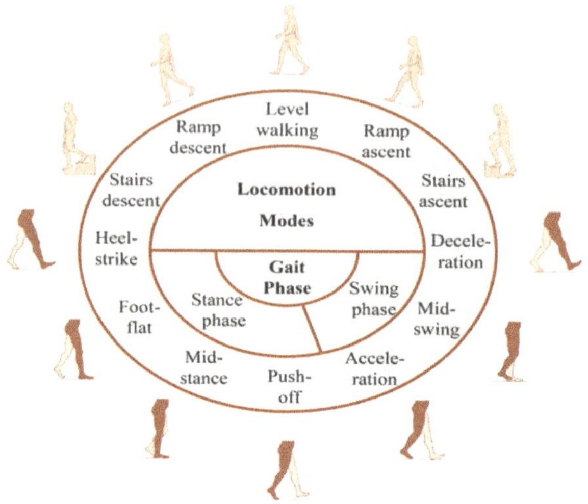

Figure 4. The two commonly studied lower-limb patterns, i.e., locomotion modes and gait phase. Five locomotion modes, along with the definition of the eight-phases gait cycle, are presented here.

3. EMG Pattern Recognition Pipeline

The differences in human body motion patterns can be reflected in EMG signals. However, the raw EMG data is usually very noisy and cannot be directly classified. Therefore, a series of processing procedures is necessary to distinguish these differences accurately. Generally, the PR procedure can be summarized in the following four steps (also depicted in Figure 5):

1. Data acquisition
2. Signal preprocessing
3. Feature extraction and reduction
4. Classification

There is no universal standard for these processing procedures yet, owing to the variability for EMG PR in different rehabilitation scenarios. Therefore, in this section, we will explain the EMG PR protocols and approaches adopted by relevant studies in detail.

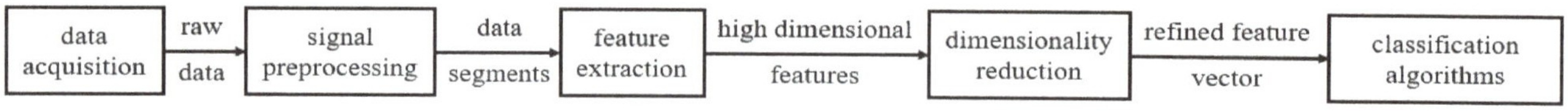

Figure 5. The pipeline of performing EMG pattern recognition.

3.1. Data Acquisition

Acquiring a high-quality EMG signal is strongly desired to ensure a satisfying recognition accuracy level, so properly designing the front-end EMG acquisition approaches is very important. In this section, we will compare the methods in front-end EMG acquisition from two aspects: the design of the EMG sensing system and the selection of muscle measurement points.

3.1.1. EMG Sensing System

The sensing system for collecting EMG signals is mainly composed of electrodes, amplifiers, microprocessors, and transmission devices. The electric signal generated by the muscle is picked up by the electrodes, amplified by the amplification circuit, and then transmitted to the host computer via the transmission device. Generally, the connection between electrodes and processor is wired while the transmission is typically wireless.

In the collection of EMG, the design of the sensor module is typically highly similar, except for the electrode. Common EMG electrodes include two main kinds of pole placement methods: monopolar electrode and bipolar electrode. Both placing methods measure the potential with reference to the electrode placed at the locations without EMG response (e.g., ankle or knee), while the Monopoles method directly measures the potential difference and bipolar method apply the differentiate amplification method [52]. Bipolar electrodes have a higher usage frequency because the common mode noise can be suppressed in real application but lack of setup flexibility when compared to monopoles. Besides, the EMG signal quality is also influenced by the distance between each electrode pole and their diameters and widths when bipolar electrodes are applied [38,52].

In addition to electrode placement, the implantation of the electrode is also reviewed here. Intramuscular EMG and surface EMG are two mainstream Electromyography signal acquisition schemes. Usually, intramuscular EMG signals are recorded using percutaneous fine wire electrodes or others made of similar materials. These electrodes need to be inserted into several muscle tissues using hypodermic needles [53]. Insertion locations are identified by palpation [54] and verified by electrical stimulation and EMG channel activity during corresponding test contractions. Different from intramuscular EMG signal collection, surface EMG (sEMG) electric potentials are acquired with electrodes placed on the skin just above the target muscle [52]. Electrodes occurring in previous experiments are usually made of silver. Typically, there are two ways for operators to contact the electrode with the skin. One is by using a silver chloride gel to achieve wet contact while the other applies dry electrodes with microneedles to record EMG signals [43].

According to the literature research, surface EMG hosts a higher usage frequency compared with intramuscular EMG [52,55–57]. The main reasons for its wide application are regarded to be non-invasive and convenient. Modern surface EMG electrodes are stuck to the surface of muscle and avoid the danger of causing potential muscle injuries to tissue, which is considered to be the critical concern in intramuscular EMG. Besides, during the use of sEMG, operators can freely select measurement points on the surface of muscle tissue and reduce the time cost to do the preparation work like disinfecting the probe points with alcohol. Nevertheless, some bold attempts in the application of intramuscular EMG have also been provided recently [53,54]. Intramuscular EMG provides another signal source to detect the human body behavior and handles some difficulties related to sEMG-based control, such as the unstable contact of the electrode with the skin. Some other additional benefits of intramuscular EMG are given in [53], for example, the ability to record deep muscle signals with little EMG crosstalk. Although the experimental results in [53,54,58] all prove that intramuscular EMG could not bring with the reduction in classification error from sEMG for single classifiers while the significant decrease of classification error for parallel classifiers can be achieved. According to the practical efforts in [53,54], the parallel configuration for simultaneous control becomes more promising via the use of intramuscular EMG, which has long been an unsolved problem in sEMG studies.

3.1.2. Muscle Site Selection

In the thesis of movement recognition, reasonable muscle group selection for EMG signal obtainment is of considerable significance for robust recognition. Various muscle groups in both the lower and upper limbs are functioning and positioned differently, and Figure 6 demonstrates the anatomical structure of the muscles.

Real muscle selection needs to consider the previous experience and specific demand in the application scenario. For example, as for prosthetic control, which is mainly designed for the amputees, experimenters commonly choose the proximal muscle groups like thigh muscle group [29,35,42] and the upper arms [59] because the distal ones are considered to be amputated. While, as for the studies oriented for non-amputees subjects, the distal muscle groups such as the shank muscle tissues and forearm and wrist muscles are often selected as targeted muscles due to their lower inter-subject variability than the proximal [43,60,61]. Gao Shuo [43] chose a pair of distal antagonistic muscles, tibialis anterior (TA) and soleus (SL) to conduct the terrain identification experiment and got satisfying results. Besides, muscle characteristic is also an important aspect to be taken into account. For example, the proximal hip muscle groups (AM, GM, and PRF) are taken into consideration in [9] due to their sensitivity to different walking speeds. It has been proved in [61] that rectus femoris (RF) and Soleus (SL) are responsible for pulling the body forward at the stance phase of the gait and therefore studies related to the recognition of uphill/upstairs behaviors demanding to overcome the gravity are more likely to choose such muscles for EMG detection [62]. The selected criterion and the specific muscle groups selected by relevant studies have been summarized in Table 1.

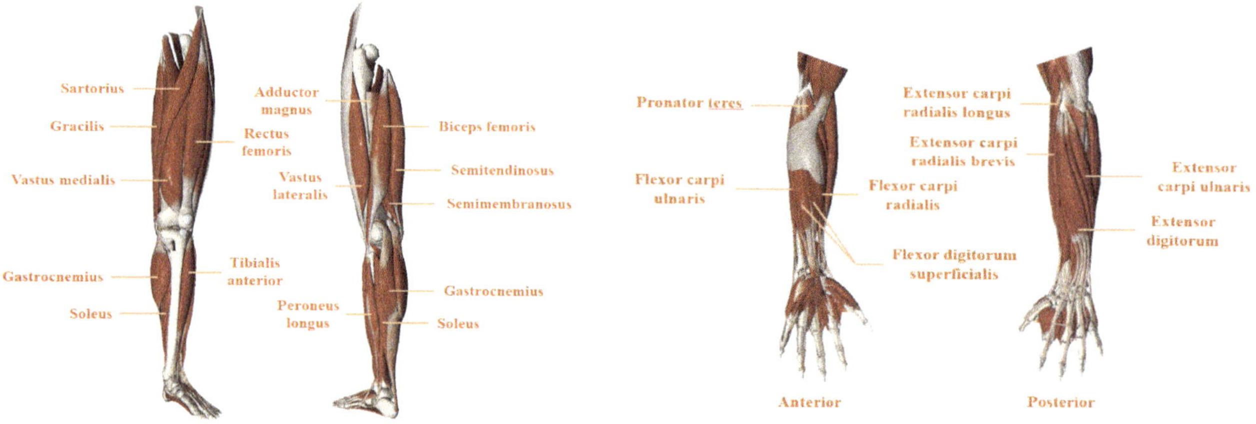

(a) (b)

Figure 6. Longitudinal representation of the muscle groups of (**a**) the lower limb (shank and thigh). (**b**) the upper limb (elbow and hand).

3.2. Signal Preprocessing

The original EMG signals obtained through the front-end acquisition equipment are generally noisy, and pattern recognition requires the use of signals of limited length for further processing. Therefore, this section will introduce filtering and windowing preprocessing methods to reduce the noise in raw data and segmenting the EMG signals.

Real EMG signals are usually mixed with various kinds of noise due to environmental disturbance and other uncontrollable factors in the experiments. Reasonable preprocessing is necessary for extracting useful features in further analysis. Filtering, normalization, and windowing are the three most common EMG data preprocessing methods. The filtering technique derives from classical signal process schemes of signal preprocessing in the frequency domain. Most of the energy of the EEG signal are mainly within the frequency range 0–500 HZ [65]. In [66,67], it is stated that high-frequency (500–1000 HZ) EMG signal is likely to be interfered with by the aliasing. As for the low-frequency region (1–10 HZ), it is mainly regarded as a kind of noise caused by the cable movement and the interface of the measurement electrode and the skin. Actually, the most commonly used EMG signal filter is essentially a finite impulse response bandpass filter with a cutoff point of 10 HZ (low) and 500 HZ (high) [68–70].

Table 1. Summary of the selected muscle group for detecting electromyography (EMG) signals.

No.	Proximal Muscle	Distal Muscle	Comments
[42]	SAR, RF, VL, VM, GRA, BFL, SEM, BFS, ADM	/	Gluteal muscles (gluteus maximus and gluteus medius) on the amputated side and the thigh muscles of the residual limb were monitored
[35]	RF, VL, VM, BFL, SEM, BTS, TFL	/	The accurate electrodes locations are adjusted according to the able-bodied subjects and transfemoral subjects
[29]	SAR, RF, VL, VM, GRA, BFL, SEM, BFS, ADM	/	It should be noted that the locations of EMG electrodes on the distal muscles were approximate
[60]	/	TA, SL	Although only two muscles are selected, the classification accuracy is still satisfying
[59]	TPA, DPA, PMC, BCL, TBL, FCR, ECR	/	One of the eight signal channels is used for the synchronization of data from the Fastrack while the left seven are utilized to collect muscle activities signal.
[27]	/	FDS, FDP, EDC, EIP, EMP	These selected muscles are responsible for controlling all fingers except the thumb.
[9]	AM, GM, PRF, VL, VM	/	The proximal hip muscle groups have higher rates of the change in EMG activation with regard to different walking speeds while the distal knee extensor muscle groups show higher rates of change for different waling slopes
[61]	GM, RF, VL, BFL	TA, GA, SL	Humans often change gait patterns to prevent overexertion and possible injury to the relatively small dorsiflexor muscles, which are walking close to maximum capacity.
[63]	RF, VL, SEM		These three thigh muscles are the most commonly used muscles to classify locomotion modes at different speeds.
[64]	BF, RF	MG, TA	To reflect the effect of gait speed and gender on joint motion of lower extremity more comprehensively, bilateral lumbar erectors spinae are also utilized besides the muscles mentioned before.

Muscles: TA = Tibialis Anterior; SL = Soleus; SAR = Sartorius; RF = rectus femoris; VL = vastus lateralis, VM = vastus medialis; GRA = gracilis; BFL = biceps femoris long head; SEM = semitendinosus; BFS = biceps femoris short head; ADM = adductor magnus.

Due to the difficulty when dealing with the long-term sensor data sequence, windowing operation is necessary to slice it into short clips for the real-time prediction task. Generally, the properties of the signal decide the window length when analyzing the EMG data. According to [71], EMG signal can be considered a wide-sense Gaussian random process. Therefore, proper window length is of great significance for information extraction. The too-long window will lead to clips with an unbearable variance, while too shot sequence may not be able to contain enough useful information for classification [72]. Huang, He et al. [29] state that the analysis window length should not exceed 200 ms, which is an ideal upper bound to control the signal variation. Research in [8,72] suggests that windows of 150–250 ms for EMG are the optimal tradeoff between the classification accuracy and the delay, while 100–250 ms windows can be used for mechanical sensors. Fast time response is also desired for continuous classification tasks in addition to high classification accuracy [29]. In [42,72], a method called overlapping analysis windows was applied to accelerate the decision update. The key aspect of this scheme lies in the careful window increment setting. The smaller the window increment step, the faster the classification result can be achieved. Furthermore, overlapping can help obtain better classification performance when processing the transition phase, such as from the sitting phase to the standing phase [42].

3.3. Feature Extraction

After the signal was preprocessed, the noise was attenuated and the window segments were obtained. However, using the entire segment as the input data is not an ideal choice due to the high computation cost and poor correlation between the input data and the target patterns, which would negatively affect the recognition performance. Therefore, it is necessary to extract some features from each window sequence. In this section, the two most commonly applied feature extraction approaches, including time-domain features, frequency domain features, and autoregressive features, are reviewed and compared.

The time-domain features of the EMG signal are based on the characteristic index of the statistical method, which regards the EMG signal as a function of time. This is an intuitive interpretation of the EMG signal. Its calculation is directly related to the magnitude of window segments, which occupies small calculation resources. In [71,73,74], Hudgins et al. proposed several time-domain features that are widely used in the following researches, including mean absolute value (MAV), mean absolute value slope, slope sign changes (SSC), waveform lengths (WL) and zero crossings (ZC). In [75], time-domain features like root mean square (RMS), waveform length (WL), number of zero-crossings(ZC), variance (VAR) and maximum(MAX) value are combined to represent the feature space.

The frequency-domain features of EMG signal are mainly to transform the time-domain signal of EMG signal into a frequency-domain signal through Fourier transform, and then analyze the spectrum characteristics or power spectrum characteristics of the signal. The advantage of this method is that it overcomes the characteristics of a time-domain signal, which is greatly affected by noise, is relatively weak, and it is easier to extract stable characteristic indexes by analyzing EMG signals in frequency-domain. Common frequency domain features are comprehensively investigated in [76]. Lots of experimental results demonstrate that mean frequency (MNF), median frequency (MDF), mean peak frequency (PKF), mean power (MNP), frequency ratio (FR), power spectrum ratio (PSR), and variance of central frequency (VCF) are not good features for EMG signal-based locomotion mode classification. Joint time-frequency domain features have been proved to be capable of effectively representing transient EMG patterns resulting from dynamic contractions [77]. The experiments comparing the time domain methods and time-frequency methods have also been conducted, and results show that the wavelet packet transform (WPT) is the best method to increase the EMG information density.

Apart from the conventional time and frequency domain feature extraction approaches, there are other ways of extracting effective features. For example, autoregressive (AR) features are usually taken into consideration in lower limb locomotion mode analysis. Huang. He et al., applied autoregression features (three-order autoregression coefficients) and time-domain features (MAV, ZC, and WL) for locomotion identification for their computation efficiency and fast time-response property.

In recent years, there are also handcrafted features that do not rely on statistical techniques. Instead, they use the prior knowledge of biomechanics to select the specific response point at the experimental curve. For example, in [43], twenty-one biomechanical features such as the peak EMG interval between two selected muscles and the duration of the EMG activation time are carefully selected. Such an extraction technique obtained an accuracy of 96.8% and is proven to outperform the traditional feature extraction technique. Although this kind of method seems lacking the general capability dealing with different scenarios, the classification performance is satisfying for the only specific task and shows less generality than the conventional features. There are also researches dedicating to improving the efficiency of the conventional feature extraction methods by designing new features. For example, in a most recent research [78], three time-domain features, including ASS,

MSR, and ASM, are specially proposed to improve the performance of EMG-PR based strategy in arm movement classification task. Experimental results showed that the new-designed features could achieve the accuracy 92.00% ± 3.11%, which is 6.49% higher than that of commonly used time-domain features [72].

3.4. Dimensionality Reduction

When the extracted feature set occupies a high-dimensional space, it may lead to the failure to correctly classify the patterns because the discriminative features are hidden in the complex feature space. Efficient data dimensionality reduction technique not only reduces the computation cost but also proves to be powerful in increasing the inter-class distance, enhancing recognition accuracy. Two commonly used dimensionality methods, i.e., feature projection and feature selection, are being discussed in this section.

3.4.1. Feature Projection

The feature projection method means projecting the original high dimension feature space into a lower-dimensional feature space. The most important characteristic of such a method is that it uses all the original features to get the reduced feature space, which will not bring any information loss. Many algorithms are proposed to accomplish this task, including approaches like principal components analysis (PCA) [77,79], Non-negative matrix factorization (NMF) [80], averaging [75], independent components analysis [81], nonlinear projection [82] and. We will mainly introduce the PCA and NMF approaches in this section.

PCA is regarded as one of the most commonly used linear dimensionality reduction techniques. It essentially takes the direction with the largest variance as the main feature and off-correlates the data in each orthogonal direction, which makes them irrelevant in different orthogonal directions. Therefore, PCA also has some limitations. For example, it can remove linear correlation very well, but there is no way for higher-order correlation. For data with high-order correlation, Kernel PCA can be considered, and the nonlinear correlation can be achieved through the Kernel function turning to linear correlation. The research in [83] illustrates the importance of having relevant embedded muscle activity features in a low-dimensional space. It is also demonstrated in this paper that the PCA technique can efficiently capture features from EMG signals in an unsupervised manner. Due to the parameterless characteristic, PCA is convenient for universal implementation but having trouble for personalized optimization itself. Besides, some other methods about the strategic combination of features have also been leveraged in recent papers, and they are improving towards the direction with higher speed and accuracy. For example, FastICA is proposed in [84] to overcome the difficulty of previously used ICA for high-density EMG signal decomposition.

Non-negative Matrix Factorization (NMF) is another dimensionality reduction technique that has also been widely studied in recent years [80,85]. D.D.Lee et al. point out in [85] that NMF reduces data dimensionality by approximately factorizing the source data into two matrices. The factorization aims to extract the latent structure from the source data to a lower-dimensional space by minimizing the predefined cost function whose value is inversely proportional to the quality of the approximation. Common cost functions include conventional least square error and Kullback-Leibler divergence. As for its application in EMG signal recognition, G.R.Naik and H.T.Nguyen first studied the identification of EMG finger movement with a nonnegative matrix factorization technique [80]. Recently, non-negative matrix factorization is also leveraged to select the subject-specific signal channel for improving the lower-limb motor imagery recognition accuracy. Apart from this, NMF is also found to be put into practice in the determination of muscle synergies while utilizing EMG signals [86].

Actually, lots of other data dimensionality reduction methods have been investigated in recent years due to the quick progress in data science, like Uncorrelated Linear Discriminant Analysis (ULDA) [87], the locality preserving projections (LPP), neighborhood preserving embedding (NPE), discriminant analysis (OFNDA) and so on. These methods provide different dimensions to increase the distinguishable information density, which will help improve recognition accuracy and processing speed.

3.4.2. Feature Selection

Feature selection means reasonably selecting a subset of features to form the new feature space, while the rest of the original features would be abandoned [88,89]. It has been proved by numerous empirical results that feature reduction can reduce data dimensionality and the computational complexity meanwhile.

A key problem in the feature selection method is that what factors should be taken into consideration to define the best EMG feature space, Zardoshti-Kermani, Mahyar, et al. [90] came up with some standards to evaluate the EMG feature space including maximum class separability, robustness, and computational complexity.

Diverse approaches have been proposed to help select more representing features from the dataset containing too much useless data. Some work derives from combining the specific physical or statistical properties. In the task like limb posture classification, deterministic approaches have been proposed to select the optimal feature-channel pairs [91]. In this work, a distance-based feature selection to determine a separability index is utilized. Besides, to measure the amount of mutual information between features and classes, a correlation-based feature selection method was applied, and both schemes were proved effective to boost the posture classification accuracy.

Evaluating relevant features is another novel approach to make feature selection proposed in recent years [92–97]. One newest work formulates the feature selection problem as the optimization problem and proposes a personal best guide binary particle swarm optimization (PBPSO) to solve the feature selection, which works by evaluating the most informative features from the original feature set [93]. In another recent paper [97], a feature selection algorithm called ReliefF is given from the heuristic angle. This algorithm first selects the random instance of one of the database classes and then searches for the k nearest neighbor instances.

3.5. Classification Algorithms

Once the features with the reduced dimensionality are determined, classification algorithms should be deployed to distinguish the different categories of the extracted feature vectors. Numerous algorithms have been proposed, and in this section, we will review some of the most frequently utilized algorithms in EMG PR, along with the comparison between them.

Traditional classification methods include linear discriminant analysis (LDA) [98], support vector machine (SVM) [99,100], k nearest neighbor (KNN) [101,102], Bayesian analysis, fuzzy logic (FL) [103] and hidden Markov models(HMM) [104] while some modern methods have also been given like artificial neural network (ANN) [105] and convolutional neural network (CNN) along with the recent progress in deep learning research. All of the above methods are effective in classifying the extracted feature space while they each have specific characteristics due to their intrinsic difference at the algorithm level. Therefore, we will briefly explain the basic principle of each type of algorithm along with the comparison of their classification performance at different rehabilitation scenarios.

LDA is one of the most simple but effective methods which has attracted great attention in recent years. Linear discriminant analysis is utilized in for lower limb prosthesis movement mode recognition and achieves competitive accuracy of 97.45% even compared with neural network classifiers while deploying a PCA reduced feature set. In another recent work [105], LDA in a One-Vs-One topology was used for non-weight bearing lower-limb movement recognition immediately after training. Nevertheless, a fatal disadvantage for the LDA model is that it is not capable of handling the linear inseparable problem even if given perfect data. At this point, ANN enjoys the ability to describe nonlinear class boundaries among different categories. MLP and Cascade are the two main structures of artificial neural networks. Identification and classification of different gait phases according to the collected EMG data is a classical linear inseparable problem. In new research focusing on this problem [104], three different MLP is deployed for the classification of two main gait phases while directly using the raw EMG data without feature extraction. The experimental comparison demonstrates that the performance of three MLP models achieves an average higher accuracy over all the popular models. On the other hand, in scenarios that some dimensionality reduction techniques like PCA have linearized the discrimination task, LDA can behave even better than the ANN methods. Besides, due to the well-defined classifier inner architecture, LDA possesses better performance stability. Nevertheless, for a given problem, it may be not easy to determine the optimal size and structure of an ANN. At last, in spite of the advantage of extracting latent features from unprocessed EMG data, the long training period is another thing that we need to take into consideration when intending to apply the ANN.

The SVM is estimated as one of the most popular approaches utilized in the movement mode classification. It is an effective data classification approach that projects the low-dimension data to the high-dimension feature space via kernel function. SVM works by finding a hyperplane to distinguish different categories in high-dimension space through the training process. It is believed that proper kernel function can help reduce the indivisible linear data to linear separable set in high-dimension space. From this, it is obvious that the most crucial problem when building the SVM model is to determine the optimal kernel function and its parameter values. Pires, Ricardo, et al. [99] uses the SVM algorithm to classify lower-extremity EMG signals during running shod/unshod with different foot strike patterns. It is also mentioned that kernel function selection, and parameter setting should depend on the specific task scenario. In [100], the SVM algorithm is utilized to develop an automatic classification system for lower limb hemiparetic patients. The empirical results demonstrate that SVM has the highest accuracy (95.2%) than KNN (89.2%) and ANN (92.3%). Particle swarm optimization (PSO) has long been a classical heuristic optimization algorithm. According to our literature review, the related works hybridizing the PSO and SVM to detect movement patterns are growing continuously in recent years. Zheng, Jiajia, et al. [106] employ PSO-optimized SVM to classify four gait phases, including initial contact, mid stance, terminal stance, and swing phase. The experimental results show that PSO-SVM exhibits the distinctive advantages on gait phase classification and improves the classification accuracy up to 32.9%–42.8% compared with the classifier based on vanilla SVM. Recently, some work compares the performance of common classifiers in different scenarios to provide references in practical application. The comparative analysis among NLR, MLP and SVM shows that for either classification performance and for the number of classification parameters, SVM attains the highest values followed by MLP, and then by NLR [107]. It should also be noted that SVM can obtain the highest classification performance while utilizing the lowest sampling rate.

Fuzzy Logic (FL) is another technique used in the classification of EMG signals, which achieves definite conclusions just from imprecise data input in a simple manner. It has been studied that FL exhibits the advantage of control techniques in biosignal processing [103]. FL can extract unrepeatable EMG features and mimic user's intent to make a decision. On the other hand, FL requires more system memory and processing time because of the use of fixed geometric-shaped membership functions in fuzzy logic limits system knowledge more in the rule base than in the membership function base [103].

The application of the hidden Markov model (HMM) is described in [108], where it is used for recognition of gait mode based on electromyographic signals. A modified Baum-Welch was used to estimate the parameter of HMM, and the Viterbi algorithm achieved the recognition of gait mode by finding the best HMM and state to assign corresponding phases to the given segments.

KNN classifier is another kind of common biosignal classifier based on traditional machine learning techniques. The authors in [101] use the K-nearest neighbor method to classify the EMG signals recorded from lower limb muscles during standing in individuals with complete spinal cord injury implanted with spinal cord epidural stimulation. Actually, most KNN-related researches in this area are correlated with other classification algorithms to find the most suitable classifiers for some certain problem. In [102], weighted KNN and SVM are both utilized as the classifier to distinguish the sEMG signals for controlling a prosthetic foot while the comparison of the accuracy of two classifies shows that weighted KNN obtains higher efficiency.

With the rapid development of deep learning technology in recent years, increasing attention has been paid to the deep feature classifier. For example, a backpropagation neural network was used in [109] to map the optimal surface EMG features to the FE angle angles. The experimental results show that the features extracted from multichannel surface EMG signals using deep belief network method proposed in this paper outperform principal components analysis (PCA), and the RMS error between the estimated joint angles and calculated ones during human walking is reduced by about 50%.

4. Multisensory Fusion

Through a series of processing, the change of movement patterns creates a stronger correlation with the EMG signal. However, due to the interactions between the lower limb movement and the external environment, as well as the low resolution of the upper limb hand fine movement in the EMG signal, the sensing strategy relying only on the EMG signal has great limitations in these two types of rehabilitation scenes. To address these issues, multisensory fusion techniques are proposed and proved to be capable of boosting pattern recognition accuracy by collecting more efficient data from different dimensions.

Generally, the EMG-centered fusion strategy can be divided into two types, i.e., fusion with kinematic sensors and fusion with kinetic sensors. The former strategy is mainly to supplement the three-dimensional motion information like human body acceleration, angular velocity, angle, etc. While the latter one is mainly to supplement the force information during the movement process. In this section, we will explain the detailed procedures of these two fusion strategies and demonstrate some successful applications using these techniques in different rehabilitation scenarios. Figure 7 demonstrates a block diagram of the above EMG-centered fusion strategy.

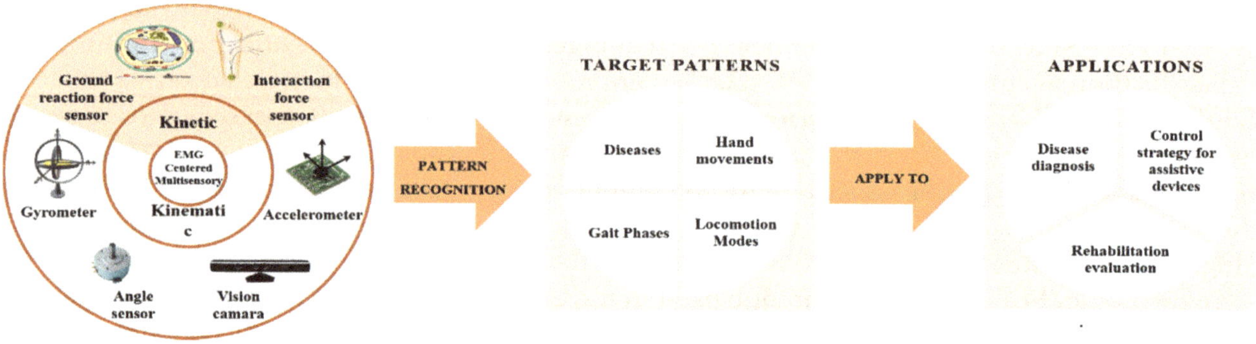

Figure 7. EMG-centered multisensory strategies and sensing blocks.

4.1. Fusion with Kinematic Sensors

Kinematic sensors are widely used in obtaining the locomotion properties of targets. In recent years, kinematic sensors have also attracted enough attention in human behavioral study combined with biosignal sensors (e.g., EMG). Kinematic information of human lower extremity describes the movements of the joints and limbs. Generally, the kinematic sensors can be divided into two main categories, inertial sensors and motion capture systems. Inertial sensors, including accelerometer, gyroscope, and magnetometer, are often used to collect kinematic data like joint angles, joint angular velocity, body orientation, and limb acceleration, etc. Motion capture systems became popular only in recent years, their biggest advantage being that they can collect locomotion information in a contactless manner.

Kinematic sensors' advantage of intuitively reflecting the 3D motion information of the limb helps compensate for the defect of EMG sensors, which only describes the whole physical process from the human nerve activity angle. Combing bioelectrical signal and motion information like acceleration has also been investigated to improve locomotion classification accuracy. Researchers in [110] especially investigate the improvement in classification error while utilizing EMG and kinematic data together rather than pure kinematic data. The empirical results demonstrate that the higher recognition rates can be obtained with combined data compared with vanilla kinematic information from the hip joint of non-dominant/impaired limb and an accelerometer.

The most successful use of the kinematics-EMG fusion strategy lies in the control of powered lower-limb prostheses. Such devices help people get rid of the disability and restore normal walking ability. Nevertheless, the adaptability of the prosthesis to other parts of the human body is still a challenging subject in which the kernel issue can be regarded as inferring human locomotion intent. Due to the restriction of the traditional recognition approach only relying on kinematic data, some recent works are making the steps to fuse EMG and mechanical information to improve the performance. The locomotion recognition system used for lower limb prosthesis control in [35] fuse the multichannel EMG signals and accelerometer measurements in feature level. The physical test shows that the empirical accuracy is over 95%, which is significantly better than traditional schemes, only applying surface Electromyography for identifying locomotion modes [29,35]. In [111], A combination of kinematic and electromyographic (EMG) signals recorded from a person's proximal humerus was used to evaluate a novel transhumeral prosthesis controller. Most especially, they trained a time-delayed artificial neural network to predict elbow flexion/extension and forearm pronation/supination from six proximal EMG signals, and humeral angular velocity and linear acceleration. Young, A. J. [15] studied the contribution of EMG data in combination with a diverse array of mechanical sensors to locomotion mode intent recognition in transfemoral amputees using powered prostheses. And this can indeed significantly reduce intent recognition errors both for transitions between locomotion modes and steady-state locomotion.

In addition, EMG centered kinematic fusion technique is also seen in applications of the hand gesture recognition. This is because the dexterous movement of the finger movements varies more significantly in the position information than the EMG information. Therefore, it is an ideal choice to combine them to obtain intention information and position information at the same time. For example, inertial measurement unit(IMU) and myoelectric units are utilized to implement the hand gesture-based control of an omnidirectional wheelchair in [112]. The system component, sensor placement, and the characteristic collected signals are demonstrated in Figure 8. In this system, the classification, which involves recognizing the activity pattern based on the periodic shape of triaxial wrist tilt angle and EMG-RMS from the two selected muscles, helps the accuracy improve to 94%.

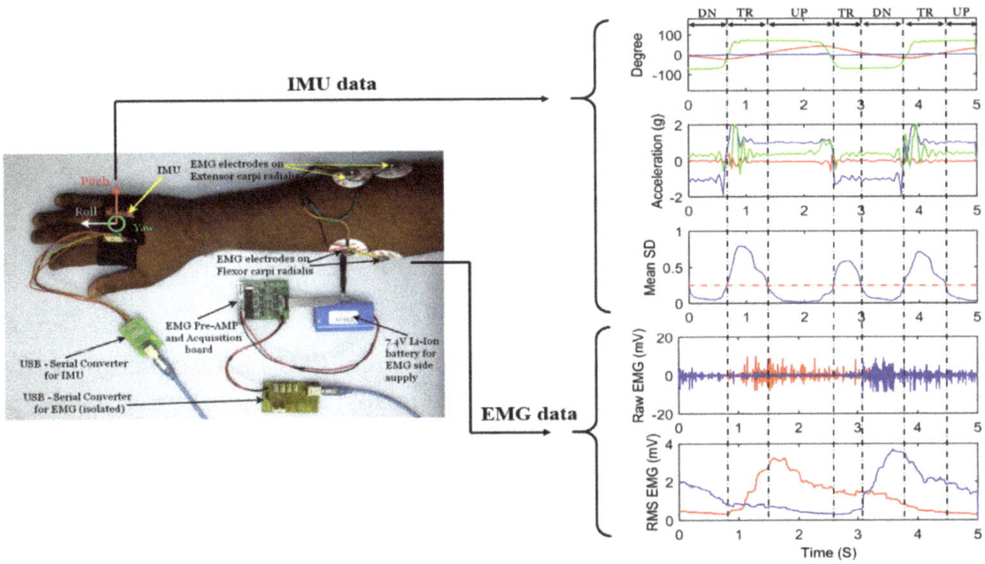

Figure 8. The fusion strategy of combining kinematics data (IMU) and EMG data, adopted from [112].

Utilizing vision technique is another effective and direct way to detect the kinematic information of human. Recently, with the vigorous development of computer vision, some researchers are trying combining the vision and EMG information for limb motion classification task. In a newly published work [113], researches implemented a framework that allows the integration of multi-sensors, EMG and visual information, to perform sensor fusion and to improve the accuracy of hand gesture recognition tasks. For embedded applications, even-based cameras were utilized to run on the limited computational resources of mobile phones. The online results of hand gesture recognition using fusion approach reached 85%, which is 13% and 11% higher than utilizing EMG and vision individually.

4.2. Fusion with Kinetic Sensors

Kinetic sensors are a kind of instrument used to measure forces and moments that are directly connected with the movement of body segments like lower limbs. Various types of force transducers, including piezoelectric [114,115], strain gauged [116,117], and capacitive transducers [118–120], have been widely used in the design of force-sensitive sensors. Joint use of kinetic sensors and electromyography sensors is believed to be able to extract human muscle reflex related information, which will help the recognition of specific body behaviors. Generally, two types of kinetic information, interaction force, and ground reaction force can both be integrated with EMG information. The following part will introduce the fusion examples with interaction force and ground reaction force, respectively.

Interaction force sensors are typically embedded in a fixed structure and then used to detect the extension or flexion of limb, which are important for interpreting the intention of the human movement. The utilization of interaction force and EMG signals are also seen in the application of the upper limb hand gesture recognition in recent years. The research in [27] showed that combining EMG and pressure data sensed only at the wrist could support the accurate classification of hand gestures. Especially, the EMG is suited to sensing finger movements, the pressure is suited to sensing wrist and forearm rotations, and their combination is significantly more accurate for a range of gestures than either technique alone. Figure 9 demonstrates the implementation of this multisensory approach in hand gesture recognition.

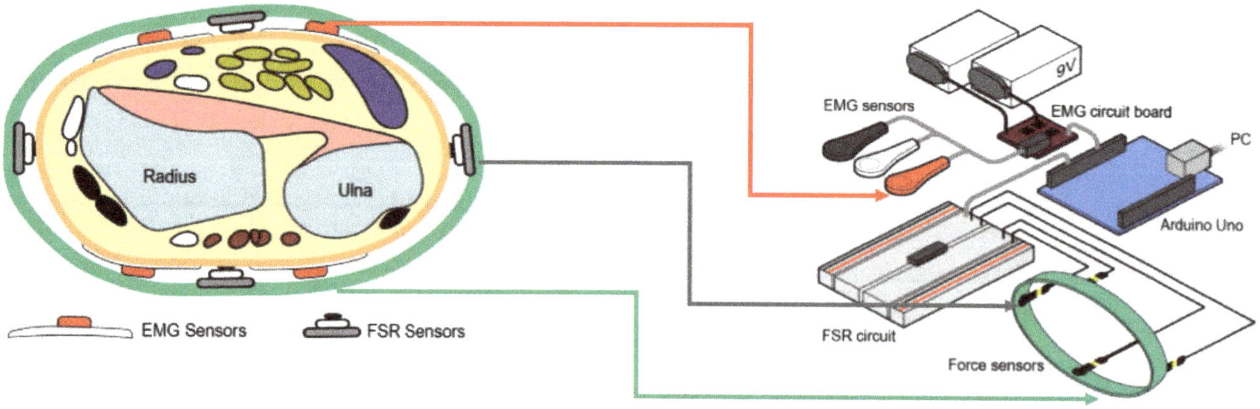

Figure 9. EMG-FSR fusion strategy and hardware diagram used to classify different hand gestures, adopted from [27].

According to our literature review, ground reaction force (GRF) is also a commonly used kinetic information, especially in lower limb rehabilitation scenarios. A typical combination pipeline focus on lower limb prosthesis is shown in Figure 10. Such integration strategy is mainly applied in the lower limb exoskeleton or prosthesis because the lower limb is mostly responsible for interaction with the ground, and many locomotion modes are closely related to the terrain changes, which is directly reflected in the GRF information. Liu, Ming. et al. [35] applied the EMG measurement results and mechanical ground reaction forces/moments recorded using a six-degree-of-freedom load cell to build an adaptive classification strategy, which further enhanced the reliability of neutrally-controlled prosthetic legs. The researchers in [60] presented a smart sensing system utilizing flexible electromyography sensors and ground reaction force sensors for locomotion mode recognition. Here, EMG and GRF information were collected from ten healthy subjects in five common locomotion modes in daily life. Rehabilitation robots is an attractive research zone which mainly helps the patients like stroke regain the locomotion ability. In [121], ground reaction forces and lower extremity electromyography are both utilized to compare inclined treadmill walking and turning conditions with its emulation on a developed balance assessment robot in order to investigate the feasibility of the existing approaches in rehabilitation.

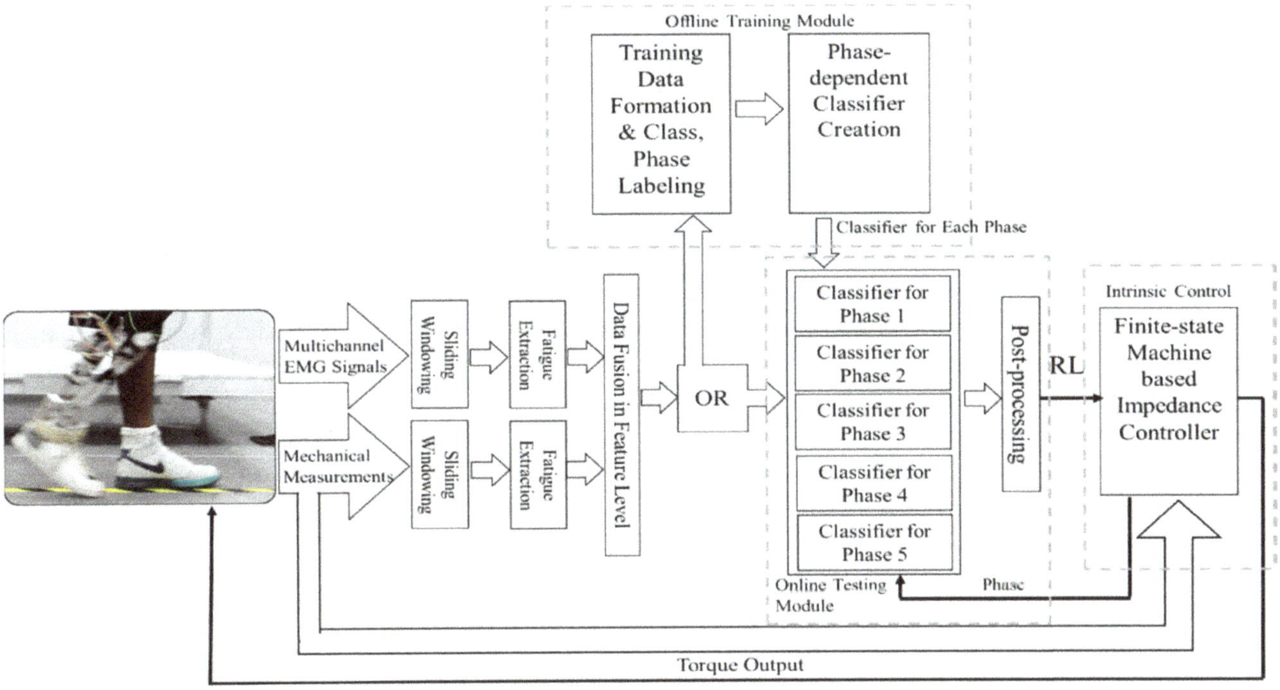

Figure 10. EMG-GRF fusion strategy and the fusion pipeline to recognize different locomotion modes adapted from [27].

4.3. *Fusion with Both Kinematics and Kinetic Sensors*

In addition to the information fusion work introduced above, we also notice some recent work combing EMG with both kinematic and kinetic data. With the improvement of processor performance and the development of machine learning algorithms to handle high dimensional data, this triple-type sensor information fusion, which used to be regarded as a difficult approach, has been implemented and outperforms existing approaches in some motion classification tasks.

Rehabilitation exoskeleton is an important application of kinematic-kinetic fusion strategy. Because this kind of equipment needs various dimensions of information to maintain the highest stability and safety, it can achieve the goal of using EMG as the subjective control input and kinematic and dynamic data as the feedback. The work in [122] used human-robot interaction force, ground reaction force, and EMG sensors to distinguish the walking environment and gait period to provide crucial information for exoskeleton control. The results obtained using an individual mechanical sensor together with sEMG showed improvement compared to the case of only using force sensors, reaching the highest accuracy of 97.8% at gait phase recognition scenarios. The sensing blocks, as well as the location of the sensors, have been demonstrated in Figure 11.

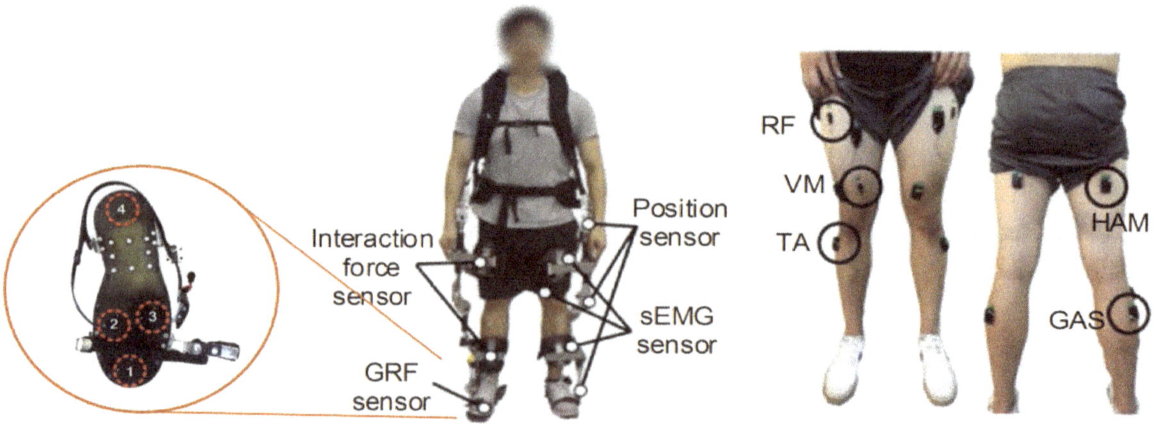

Figure 11. Multisensory fusion strategy using EMG, kinematic sensors, and kinetic sensors together for the application of rehabilitation exoskeleton, adopted from [122].

Gait pattern analysis has also been widely used to assist in the diagnosis of muscle diseases. By multi-sensor data fusion, gait analysis gives objective and quantitative information about the gait pattern and the deviation due to the muscular situation of these patients, which are of great significance to the clinical research. Cui, Chengkun, et al. [121] conducted the simultaneous recognition and assessment of post-stroke hemiparetic gait by fusing kinematic, kinetic, and electrophysiological data. In [123], researchers investigated the gait pattern of 10 patients with myotonic dystrophy (Steinert disease) compared to 20 healthy controls through manual muscle test and gait analysis in terms of kinematic, kinetic and EMG data.

Table 2 summarizes the fusion strategy, targeted recognition classes, extracted features, proposed classifiers, and the final accuracy results of the multisensory application in different scenarios of rehabilitation.

Table 2. Summary of the pattern recognition techniques applied in relevant studies.

No.	Applied Sensors	Classes	Feature	Classifier	Accuracy
[35]	EMG + GRF	Five common locomotion modes (W, RA, RD, SA, SD) and eight task transitions: W->SA, W->SD, W->RA, W->RD, SA->W, SD->W, RA->W and RD->W	EMG data feature: MAV, SL, SSC and ZC, mechanical signals: maximum, minimum, mean value and standard deviation	Entropy-based adaptation (EBA), Learning form testing data (LIFT) and Transductive Support Vector Machine (TSVM)	EBA: 95%, LIFT: 95% and TSVM: 96.25%, vanilla SVM: 87.5%
[42]	EMG + GRF	Locomotion modes: LW, SO, SA, SD, RA and RD and related transitions: W->sA, W->RA, W->O, SD->W, RD->W, SA/RA->W, W->SD/RD	EMG time-domain feature: MAV, SSC, WL, ZC, Mechanical signal features: maximum, minimum, mean value of each direction of force and moment	SVM	99% or higher accuracy in the stance phase and 95% accuracy in the swing phase

Table 2. *Cont.*

No.	Applied Sensors	Classes	Feature	Classifier	Accuracy
[122]	Position sensors, GRF, interaction force EMG	Five walking environments: LW, RA, RD, SA, and SD Seven gait periods: LS, MST, TST, PS, IS, MS and TS	GRF feature: four positions in the foot for four time periods, position feature: three joint angles for four time periods. Interaction force feature: two points in the link for four time periods, sEMG feature: MAV, ZC, SSC and WL	BLDA	96.1%(environment classification accuracy) 97.8%(gait period classification period)
[27]	EMG sensor, pressure force sensor	Finger gestures, wrist gestures, and other gestures	Root mean square (RMS), standard deviation (SD) and peak amplitude	SVM	95.8%
[112]	IMU, EMG sensor	Six hand gestures (forward, clockwise, left, backward, anticlockwise, right)	Nine IMU features extracted from wrist Euler angle and six EMG features extracted from EMG RMS signal	DSVM	Real-time recognition accuracy 90.5%
[124]	EMG signal acquisition system, data glove	Thumb flexion, finger flexion, thumb opposition, middle/ring/little finger flexion, long fingers flexion, tradigital grasp, lateral grip/key grip	MAV (mean of absolute value)	Locally weighted learning	79% for amputee and 89% for non-disabled participants

Classes: LW = level-ground walking; RA = ramp ascent; RD = ramp descent; SA = stairs ascent; SD = stairs descent; SO = stepping over an obstacle; IT = ipsilateral turning; CT = contralateral turning; SS = standing still; LP = loading response; MST = midstance; TST = terminal stance; PS = pre-swing; IS = initial swing; MS = mid-swing; TS = terminal swing. Feature: MAV = mean absolute value; ZC = zero crossing; SSC = slope sign changes; WL = waveform length; SL = signal length.

5. Challenges and Future Development

Currently, fruitful results have been achieved by EMG-centered multisensory pattern recognition methods in the rehabilitation field. However, there are still limitations in terms of accuracy, robustness, data volume, and flexibility when current approaches are applied to practical applications. In this section, we will explain the main issues and potential solutions and research directions of multisensory EMG PR.

5.1. Low Data Quality

Low data quality is a pressing problem in EMG detection, especially under a multisensory fusion scenario. Because the data quality of each dimension can significantly affect the final recognition accuracy. Since bioelectrical signals are generally more susceptible to noise interference, in EMG centered multisensory fusion, the data quality of EMG signals is the most important influential factor.

In Section 3, we explain the preprocessing of the EMG signal, whose purpose is mainly to reduce the noise in the raw EMG signal. Although by the preprocessing technique, the deterministic noise, e.g., charger noise, can be filtered and stochastic noise such as white noise can be compressed, interference comes from the source of the bioelectric signal that is challenging to be removed by data processing technique. First, the EMG crosstalk effect is an inevitable interference in EMG detection [22].

It means that the amplitude of the EMG signal is not only contributed by the targeted muscle but also influenced by the adjacent and surrounding muscles, hindering precise detection of the muscle activity. Second, electrode shift also results in severe EMG signal misregistration, since the traditional electrochemical gel electrode suffers difficulty in firmly attaching to the skin; a shift of merely 1 cm would reduce the classification accuracy by 5% to 20% [125]. Third, even when the patient performs the same locomotion under the same environment, the applied muscle force may slightly change due to the impossibility in perfectly controlling the body, resulting in the variations of the EMG signals of the selected muscles, and reducing the data quality [19].

Advanced sensing and detecting means could be possible solutions to the problem of low-quality data. With the integration and miniaturization of sensory circuits, high-density EMG (HD-EMG) has become a promising sensing approach. This type of sensing technique increases the coverage and density of the electrodes. Hundreds of electrodes are integrated with a small size overlying a restricted area of the skin [126,127]. The most significant benefit of HD-EMG is that the possibility of subtracting information at the motor unit level greatly improved compared with conventional EMG, minimizing the effect of EMG crosstalk at this precision level. The multiple electrodes are arranged in the form of a two-dimensional array, for example, in the shape of 8×24 [127] or 8×16 [126], which will produce an "EMG image". The EMG image presents a comprehensive view of EMG signals both in the time domain and spatial domain, providing far richer information than the conventional EMG electrode placement method of implementing one or two electrodes at a single muscle. For example, the HD-EMG arrays attached to the elbow area were used for the precise hand gesture recognition, reaching the accuracy as high as 99.0% in classifying twenty-seven gestures [126]. A typical procedure of utilizing the "EMG image" generated by the HD-EMG to conduct pattern recognition is demonstrated in Figure 12. Even though abundant information can be extracted with the help of HD-EMG, it also increased the burden of the acquisition and processing hardware. Because the sampling rate of EMG signals requires at least 1000 Hz at each channel, an 128 channel HD-EMG system will produce over 128,000 observations in one second, which would make the data scale enormous and lead to challenges in real-time processing.

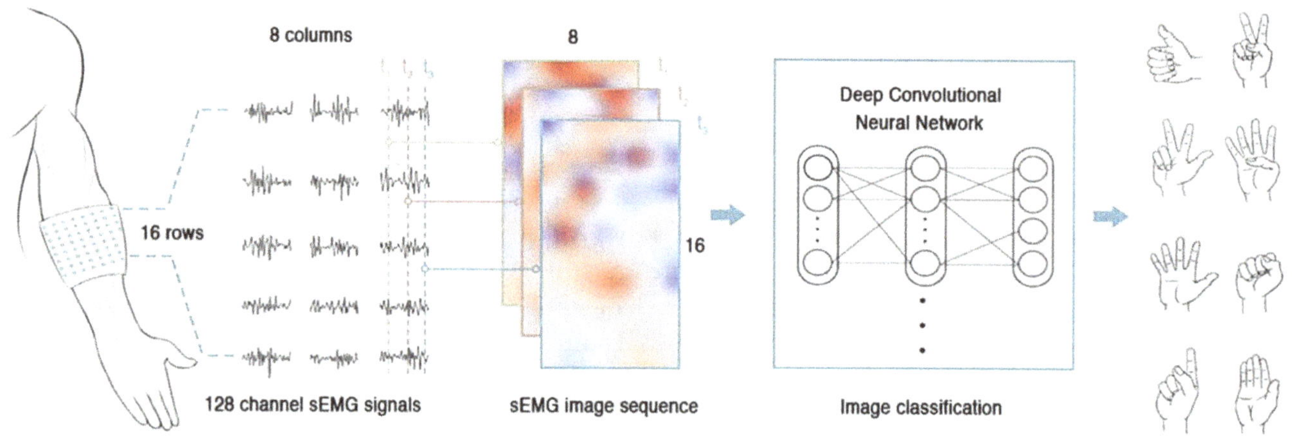

Figure 12. The procedure of applying High-Density EMG (HD-EMG) in discriminating hand gestures, adopted from [126].

5.2. *Inadequate and Undisclosed Data*

High-quality data acquisition is the premise of high-precision multisensory pattern recognition. Meanwhile, for multi-sensor fusion, due to the large variability in the patient's muscle and physical condition and the difficulty in obtaining high-quality multisensory data, adequate and open-source data is of equal importance. This section will explain the necessity of establishing a big and open sensor data library in detail, and review some currently developing databases.

Currently, most of the current EMG researches were recruiting a relatively small volume of the volunteers to collect EMG signals, such as 5–20 healthy individuals or no more than five patients. The relatively small size is owing to the limited access to experimental resources due to the insufficient funding budget. Therefore, recruiting tens of participants is a balanced choice for verifying the proposed algorithms for most research groups. Nevertheless, there are a few concerns about this choice.

Firstly, the variation of the EMG signal is usually significant in different individuals. A strong correlation between EMG signals and the age, height, weight, exercise habits, and health status of individuals are found in relevant studies [128]. The sample size of tens of experimenters is often difficult to cover all these differences between various populations. Besides, researchers usually adopt their experimental protocols and different sensing equipment, and it is not easy to investigate the generality of the method proposed by one work across these influential factors.

Furthermore, the requirement of sensing equipment for robust EMG acquisition is quite high, and the collection system is typically expensive. It may potentially hinder some labs or researchers who do not have the experimental conditions from investigating EMG signals on the algorithm level.

An important approach for solving the above problem is to promote the concept of "big data-based EMG," which means that the verification method of EMG pattern recognition should shift from the verification in small sample experimental data to the performance of the proposed algorithm based on big data in different populations. Well-established datasets not only allows researchers to examine the quality and correctness of their acquired data more conveniently but testing the generality of their proposed methods in different datasets. In addition, larger datasets enable the application of some advanced algorithms such as deep learning in digging the underlying information in EMG signals [129].

In the past, the experiment data of EMG were mostly stored within the laboratories of individual researchers rather than publishing online, which made it hard to gather multiple datasets. In recent years, with the occurrence of "data paper," researchers are encouraged to publish their experimental data as an individual publication [130]. Such scientific publications promote the transparency of the raw data, and thus more EMG datasets are being available. In addition, there are also studies dedicated to establishing a standard dataset, trying to provide a standard experimental procedure and cover as many different muscles, movements, and population as possible. A few influential datasets such as Surface Electromyography for the Non-Invasive Assessment of Muscles (SENIAM), The Ninapro project [131] have emerged in recent years. However, there is still a long way to go in reaching the consensus of a widely accepted protocol and establishing a thorough dataset.

5.3. Discrete Interpretation of Continuous Movements

The development of the data quality and quantity offers the possibility to develop more effective processing techniques, especially in improving the simultaneity and continuity of the EMG-PR-based control strategy, which are two key drawbacks at the state of the art technique. In this section, we will explain how simultaneity and continuity problem is affecting the EMG PR performance, and provide possible solutions and research directions in the light of the multisensory technique.

As mentioned earlier, the EMG PR technique is widely used in the real-time Human-Machine Interface system (HMI). However, the broad use of clinical viable EMG based robots are still not reported yet. The potential problem is that a complete pipeline, including sensing, signal transmission, and processing, has to be done in order to recognize the current pattern. There is a time delay in this procedure, and it is acceptable in some scenarios, such as sign language recognition, when only static patterns like hand gestures are to be recognized. However, the patterns relevant to lower limbs are mostly dynamic and require real-time and instant recognition, and therefore the time delay may greatly influence the application of conventional PR technique in lower limb HMI devices.

There are several attempts to resolve the problem of discrete interpretation. One of them is to design the transition logic between two consecutive patterns skillfully, and some pioneers studies are trying to design the transition strategy. In [42], overlapped windows are utilized to overcome the time delay problem, and the comparison between the overlapped windows and non-overlapping windows are depicted in Figure 13. The increment of two consecutive and the overlapped window is only 12 ms, generating approximate continuous decision flow. The majority vote method is used to prevent misjudging problem. In addition, because the EMG signal is generated before the actual motion, there are also studies using the currently collected signals to predict the patterns in the next moment so that the robotic actuators could react in advance to adapt to the changing patterns [132,133]. However, the prediction method is only applicable in the periodical movement like gait, and still have difficulties in predicting more complicated motions. So far, there is still no consensus on the best transition method among EMG patterns, and the robust transition is a research interest in the EMG PR field.

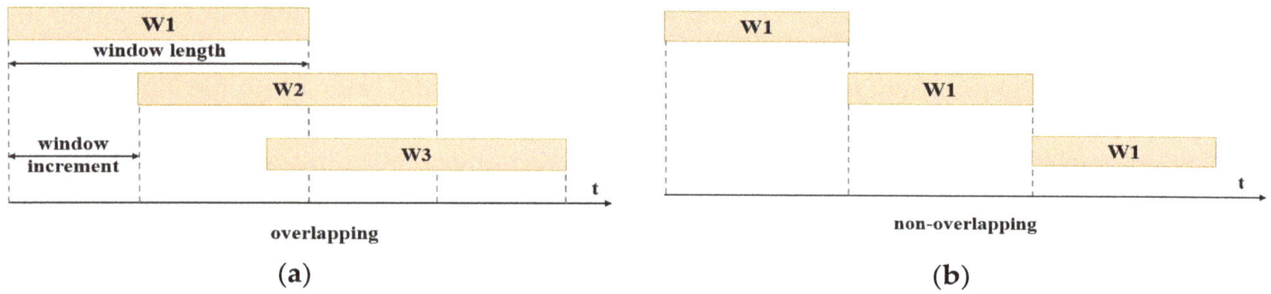

Figure 13. A conceptual depiction of: (**a**) the overlapping windowing method. (**b**) the non-overlapping windowing method.

With the development of multisensory fusion and the increasingly thorough study of human body motion, the method of combining the biomechanical model with pattern recognition is also attracting increasing attention. Some open-source software, like OpenSim, is developed to provide present biomechanical models. With the help of the multisensory fusion, both the EMG signals and other mechanical signals collected from the patient's body can be used to calibrate and specialize the raw biomechanical models. After that, with proper mapping strategies, these models can be driven by EMG signals and, therefore, intuitively simulate the movement of human extremities, providing crucial information for continuous control of HMI systems. For example, a model-based control strategy is proposed in [134], using the EMG signal as the input for the carefully tuned and calibrated hand-finger biomechanic model, and managed to continuously control a prosthesis hand to finish the task of gripping in the response time of 16.2 ms per loop. The control schemes and multisensory strategy is demonstrated in Figure 14. Nevertheless, the model-based method requires tedious procedures to calibrate and tune the model, and it is proved difficult to separate the EMG signals into distinct functional movements for the subject with small arms. At present, it is still in the laboratory research stage.

5.4. Future Analysis

In the above three sections, we explain the challenges of multisensory EMG PR and the emerging technologies potentially capable to solve these challenges. We believe that in the foreseeable future, multisensory EMG PR has high possibility to develop in these three directions for the following reasons. Firstly, the application of the novel EMG sensing technique, e.g., High-Density EMG, will greatly improve the EMG signal's quality. Besides, the spatial resolution of the EMG signals will also be enhanced from the level of distinguishing different muscle tissues to the level of distinguishing single cells, making it possible for EMG signals to apply in detection of very fine movements. Secondly, more open source databases with high data quality, complete muscle measurement points and rich application scenarios will be built, which will further reduce the obstacles of self-designed experiments and attract more researchers to join the field of EMG signal analysis. Thirdly, with the reduction of EMG research barriers, the research of EMG analysis algorithm will continue to increase, and more advanced algorithms to solve the traditional PR problem, such as the overlapping window and biomechanical model mentioned in this paper, will be proposed and verified.

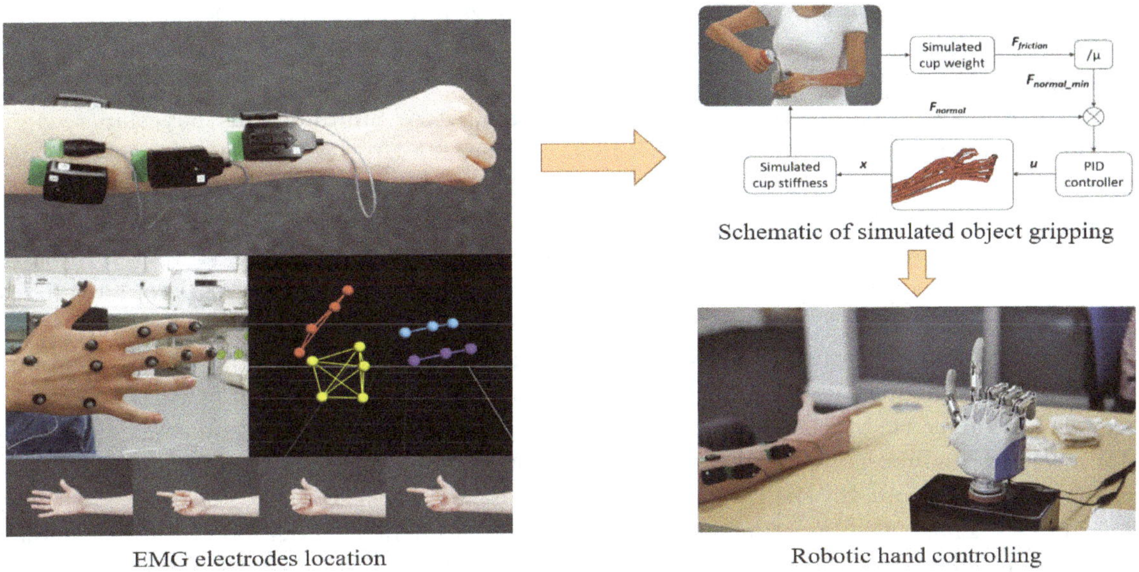

Figure 14. The schematic of utilizing biomechanical based and EMG centered multisensory technique in controlling a robotic hand, adopted from [134].

6. Conclusions

Employing electromyography (EMG) centered multisensory integration pattern recognition (PR) techniques demonstrates strong potential in precisely interpreting patients' intentions and locomotion modes, which are of significance for analyzing the progress of rehabilitation status. However, commercialized products widely applied in hospitals or home-based internet of health things (IoHT) have not been reported yet. This article aims to reveal the reason behind this phenomenon by thoroughly reviewing the state-of-the-art research outcomes and providing a comprehensive analysis of limitations. The content provided here not only allows readers to have a full picture view of this area but also shows potential directions in further enhancing the development of applying EMG centered multisensory fusion PR techniques in rehabilitation associated applications.

Author Contributions: Conceptualization, C.F., and S.G.; methodology, C.F. and B.H.; validation, C.F., B.H., and S.G.; investigation, B.H.; resources, S.G., J.C.; data curation, B.H.; writing—original draft preparation, B.H.; writing—review and editing, C.F.; visualization, Y.W.; supervision, S.G.; project administration, C.F.; funding acquisition, S.G. All authors have read and agreed to the published version of the manuscript.

References

1. Bisio, I.; Delfino, A.; Lavagetto, F.; Sciarrone, A. Enabling IoT for in-home rehabilitation: Accelerometer signals classification methods for activity and movement recognition. *IEEE Internet Things J.* **2016**, *4*, 135–146. [CrossRef]
2. Moore, Z.; Sifferman, C.; Tullis, S.; Ma, M.; Proffitt, R.; Skubic, M. Depth Sensor-Based In-Home Daily Activity Recognition and Assessment System for Stroke Rehabilitation. In Proceedings of the 2019 IEEE International Conference on Bioinformatics and Biomedicine (BIBM), San Diego, CA, USA, 18–21 November 2019; pp. 1051–1056.

3. Nazmi, N.; Rahman, M.A.A.; Yamamoto, S.I.; Ahmad, S.A. Walking gait event detection based on electromyography signals using artificial neural network. *Biomed. Signal. Process. Control.* **2019**, *47*, 334–343. [CrossRef]
4. Joshi, D.; Hahn, M.E. Terrain and Direction Classification of Locomotion Transitions Using Neuromuscular and Mechanical Input. *Ann. Biomed. Eng.* **2016**, *44*, 1275–1284. [CrossRef] [PubMed]
5. Tao, W.; Liu, T.; Zheng, R.; Feng, H. Gait Analysis Using Wearable Sensors. *Sensors* **2012**, *12*, 2255–2283. [CrossRef] [PubMed]
6. Martinez-Hernandez, U.; Mahmood, I.; Dehghani-Sanij, A.A. Simultaneous Bayesian recognition of locomotion and gait phases with wearable sensors. *IEEE Sens. J.* **2017**, *18*, 1282–1290. [CrossRef]
7. Young, A.J.; Ferris, D.P. State of the Art and Future Directions for Lower Limb Robotic Exoskeletons. *IEEE Trans. Neural Syst. Rehabil. Eng.* **2017**, *25*, 171–182. [CrossRef]
8. Long, Y.; Du, Z.-J.; Wang, W.-D.; Zhao, G.-Y.; Xu, G.-Q.; He, L.; Mao, X.-W.; Dong, W. PSO-SVM-based online locomotion mode identification for rehabilitation robotic exoskeletons. *Sensors* **2016**, *16*, 1408. [CrossRef]
9. Kang, I.; Kunapuli, P.; Hsu, H.; Young, A.J. Electromyography (EMG) Signal Contributions in Speed and Slope Estimation Using Robotic Exoskeletons. In Proceedings of the 2019 IEEE 16th International Conference on Rehabilitation Robotics (ICORR), Toronto, ON, Canada, 24–28 June 2019; pp. 548–553.
10. Ziegier, J.; Gattringer, H.; Mueller, A. Classification of gait phases based on bilateral emg data using support vector machines. In Proceedings of the 2018 7th IEEE International Conference on Biomedical Robotics and Biomechatronics (Biorob), Enschede, The Netherlands, 26–29 August 2018; pp. 978–983.
11. Gui, K.; Liu, H.; Zhang, D. A Practical and Adaptive Method to Achieve EMG-Based Torque Estimation for a Robotic Exoskeleton. *IEEE Asme Trans. Mechatron.* **2019**, *24*, 483–494. [CrossRef]
12. Setiawan, J.D.; Ariyanto, M.; Munadi, M.; Mutoha, M.; Glowacz, A.; Caesarendra, W. Grasp Posture Control of Wearable Extra Robotic Fingers with Flex Sensors Based on Neural Network. *Electronics* **2020**, *9*, 905. [CrossRef]
13. Kańtoch, E. Recognition of sedentary behavior by machine learning analysis of wearable sensors during activities of daily living for telemedical assessment of cardiovascular risk. *Sensors* **2018**, *18*, 3219. [CrossRef]
14. Jin, D.; Yang, J.; Zhang, R.; Wang, R.; Zhang, J. Terrain identification for prosthetic knees based on electromyographic signal features. *Tsinghua Sci. Technol.* **2006**, *11*, 74–79. [CrossRef]
15. Young, A.; Kuiken, T.; Hargrove, L. Analysis of using EMG and mechanical sensors to enhance intent recognition in powered lower limb prostheses. *J. Neural Eng.* **2014**, *11*, 056021. [CrossRef]
16. Chen, X.; Zeng, Y.; Yin, Y.H. Improving the Transparency of an Exoskeleton Knee Joint Based on the Understanding of Motor Intent Using Energy Kernel Method of EMG. *IEEE Trans. Neural Syst. Rehabil. Eng.* **2017**, *25*, 577–588. [CrossRef] [PubMed]
17. Kilicarslan, A.; Prasad, S.; Grossman, R.G.; Contreras-Vidal, J.L. High accuracy decoding of user intentions using EEG to control a lower-body exoskeleton. Proceedings of THE 2013 35th annual international conference of the IEEE Engineering in Medicine and Biology Society (EMBC), Osaka, Japan, 3–7 July 2013; pp. 5606–5609.
18. Scheme, E.; Englehart, K. Electromyogram pattern recognition for control of powered upper-limb prostheses: State of the art and challenges for clinical use. *J. Rehabil. Res. Dev.* **2011**, *48*, 643–660. [CrossRef] [PubMed]
19. Samuel, O.W.; Asogbon, M.G.; Geng, Y.; Al-Timemy, A.H.; Pirbhulal, S.; Ji, N.; Chen, S.; Fang, P.; Li, G. Intelligent EMG pattern recognition control method for upper-limb multifunctional prostheses: Advances, current challenges, and future prospects. *IEEE Access* **2019**, *7*, 10150–10165. [CrossRef]
20. Kawamoto, H.; Taal, S.; Niniss, H.; Hayashi, T.; Kamibayashi, K.; Eguchi, K.; Sankai, Y. Voluntary Motion Support Control of Robot Suit HAL Triggered by Bioelectrical Signal for Hemiplegia. In Proceedings of the 2010 Annual International Conference of the IEEE Engineering in Medicine and Biology Society, Buenos Aires, Argentina, 31 August–4 September 2010; IEEE: New York, NY, USA, 2010; pp. 462–466. [CrossRef]
21. Kawamoto, H.; Lee, S.; Kanbe, S.; Sankai, Y. Power assist method for HAL-3 using EMG-based feedback controller. In Proceedings of the 2003 IEEE International Conference on Systems, Man and Cybernetics, Washington, DC, USA, 5–8 October 2003; pp. 1648–1653.
22. Solomonow, M.; Baratta, R.; Bernardi, M.; Zhou, B.; Lu, Y.; Zhu, M.; Acierno, S. Surface and wire EMG crosstalk in neighbouring muscles. *J. Electromyogr. Kinesiol.* **1994**, *4*, 131–142. [CrossRef]

23. Al-Timemy, A.H.; Khushaba, R.N.; Bugmann, G.; Escudero, J. Improving the performance against force variation of EMG controlled multifunctional upper-limb prostheses for transradial amputees. *IEEE Trans. Neural Syst. Rehabil. Eng.* **2015**, *24*, 650–661. [CrossRef]
24. Sadikoglu, F.; Kavalcioglu, C.; Dagman, B. Electromyogram (EMG) signal detection, classification of EMG signals and diagnosis of neuropathy muscle disease. *Procedia Comput. Sci.* **2017**, *120*, 422–429. [CrossRef]
25. Scheme, E.; Fougner, A.; Stavdahl, Ø.; Chan, A.D.; Englehart, K. Examining the adverse effects of limb position on pattern recognition based myoelectric control. In Proceedings of the 2010 Annual International Conference of the IEEE Engineering in Medicine and Biology, Buenos Aires, Argentina, 31 August–4 September 2010; pp. 6337–6340.
26. Arozi, M.; Caesarendra, W.; Ariyanto, M.; Munadi, M.; Setiawan, J.D.; Glowacz, A. Pattern Recognition of Single-Channel sEMG Signal Using PCA and ANN Method to Classify Nine Hand Movements. *Symmetry* **2020**, *12*, 541. [CrossRef]
27. McIntosh, J.; McNeill, C.; Fraser, M.; Kerber, F.; Löchtefeld, M.; Krüger, A. EMPress: Practical hand gesture classification with wrist-mounted EMG and pressure sensing. In Proceedings of the 2016 CHI Conference on Human Factors in Computing Systems, San Jose, CA, USA, 7–12 May 2016; pp. 2332–2342.
28. Shultz, A.H.; Goldfarb, M. A Unified Controller for Walking on Even and Uneven Terrain With a Powered Ankle Prosthesis. *IEEE Trans. Neural Syst. Rehabil. Eng.* **2018**, *26*, 788–797. [CrossRef]
29. Huang, H.; Kuiken, T.A.; Lipschutz, R.D. A strategy for identifying locomotion modes using surface electromyography. *IEEE Trans. Biomed. Eng.* **2008**, *56*, 65–73. [CrossRef] [PubMed]
30. Gavin, J.P.; Immins, T.; Wainwright, T. Stair negotiation as a rehabilitation intervention for enhancing recovery following total hip and knee replacement surgery. *Int. J. Orthop. Trauma Nurs.* **2017**, *25*, 3–10. [CrossRef] [PubMed]
31. Rissanen, S.M.; Kankaanpää, M.; Meigal, A.; Tarvainen, M.P.; Nuutinen, J.; Tarkka, I.M.; Airaksinen, O.; Karjalainen, P.A. Surface EMG and acceleration signals in Parkinson's disease: Feature extraction and cluster analysis. *Med. Biol. Eng. Comput.* **2008**, *46*, 849–858. [CrossRef]
32. Jenkins, M.; Almeida, Q.; Spaulding, S.; Van Oostveen, R.; Holmes, J.; Johnson, A.M.; Perry, S. Plantar cutaneous sensory stimulation improves single-limb support time, and EMG activation patterns among individuals with Parkinson's disease. *Parkinsonism Relat. Disord.* **2009**, *15*, 697–702. [CrossRef] [PubMed]
33. Fang, Y.; Liu, H.; Li, G.; Zhu, X. A multichannel surface EMG system for hand motion recognition. *Int. J. Hum. Robot.* **2015**, *12*, 1550011. [CrossRef]
34. Yoshikawa, M.; Mikawa, M.; Tanaka, K. Real-time hand motion estimation using EMG signals with support vector machines. In Proceedings of the 2006 SICE-ICASE International Joint Conference, Busan, Korea, 18–21 October 2006; pp. 593–598.
35. Ming, L.; Fan, Z.; Helen, H.H. An Adaptive Classification Strategy for Reliable Locomotion Mode Recognition. *Sensors* **2017**, *17*, 2020. [CrossRef] [PubMed]
36. Chen, B.J.; Wang, Q.N.; Wang, L. Adaptive Slope Walking With a Robotic Transtibial Prosthesis Based on Volitional EMG Control. *IEEE Asme Trans. Mechatron.* **2015**, *20*, 2146–2157. [CrossRef]
37. Bhattacharyya, A.; Roy, S.; Sarkar, A.D. Active Exoskeleton Hand Exerciser Using Multisensory Feed Back. *Int. J. Ind. Eng. Manag.* **2017**, *2*, 33–36. [CrossRef]
38. Nazmi, N.; Rahman, A.; Azizi, M.; Yamamoto, S.-I.; Ahmad, S.A.; Zamzuri, H.; Mazlan, S.A. A review of classification techniques of EMG signals during isotonic and isometric contractions. *Sensors* **2016**, *16*, 1304. [CrossRef]
39. Farina, D.; Merletti, R.; Stegeman, D. Biophysics of the generation of EMG signals. *Electromyogr. Physiol. Eng. Noninvasive Appl.* **2004**, *4*, 81–105.
40. Ibrahim, A.; Gannapathy, V.; Chong, L.; Isa, I. Analysis of electromyography (EMG) signal for human arm muscle: A review. In *Advanced Computer and Communication Engineering Technology*; Springer: Berlin/Heidelberg, Germany, 2016; pp. 567–575.
41. David, A.W. *The Biomechanics and Motor Control of Human Gait*; University of Waterloo Press: Waterloo, ON, Canada, 1988.
42. Huang, H.; Zhang, F.; Hargrove, L.J.; Dou, Z.; Rogers, D.R.; Englehart, K.B. Continuous locomotion-mode identification for prosthetic legs based on neuromuscular–mechanical fusion. *IEEE Trans. Biomed. Eng.* **2011**, *58*, 2867–2875. [CrossRef] [PubMed]

43. Gao, S.; Wang, Y.; Fang, C.; Xu, L. A Smart Terrain Identification Technique Based on Electromyography, Ground Reaction Force, and Machine Learning for Lower Limb Rehabilitation. *Appl. Sci.* **2020**, *10*, 2638. [CrossRef]
44. Lay, A.N.; Hass, C.J.; Nichols, T.R.; Gregor, R.J. The effects of sloped surfaces on locomotion: An electromyographic analysis. *J. Biomech.* **2007**, *40*, 1276–1285. [CrossRef] [PubMed]
45. Alexander, N.; Schwameder, H. Effect of sloped walking on lower limb muscle forces. *Gait Posture* **2016**, *47*, 62–67. [CrossRef] [PubMed]
46. Ma, L.; Yang, Y.; Chen, N.; Song, R.; Li, L. Effect of different terrains on onset timing, duration and amplitude of tibialis anterior activation. *Biomed. Signal. Process. Control.* **2015**, *19*, 115–121. [CrossRef]
47. Li, B.; Gui, Q.; Ali, H.B.; Li, H.; Jin, Z. A wearable sit-to-stand detection system based on angle tracking and lower limb EMG. In Proceedings of the 2016 IEEE Signal Processing in Medicine and Biology Symposium (SPMB), Philadelphia, PA, USA, 3 December 2016; pp. 1–6.
48. Pappas, I.P.; Popovic, M.R.; Keller, T.; Dietz, V.; Morari, M. A reliable gait phase detection system. *IEEE Trans. Neural Syst. Rehabil. Eng.* **2001**, *9*, 113–125. [CrossRef]
49. Perry, J.; Davids, J.R. Gait analysis: Normal and pathological function. *J. Pediatr. Orthop.* **1992**, *12*, 815. [CrossRef]
50. Jung, J.Y.; Heo, W.; Yang, H.; Park, H. A Neural Network-Based Gait Phase Classification Method using Sensors Equipped on Lower Limb Exoskeleton Robots. *Sensors* **2015**, *15*, 27738–27759. [CrossRef]
51. Abdulhay, E.; Arunkumar, N.; Narasimhan, K.; Vellaiappan, E.; Venkatraman, V. Gait and tremor investigation using machine learning techniques for the diagnosis of Parkinson disease. *Future Gener. Comput. Syst.* **2018**, *83*, 366–373. [CrossRef]
52. Simão, M.; Mendes, N.; Gibaru, O.; Neto, P. A review on electromyography decoding and pattern recognition for human-machine interaction. *IEEE Access* **2019**, *7*, 39564–39582. [CrossRef]
53. Smith, L.H.; Hargrove, L.J. Comparison of surface and intramuscular EMG pattern recognition for simultaneous wrist/hand motion classification. In Proceedings of the 2013 35th annual international conference of the IEEE engineering in medicine and biology society (EMBC), Osaka, Japan, 3–7 July 2013; pp. 4223–4226.
54. Smith, L.H.; Kuiken, T.A.; Hargrove, L.J. Real-time simultaneous and proportional myoelectric control using intramuscular EMG. *J. Neural Eng.* **2014**, *11*, 066013. [CrossRef] [PubMed]
55. Leonard, C.T.; Brown, J.S.; Price, T.R.; Queen, S.A.; Mikhailenok, E.L. Comparison of surface electromyography and myotonometric measurements during voluntary isometric contractions. *J. Electromyogr. Kinesiol.* **2004**, *14*, 709–714. [CrossRef] [PubMed]
56. Samadani, A.-A.; Kulic, D. Hand gesture recognition based on surface electromyography. In Proceedings of the 2014 36th Annual International Conference of the IEEE Engineering in Medicine and Biology Society, Chicago, IL, USA, 26–30 August 2014; pp. 4196–4199.
57. Du, Y.-C.; Lin, C.-H.; Shyu, L.-Y.; Chen, T. Portable hand motion classifier for multi-channel surface electromyography recognition using grey relational analysis. *Expert Syst. Appl.* **2010**, *37*, 4283–4291. [CrossRef]
58. Farrell, T.R. A comparison of the effects of electrode implantation and targeting on pattern classification accuracy for prosthesis control. *IEEE Trans. Biomed. Eng.* **2008**, *55*, 2198–2211. [CrossRef]
59. Martelloni, C.; Carpaneto, J.; Micera, S. Classification of upper arm EMG signals during object-specific grasp. In Proceedings of the Conference proceedings: Annual International Conference of the IEEE Engineering in Medicine and Biology Society, Vancouver, BC, Canada, 21–24 August 2008; pp. 5061–5064.
60. Fang, C.; Wang, Y.; Gao, S. Flexible and Wearable GRF and EMG Sensors Enabled Locomotion Mode Recognition for IoHT Based In-Home Rehabilitation. Available online: https://www.techrxiv.org/articles/Flexible_and_Wearable_GRF_and_EMG_Sensors_Enabled_Locomotion_Mode_Recognition_for_IoHT_Based_In-home_Rehabilitation/11987994/1 (accessed on 21 March 2020).
61. Li, L.; Ogden, L.L. Muscular activity characteristics associated with preparation for gait transition. *J. Sport Health Sci.* **2012**, *1*, 27–35. [CrossRef]
62. Yousif, A.E.; Aziz, M.Y. Biomechanical analysis of the human femur bone during going upstairs and sitting down. In Proceedings of the 2012 First National Conference for Engineering Sciences (FNCES 2012), Baghdad, Iraq, 7–8 November 2012; pp. 1–7.

63. Pati, S.; Joshi, D.; Mishra, A. Locomotion classification using EMG signal. In Proceedings of the 2010 International Conference on Information and Emerging Technologies, Karachi, Pakistan, 14–16 June 2010; pp. 1–6.
64. Chiu, M.-C.; Wang, M.-J. The effect of gait speed and gender on perceived exertion, muscle activity, joint motion of lower extremity, ground reaction force and heart rate during normal walking. *Gait Posture* **2007**, *25*, 385–392. [CrossRef]
65. Komi, P.V.; Tesch, P. EMG frequency spectrum, muscle structure, and fatigue during dynamic contractions in man. *Eur. J. Appl. Physiol. Occup. Physiol.* **1979**, *42*, 41–50. [CrossRef]
66. Larsson, B.; Månsson, B.; Karlberg, C.; Syvertsson, P.; Elert, J.; Gerdle, B. Reproducibility of surface EMG variables and peak torque during three sets of ten dynamic contractions. *J. Electromyogr. Kinesiol.* **1999**, *9*, 351–357. [CrossRef]
67. Wang, J.; Tang, L.; Bronlund, J.E. Surface EMG signal amplification and filtering. *Int. J. Comput. Appl.* **2013**, *82*, 15–22. [CrossRef]
68. Barzilay, O.; Wolf, A. A fast implementation for EMG signal linear envelope computation. *J. Electromyogr. Kinesiol.* **2011**, *21*, 678–682. [CrossRef]
69. Dutta, A.; Khattar, B.; Banerjee, A. Nonlinear Analysis of Electromyogram Following Neuromuscular Electrical Stimulation-Assisted Gait Training in Stroke Survivors. In *Converging Clinical and Engineering Research on Neurorehabilitation*; Springer: Berlin/Heidelberg, Germany, 2013; pp. 53–57.
70. Barsakcioglu, D.Y.; Farina, D. A real-time surface emg decomposition system for non-invasive human-machine interfaces. In Proceedings of the 2018 IEEE Biomedical Circuits and Systems Conference (BioCAS), Cleveland, OI, USA, 17–19 October 2018; pp. 1–4.
71. Hudgins, B.; Parker, P.; Scott, R.N. A new strategy for multifunction myoelectric control. *IEEE Trans. Biomed. Eng.* **1993**, *40*, 82–94. [CrossRef] [PubMed]
72. Englehart, K.; Hudgins, B. A robust, real-time control scheme for multifunction myoelectric control. *IEEE Trans. Biomed. Eng.* **2003**, *50*, 848–854. [CrossRef] [PubMed]
73. Zardoshti-Kermani, M.; Wheeler, B.C.; Badie, K.; Hashemi, R.M. EMG feature evaluation for movement control of upper extremity prostheses. *IEEE Trans. Rehabil. Eng.* **1995**, *3*, 324–333. [CrossRef]
74. Englehart, K.; Hugdins, B.; Parker, P. *Multifunction Control of Prostheses Using the Myoelectric Signal*; CRC Press: New York, NY, USA, 2000; pp. 153–208.
75. Afzal, T.; Iqbal, K.; White, G.; Wright, A.B. A method for locomotion mode identification using muscle synergies. *IEEE Trans. Neural Syst. Rehabil. Eng.* **2016**, *25*, 608–617. [CrossRef]
76. Phinyomark, A.; Phukpattaranont, P.; Limsakul, C. Feature reduction and selection for EMG signal classification. *Expert Syst. Appl.* **2012**, *39*, 7420–7431. [CrossRef]
77. Englehart, K.; Hudgins, B.; Parker, P.A.; Stevenson, M. Classification of the myoelectric signal using time-frequency based representations. *Med. Eng. Phys.* **1999**, *21*, 431–438. [CrossRef]
78. Samuel, O.W.; Zhou, H.; Li, X.; Wang, H.; Zhang, H.; Sangaiah, A.K.; Li, G. Pattern recognition of electromyography signals based on novel time domain features for amputees' limb motion classification. *Comput. Electr. Eng.* **2018**, *67*, 646–655. [CrossRef]
79. Hargrove, L.J.; Li, G.; Englehart, K.B.; Hudgins, B.S. Principal components analysis preprocessing for improved classification accuracies in pattern-recognition-based myoelectric control. *IEEE Trans. Biomed. Eng.* **2008**, *56*, 1407–1414. [CrossRef]
80. Naik, G.R.; Nguyen, H.T. Nonnegative matrix factorization for the identification of EMG finger movements: Evaluation using matrix analysis. *IEEE J. Biomed. Health Inform.* **2014**, *19*, 478–485. [CrossRef]
81. Naik, G.R.; Kumar, D.K.; Palaniswami, M. Surface EMG based hand gesture identification using semi blind ICA: Validation of ICA matrix analysis. *Electromyogr. Clin. Neurophysiol.* **2008**, *48*, 169–180.
82. Gallant, P.; Morin, E.; Peppard, L. Feature-based classification of myoelectric signals using artificial neural networks. *Med. Biol. Eng. Comput.* **1998**, *36*, 485–489. [CrossRef] [PubMed]
83. Naik, G.R.; Selvan, S.E.; Gobbo, M.; Acharyya, A.; Nguyen, H.T. Principal component analysis applied to surface electromyography: A comprehensive review. *IEEE Access* **2016**, *4*, 4025–4037. [CrossRef]
84. Chen, M.; Zhou, P. A novel framework based on FastICA for high density surface EMG decomposition. *IEEE Trans. Neural Syst. Rehabil. Eng.* **2015**, *24*, 117–127. [CrossRef] [PubMed]
85. Lee, D.D.; Seung, H.S. Algorithms for non-negative matrix factorization. In Proceedings of the Advances in neural information processing systems, Vancouver, BC, Canada, 3–8 December 2001; pp. 556–562.

86. Farina, D.; Jiang, N.; Rehbaum, H.; Holobar, A.; Graimann, B.; Dietl, H.; Aszmann, O.C. The extraction of neural information from the surface EMG for the control of upper-limb prostheses: Emerging avenues and challenges. *IEEE Trans. Neural Syst. Rehabil. Eng.* **2014**, *22*, 797–809. [CrossRef]
87. Liu, J.; Zhou, P. A novel myoelectric pattern recognition strategy for hand function restoration after incomplete cervical spinal cord injury. *IEEE Trans. Neural Syst. Rehabil. Eng.* **2012**, *21*, 96–103. [CrossRef]
88. Zhou, P.; Lowery, M.M.; Englehart, K.B.; Huang, H.; Li, G.; Hargrove, L.; Dewald, J.P.; Kuiken, T.A. Decoding a new neural–machine interface for control of artificial limbs. *J. Neurophysiol.* **2007**, *98*, 2974–2982. [CrossRef]
89. Nazarpour, K.; Sharafat, A.; Firoozabadi, S. Surface EMG signal classification using a selective mix of higher order statistics. In Proceedings of the 2005 IEEE Engineering in Medicine and Biology 27th Annual Conference, Shanghai, China, 1–4 September 2005; pp. 4208–4211.
90. Chowdhury, R.H.; Reaz, M.B.I.; Ali, M.A.B.; Bakar, A.A.A.; Chellappan, K.; Chang, T.G. Surface Electromyography Signal Processing and Classification Techniques. *Sensors* **2013**, *13*, 12431–12466. [CrossRef]
91. Al-Angari, H.M.; Kanitz, G.; Tarantino, S.; Cipriani, C. Distance and mutual information methods for EMG feature and channel subset selection for classification of hand movements. *Biomed. Signal. Process. Control.* **2016**, *27*, 24–31. [CrossRef]
92. Boostani, R.; Moradi, M.H. Evaluation of the forearm EMG signal features for the control of a prosthetic hand. *Physiol. Meas.* **2003**, *24*, 309. [CrossRef]
93. Too, J.; Abdullah, A.R.; Mohd Saad, N.; Tee, W. Emg feature selection and classification using a pbest-guide binary particle swarm optimization. *Computation* **2019**, *7*, 12. [CrossRef]
94. Phinyomark, A.; Hirunviriya, S.; Limsakul, C.; Phukpattaranont, P. Evaluation of EMG feature extraction for hand movement recognition based on Euclidean distance and standard deviation. In Proceedings of the ECTI-CON2010: The 2010 ECTI International Confernce on Electrical Engineering/Electronics, Computer, Telecommunications and Information Technology, Chiang Mai, Thailand, 19–21 May 2010; pp. 856–860.
95. Huang, H.; Xie, H.-B.; Guo, J.-Y.; Chen, H.-J. Ant colony optimization-based feature selection method for surface electromyography signals classification. *Comput. Biol. Med.* **2012**, *42*, 30–38. [CrossRef] [PubMed]
96. Liu, J.; Li, X.; Li, G.; Zhou, P. EMG feature assessment for myoelectric pattern recognition and channel selection: A study with incomplete spinal cord injury. *Med. Eng. Phys.* **2014**, *36*, 975–980. [CrossRef] [PubMed]
97. Benazzouz, A.; Guilal, R.; Amirouche, F.; Slimane, Z.E.H. EMG Feature Selection for Diagnosis of Neuromuscular Disorders. In Proceedings of the 2019 International Conference on Networking and Advanced Systems (ICNAS), Annaba, Algeria, 26–27 June 2019; pp. 1–5.
98. Gupta, R.; Agarwal, R. Single channel EMG-based continuous terrain identification with simple classifier for lower limb prosthesis. *Biocybern. Biomed. Eng.* **2019**, *39*, 775–788. [CrossRef]
99. Pires, R.; Falcari, T.; Campo, A.B.; Pulcineli, B.C.; Hamill, J.; Ervilha, U.F. Using a Support Vector Machine Algorithm to Classify Lower-Extremity EMG Signals During Running Shod/Unshod With Different Foot Strike Patterns. *J. Appl. Biomech.* **2019**, *35*, 87–90. [CrossRef]
100. Li, H.-T.; Han, S.-L.; Pan, M.-C. Lower-limb motion classification for hemiparetic patients through IMU and EMG signal processing. In Proceedings of the 2016 International Conference on Biomedical Engineering (BME-HUST), Hanoi, Vietnam, 4–6 October 2016; pp. 113–118.
101. Mesbah, S.; Gonnelli, F.; El-baz, A.; Angeli, C.; Harkema, S.; Rejc, E. Spectral analysis of lower limb EMG activity in individuals with motor complete SCI during standing with epidural stimulation. In Proceedings of the 2018 IEEE International Symposium on Signal Processing and Information Technology (ISSPIT), Louisville, KY, USA, 6–8 December 2018; pp. 1–5.
102. Prasad, C.; Balakandan, V.K.; Moorthy, P.; Kochuvila, S. Classification of sEMG Signals for Controlling of a Prosthetic foot using SVM and KNN. In Proceedings of the 2019 International Conference on Intelligent Computing and Control Systems (ICCS), Madurai, India, 15–17 May 2019; pp. 454–458.
103. Xie, H.-B.; Guo, T.; Bai, S.; Dokos, S. Hybrid soft computing systems for electromyographic signals analysis: A review. *Biomed. Eng. Online* **2014**, *13*, 8. [CrossRef]
104. Meng, M.; Luo, Z.; She, Q.; Ma, Y. Automatic recognition of gait mode from EMG signals of lower limb. In Proceedings of the 2010 The 2nd International Conference on Industrial Mechatronics and Automation, HongKong, China, 30 May 2010; pp. 282–285.

105. Morbidoni, C.; Principi, L.; Mascia, G.; Strazza, A.; Verdini, F.; Cucchiarelli, A.; Di Nardo, F. Gait phase classification from surface EMG signals using Neural Networks. In *Mediterranean Conference on Medical and Biological Engineering and Computing*; Springer: Cham, Switzerland, 2019; pp. 75–82.
106. Lendaro, E.; Mastinu, E.; Håkansson, B.; Ortiz-Catalan, M. Real-time classification of non-weight bearing lower-limb movements using EMG to facilitate phantom motor execution: Engineering and case study application on phantom limb pain. *Front. Neurol.* **2017**, *8*, 470. [CrossRef]
107. Zheng, J.; Chen, J.; Yang, M.; Chen, S. PSO-SVM-based gait phase classification during human walking on unstructured terrains: Application in lower-limb exoskeleton. *Proc. Inst. Mech. Eng. Part. C J. Mech. Eng. Sci.* **2019**, *233*, 7144–7154. [CrossRef]
108. Bellingegni, A.D.; Gruppioni, E.; Colazzo, G.; Davalli, A.; Sacchetti, R.; Guglielmelli, E.; Zollo, L. NLR, MLP, SVM, and LDA: A comparative analysis on EMG data from people with trans-radial amputation. *J. Neuroeng. Rehabil.* **2017**, *14*, 82. [CrossRef]
109. Chen, J.; Zhang, X.; Cheng, Y.; Xi, N. Surface EMG based continuous estimation of human lower limb joint angles by using deep belief networks. *Biomed. Signal. Process. Control.* **2018**, *40*, 335–342. [CrossRef]
110. Afzal, T.; White, G.; Wright, A.B.; Iqbal, K. Locomotion mode identification for lower limbs using neuromuscular and joint kinematic signals. In Proceedings of the 2014 36th Annual International Conference of the IEEE Engineering in Medicine and Biology Society, Chicago, IL, USA, 27–31 August 2014; pp. 4071–4074.
111. Blana, D.; Kyriacou, T.; Lambrecht, J.M.; Chadwick, E.K. Feasibility of using combined EMG and kinematic signals for prosthesis control: A simulation study using a virtual reality environment. *J. Electromyogr. Kinesiol.* **2016**, *29*, 21–27. [CrossRef]
112. Kundu, A.S.; Mazumder, O.; Lenka, P.K.; Bhaumik, S. Hand gesture recognition based omnidirectional wheelchair control using IMU and EMG sensors. *J. Intell. Robot. Syst.* **2018**, *91*, 529–541. [CrossRef]
113. Ceolini, E.; Taverni, G.; Khacef, L.; Payvand, M.; Donati, E. Sensor fusion using EMG and vision for hand gesture classification in mobile applications. In Proceedings of the 2019 IEEE Biomedical Circuits and Systems Conference (BioCAS), Nara, Japan, 17–19 October 2019; pp. 1–4.
114. Pedotti, A.; Assente, R.; Fusi, G.; De Rossi, D.; Dario, P.; Domenici, C. Multisensor piezoelectric polymer insole for pedobarography. *Ferroelectrics* **1984**, *60*, 163–174. [CrossRef]
115. Hidler, J. Robotic-assessment of walking in individuals with gait disorders. In Proceedings of the 26th Annual International Conference of the IEEE Engineering in Medicine and Biology Society, San Francisco, CA, USA, 1–4 September 2004; pp. 4829–4831.
116. Riener, R.; Rabuffetti, M.; Frigo, C.; Quintern, J.; Schmidt, G. Instrumented staircase for ground reaction measurement. *Med. Biol. Eng. Comput.* **1999**, *37*, 526–529. [CrossRef] [PubMed]
117. Faivre, A.; Dahan, M.; Parratte, B.; Monnier, G. Instrumented shoes for pathological gait assessment. *Mech. Res. Commun.* **2004**, *31*, 627–632. [CrossRef]
118. Lacković, I.; Bilas, V.; Šantić, A.; Nikolić, V. Measurement of gait parameters from free moving subjects. *Measurement* **2000**, *27*, 121–131. [CrossRef]
119. Šantić, A.; Bilas, V.; Lacković, I. A system for measurement forces in feet and crutches during normal na pathological gait. *Period. Biol.* **2002**, *104*, 305–310.
120. Hennig, E.M.; Staats, A.; Rosenbaum, D. Plantar pressure distribution patterns of young school children in comparison to adults. *Foot Ankle Int.* **1994**, *15*, 35–40. [CrossRef]
121. Zadravec, M.; Olenšek, A.; Matjačić, Z. Emulation of hill walking and turning on Balance Assessment Robot: A preliminary study. In Proceedings of the 2019 IEEE 16th International Conference on Rehabilitation Robotics (ICORR), Toronto, ON, Canada, 24–28 June 2019; pp. 7–12.
122. KYEONG, S.; SHIN, W.; YANG, M.; HEO, U.; FENG, J.-r.; KIM, J. Recognition of walking environments and gait period by surface electromyography. *Front. Inf. Technol. Electron. Eng.* **2019**, *20*, 342–352. [CrossRef]
123. Galli, M.; Cimolin, V.; Crugnola, V.; Priano, L.; Menegoni, F.; Trotti, C.; Milano, E.; Mauro, A. Gait pattern in myotonic dystrophy (Steinert disease): A kinematic, kinetic and EMG evaluation using 3D gait analysis. *J. Neurol. Sci.* **2012**, *314*, 83–87. [CrossRef]
124. Cipriani, C.; Antfolk, C.; Controzzi, M.; Lundborg, G.; Rosén, B.; Carrozza, M.C.; Sebelius, F. Online myoelectric control of a dexterous hand prosthesis by transradial amputees. *IEEE Trans. Neural Syst. Rehabil. Eng.* **2011**, *19*, 260–270. [CrossRef]

125. Young, A.; Hargrove, L. Strategies to reduce myoelectric pattern recognition sensitivity to electrode shift. In Proceedings of the 18th Congress of the International Society of Electrophysiology and Kinesiology, Aalborg, Denmark, 17–19 June 2010; pp. 16–19.
126. Geng, W.; Du, Y.; Jin, W.; Wei, W.; Hu, Y.; Li, J. Gesture recognition by instantaneous surface EMG images. *Sci. Rep.* **2016**, *6*, 36571. [CrossRef] [PubMed]
127. Amma, C.; Krings, T.; Böer, J.; Schultz, T. Advancing muscle-computer interfaces with high-density electromyography. In Proceedings of the 33rd Annual ACM Conference on Human Factors in Computing Systems, Seoul, Korea, 18–23 April 2015; pp. 929–938.
128. Winter, D.A.; Yack, H. EMG profiles during normal human walking: Stride-to-stride and inter-subject variability. *Electroencephalogr. Clin. Neurophysiol.* **1987**, *67*, 402–411. [CrossRef]
129. Phinyomark, A.; Scheme, E. EMG pattern recognition in the era of big data and deep learning. *Big Data Cogn. Comput.* **2018**, *2*, 21. [CrossRef]
130. Gorgolewski, K.; Margulies, D.S.; Milham, M.P. Making data sharing count: A publication-based solution. *Front. Neurosci.* **2013**, *7*, 9. [CrossRef]
131. Atzori, M.; Gijsberts, A.; Heynen, S.; Hager, A.-G.M.; Deriaz, O.; Van Der Smagt, P.; Castellini, C.; Caputo, B.; Müller, H. Building the Ninapro database: A resource for the biorobotics community. In Proceedings of the 2012 4th IEEE RAS & EMBS International Conference on Biomedical Robotics and Biomechatronics (BioRob), Rome, Italy, 24–27 June 2012; pp. 1258–1265.
132. Young, A.J.; Simon, A.M.; Hargrove, L.J. A Training Method for Locomotion Mode Prediction Using Powered Lower Limb Prostheses. *IEEE Trans. Neural Syst. Rehabil. Eng.* **2014**, *22*, 671–677. [CrossRef]
133. Martinez-Hernandez, U.; Rubio-Solis, A.; Panoutsos, G.; Dehghani-Sanij, A.A. A combined adaptive neuro-fuzzy and bayesian strategy for recognition and prediction of gait events using wearable sensors. In Proceedings of the 2017 IEEE International Conference on Fuzzy Systems (FUZZ-IEEE), Naples, Italy, 9–12 July 2017; pp. 1–6.
134. Blana, D.; Van Den Bogert, A.J.; Murray, W.M.; Ganguly, A.; Krasoulis, A.; Nazarpour, K.; Chadwick, E.K. Model-based control of individual finger movements for prosthetic hand function. *IEEE Trans. Neural Syst. Rehabil. Eng.* **2020**, *28*, 612–620. [CrossRef]

11

Optical-Resolution Photoacoustic Microscopy Using Transparent Ultrasound Transducer

Haoyang Chen [1], Sumit Agrawal [1], Ajay Dangi [1], Christopher Wible [1], Mohamed Osman [1], Lidya Abune [1], Huizhen Jia [1], Randall Rossi [2], Yong Wang [1] and Sri-Rajasekhar Kothapalli [1,3,4,*]

1 Department of Biomedical Engineering, The Pennsylvania State University, State College, PA 16802, USA; haoyangchen@psu.edu (H.C.); sua347@psu.edu (S.A.); axd571@psu.edu (A.D.); clw5710@psu.edu (C.W.); mqo5163@psu.edu (M.O.); lua28@psu.edu (L.A.); huj202@psu.edu (H.J.); yxw30@psu.edu (Y.W.)

2 Huck Institutes of the Life Sciences, The Pennsylvania State University, State College, PA 16802, USA; rmr29@psu.edu

3 Penn State Cancer Institute, The Pennsylvania State University, Hershey, PA 17033, USA

4 Graduate Program in Acoustics, The Pennsylvania State University, State College, PA 16802, USA

* Correspondence: srkothapalli@psu.edu

Abstract: The opacity of conventional ultrasound transducers can impede the miniaturization and workflow of current photoacoustic systems. In particular, optical-resolution photoacoustic microscopy (OR-PAM) requires the coaxial alignment of optical illumination and acoustic-detection paths through complex beam combiners and a thick coupling medium. To overcome these hurdles, we developed a novel OR-PAM method on the basis of our recently reported transparent lithium niobate ($LiNbO_3$) ultrasound transducer (Dangi et al., Optics Letters, 2019), which was centered at 13 MHz ultrasound frequency with 60% photoacoustic bandwidth. To test the feasibility of wearable OR-PAM, optical-only raster scanning of focused light through a transducer was performed while the transducer was fixed above the imaging subject. Imaging experiments on resolution targets and carbon fibers demonstrated a lateral resolution of 8.5 μm. Further, we demonstrated vasculature mapping using chicken embryos and melanoma depth profiling using tissue phantoms. In conclusion, the proposed OR-PAM system using a low-cost transparent $LiNbO_3$ window transducer has a promising future in wearable and high-throughput imaging applications, e.g., integration with conventional optical microscopy to enable a multimodal microscopy platform capable of ultrasound stimulation.

Keywords: photoacoustic microscopy; ultrasonic transducer; optical-resolution photoacoustic microscopy; transparent ultrasound transducer; ultrasound stimulation

1. Introduction

Optical-resolution photoacoustic microscopy (OR-PAM) has recently gained significant attention from the biomedical-imaging community as it provides labelfree optical contrast from physiologically relevant tissue chromophores that are located a few millimeters deep, with subcellular spatial resolution [1–5]. In OR-PAM, a tightly focused laser pulse illuminates the tissue and generates wideband acoustic waves from light-absorbing chromophores that are then detected by an acoustic transducer. Time-resolved photoacoustic waves, in combination with the two-dimensional raster scanning along the x-y plane (lateral dimension), generate three-dimensional data from which maximum amplitude projection (MAP) and volume-rendered photoacoustic images can be created.

Conventional OR-PAM setups use complex imaging geometries to coaxially align optical illumination and acoustic detection paths. In early OR-PAM setups [6], coaxial alignment was achieved using an acoustic-optic prism combiner consisting of one right-angle prism and one rhomboid prism pressed tightly to a thin layer of silicone oil. The laser light was focused by a system of optical lenses and then passed through the prism combiner before irradiating the tissue. A correction lens was attached to the prism combiner to refocus the light that was defocused through the combiner. Tissue-generated photoacoustic waves propagated through the rhomboid prism and were reflected by the silicone oil layer into the ultrasound detector attached to the prism. Since the entire imaging head, consisting of the above acoustic-optic prism combiner, the transducer, and the focused light, was moved to scan the subject, these systems exhibited slow acquisition speed, limited field of view (FOV), and significant acoustic loss.

The current generation of OR-PAMs reflect the light, instead of the acoustic waves, by sandwiching an aluminium foil in the acoustic-optic combiner. This allows dual axis optic only scanning using a two dimensional galvo mirror to improve the image acquisition speed and generate a wide FOV [7]. The entire imaging head, including the galvo mirror, is submerged in a large volume ($70 \times 40 \times 20$ mm^3) of a nonconducting liquid coupling medium that rests above the imaged subject. Such a bulky imaging head limits high throughput and wearable imaging applications because it constrains animal imaging performed under anesthesia and causes discomfort to living subjects. Moreover, acoustic loss here is still significant because acoustic waves travel through the large coupling medium and the prism combiner before being detected by the transducer.

Alternatively, some OR-PAMs include a ring-shaped single-element ultrasound transducer to eliminate the off-axis alignment problems of optical illumination and acoustic detection. The focused light is directly delivered through a hole at the center of the transducer, or coupled using a single-mode fiber integrated with a gradient-index (GRIN) lens. The imaging head is then two-dimensionally raster-scanned using mechanical stages to generate volumetric images [8–12]. Although the imaging head is miniaturized in these OR-PAM systems, the FOV, numerical aperture, and imaging speed (due to physical scanning of the imaging head) are still limited. Besides, they still require a-few-milimeter thick water coupling medium above the imaged subject due to long working distances.

The above drawbacks of conventional OR-PAM systems can be addressed if ultrasound detectors are transparent to light. To achieve this, all-optical ultrasound detection technologies, such as Fabry–Pérot etalons [13], microring resonators [14], and other photonic integrated circuits [15] were studied for PAM. Although these are transparent technologies offering high photoacoustic sensitivity, they require complex fiber integration with an additional laser source and other optical-detection instruments. More importantly, they lack ultrasound excitation capabilities for applications that require combined ultrasound sensing and ultrasound tissue stimulation [16,17]. Recently, transparent capacitive micromachined ultrasonic transducers (CMUTs) were developed [18,19]. However, CMUTs need specialized front-end application-specific integrated circuits (ASICs), and involve a complicated fabrication process inside a cleanroom.

In order to address all the above limitations, we recently reported a photoacoustic-imaging technique using an optically transparent bulk piezoelectric lithium niobate ($LiNbO_3$) ultrasound transducer [20]. $LiNbO_3$ offers several advantages over other piezoelectric materials:

1. It exhibits a good electromechanical coupling coefficient (53%);
2. It demonstrates a high Curie temperature (>1100 °C), making it easy to process through high-temperature sputtering without losing poling [21];
3. It shows promising results in high-frequency ultrasound and PAM applications [22–24].

On the basis of these advantages, our previous work [20] introduced two transparent photoacoustic-imaging schematics, one that directly integrated a multimode optical fiber with the transparent $LiNbO_3$ transducer, and the other that involved the optical-only scanning of the laser spot over a 10×10 mm^2 $LiNbO_3$ window transducer.

Extending the window-transducer approach, here we present a novel OR-PAM that allows the optical-only scanning of a tightly focused light beam through a 10×10 mm^2 single-element $LiNbO_3$ transparent-ultrasound-transducer (TUT) window and demonstrates its applicability to image biological samples. The spatial resolution and signal-to-noise ratio (SNR) of the OR-PAM system were characterized using imaging experiments on resolution test targets and carbon-fiber phantoms. The biological imaging capabilities of the OR-PAM were studied using *ex ovo* chick-embryo chorioallantoic-membrane (CAM) vasculature and imaging melanoma phantoms through a piece of mouse skin.

The proposed TUT-based OR-PAM approach simplifies the coaxial alignment of optic and acoustic paths without the need for additional optical components (such as acoustic-optic prism combiners and correction lenses) and a large acoustic-coupling medium. Our approach provides other advantages:

1. The TUT can be fixed onto the imaging object (such as the skull of a mouse) to facilitate wearable imaging without a thick coupling medium. In the future, this will likely help in imaging the brains of freely behaving or awake mice in combination with ultrasound stimulation;
2. Depending on the size of the TUT, it enables the high-speed scanning of large areas with single-channel data acquisition.
3. In the future, our TUT approach can also be integrated into conventional optical microscopes to realize a multimodal microscopy platform with ultrasound-stimulation capabilities.

The rest of this paper is organized as follows. Section 2 describes the process of TUT fabrication and a schematic representation of the OR-PAM setup. TUT characterization and validation studies, including carbon-fiber imaging, CAM vasculature, and melanoma depth profiling, are presented in Section 3. The advantages of the proposed TUT-based OR-PAM system, the limitations, and its future directions are discussed in Section 4.

2. Materials and Methods

2.1. Transducer-Fabrication Processes

As reported in our recent work [20], a 250 μm thick Y-cut 36° $LiNbO_3$ wafer was sputtered with 200 nm thick indium tin oxide (ITO) on both sides and then diced into square pieces of 10×10 mm^2, which resulted in ~80% optical transparency in the visible and near-infrared optical-wavelength regions. Square tubing (0.5 in. width, 0.032 in. wall thickness, and 10 mm height) was used as a conductive housing. The bottom electrode and brass tubing were connected using a conductive silver epoxy (E-solder 3022, Von Roll Isola Inc., New Haven, CT, USA) that outlined the 4 edges of the bottom electrode. The conductive silver epoxy had 1 mm thickness and 2 mm total width, with 1 mm covering the bottom electrode. This resulted in an FOV of 9×9 mm^2. The conductive epoxy also acted as an absorber for the surface-acoustic waves generated by the $LiNbO_3$ in response to pulsed-light incidence.

The top electrode was connected to an SMA to BNC connector using a microstranded wire. A nonconducting and transparent epoxy (Epotek-301, Epoxy Technologies Inc., Billerica, MA, USA) was poured until it filled the brass housing. This epoxy was used as the backing layer that would reduce the ringing effect by absorbing vibrational energy, and improve bandwidth [25]. Extra care was taken to ensure that no particles were trapped in the epoxy that may have diffracted the light or caused a shadowing effect.

The epoxy is known to shrink during the curing process that can lead to a curved surface inside the brass housing. This curvature can lead to light diffractions and aberrations. In order to ameliorate this effect, a microglass slide with 150 μm thickness was placed on top of the transducer to form a flat surface. A cross-sectional schematic view of the TUT is shown in Figure 1a. Figure 1b shows a photograph of the TUT on top of a Nittany Lion mascot.

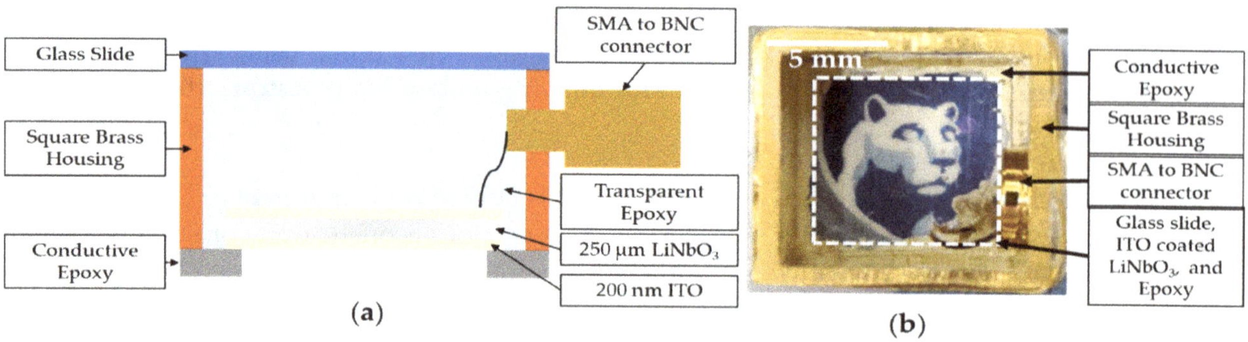

Figure 1. Transparent-ultrasound-transducer (TUT) design based on piezoelectric lithium niobate ($LiNbO_3$) material. (**a**) Schematic cross-sectional view of fabricated TUT, which had 10 mm height and 9×9 mm^2 field of view. ITO: Indium tin oxide; (**b**) Photograph of fabricated TUT clearly showing Nittany Lion mascot underneath.

2.2. Optical-Resolution Photoacoustic-Microscopy Experiment Setup

A schematic representing the top-down view of the OR-PAM setup is shown in Figure 2. The system employed a high-speed pulsed laser (GLPM-10, IPG Photonics; 532 nm wavelength; 1.4 ns pulse duration; tunable pulse-repetition rate in the range of 10–600 kHz; tunable pulse energy between 1.6 and 19 μJ). The 4 mm diameter laser beam passed through a beam sampler (BSF10-A, Thorlabs Inc., Newton, NJ, USA) that diverted 10% of its energy to a photodiode (DET10A, Thorlabs Inc.) used to synchronize with a high-speed (1 gigasample per second) 16 bit data-acquisition system (Razormax-16, Dynamic Signals LLC, Lockport, IL, USA) connected to a computer.

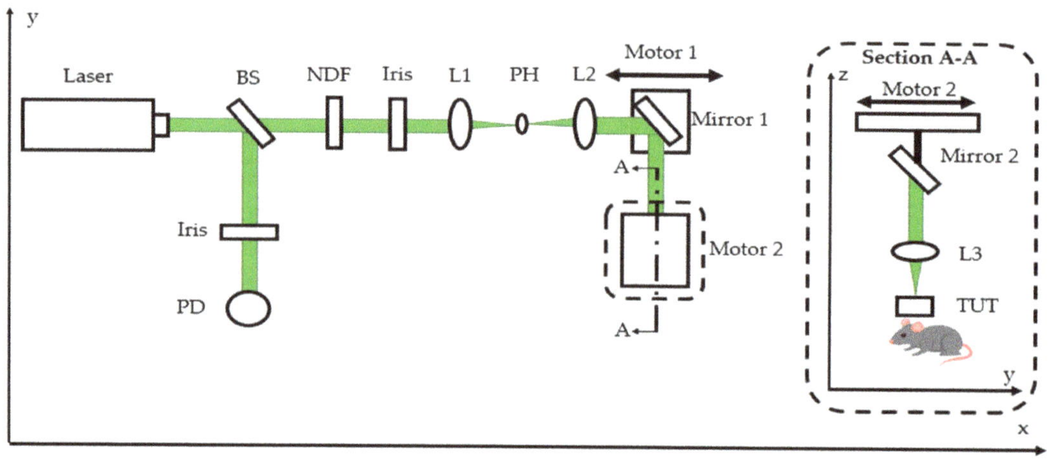

Figure 2. Top-down view schematic of optical-resolution photoacoustic-microscopy (OR-PAM) setup. Raster scanning achieved by Motor 1 moving Mirror 1 to perform x-axis scan. Motor 2 moved Mirror 2 and L3 to perform y-axis scan. BS: beam sampler; NDF: neutral density filter; PD: photodiode; PH: pinhole; L1, L2, L3: planoconvex lenses with 50, 75, and 50 mm focal lengths, respectively.

The remaining 90% of the beam energy passed through a neutral density filter (NDC-50C-4M, Thorlabs Inc., Newton, NJ, USA) and an iris before entering a spatial filter system. A 20 μm pinhole (P20D, Thorlabs Inc., Newton, NJ, USA) and 2 lenses, with focal lengths 50 (LA1131-A, Thorlabs Inc., Newton, NJ, USA) and 75 mm (LA1608, Thorlabs Inc., Newton, NJ, USA) respectively, were then used to filter and collimate the beam. In order to raster-scan the sample for imaging, 2 motorized stages (NRT-1000, Thorlabs Inc., Newton, NJ, USA) were used to guide the light along the x and y axes for scanning (Figure 2). A 45° mirror was mounted onto Motor-1, which moved along the x-axis. Motor-2 was mounted on a vertical stage (on the z-axis) and drove another 45° mirror and a 50 mm focal-length planoconvex lens (LA1131-A, Thorlabs Inc., Newton, NJ, USA) along the y-axis. The focused light passed through the TUT mounted just above the imaging sample. A thin layer (~1 mm) of deionized water was used as a coupling medium to receive photoacoustic waves generated from the tissue.

3. Results and Discussion

3.1. System and Transducer Characterization

First, the transducer was evaluated by analyzing its electrical impedance using a vector network analyzer (Agilent E5100A, Keysight Technologies, Inc., Santa Rosa, CA, USA). Impedance measurements are used to estimate the effective electromechanical coupling coefficient, k_{eff}, of the transducer, which represents its efficiency to convert between electrical and mechanical energy [26]. As seen in Figure 3a, the resonance and antiresonance frequencies were measured to be 12.05 and 14.22 MHz, respectively, with a resultant k_{eff} of ~0.53.

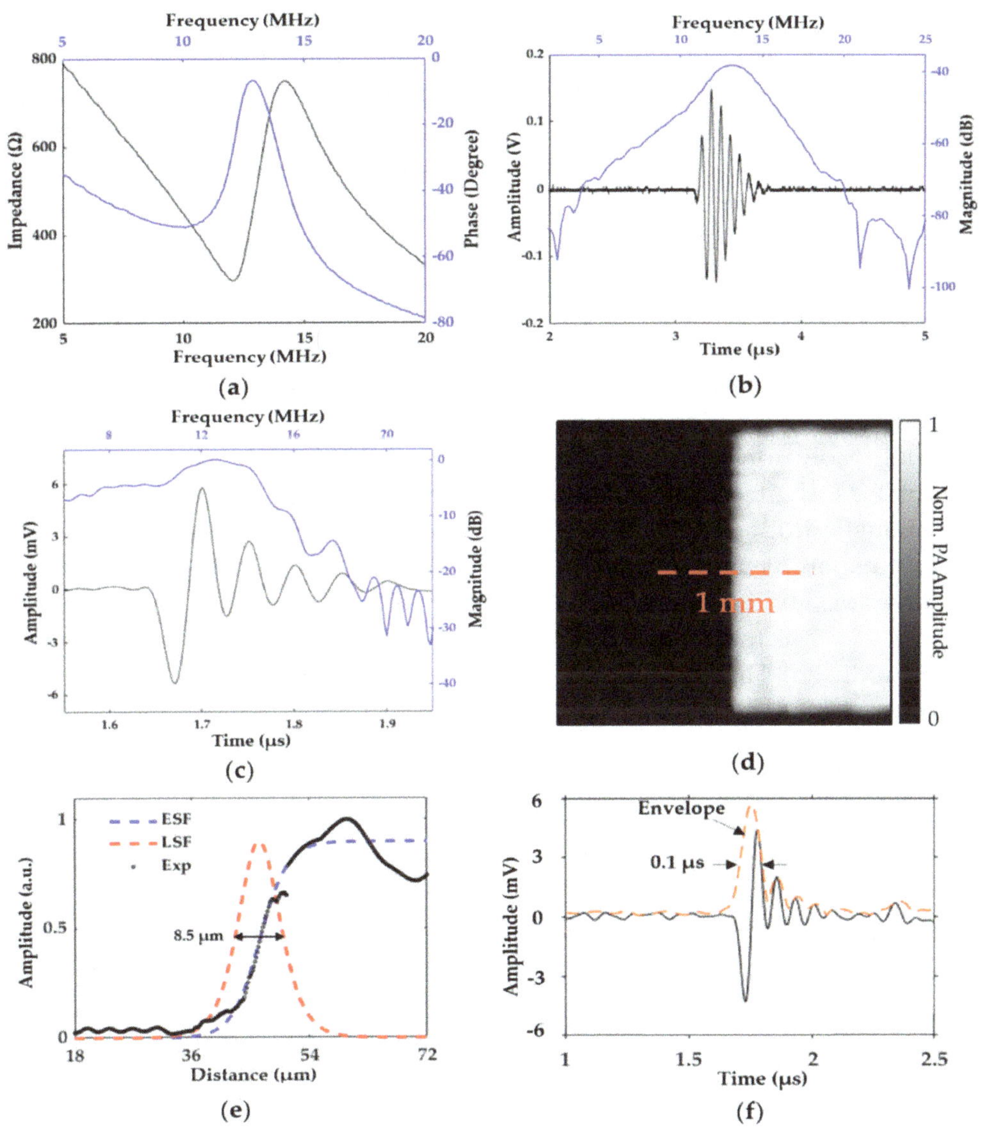

Figure 3. Results of transparent lithium niobate ultrasound-transducer-based OR-PAM system characterization. (**a**) Measured electrical impedance results; (**b**) Pulse-echo response; (**c**) Photoacoustic pulse response of USAF resolution test target; (**d**) Maximum-amplitude-projection (MAP) image of target via edge scanning. PA: photoacoustic; (**e**) Edge-response data and fitted line-spread-function (LSF) curve showed 8.5 μm lateral resolution. ESF: edge spread function; (**f**) Gaussian enveloped curve fitted profile showed 150 μm axial resolution.

Next, we performed pulse-echo and hydrophone measurements on the TUT using the methods described in our earlier work [20]. Pulse-echo measurement showed a center frequency of 13 MHz and a fractional bandwidth of 25%, as seen in Figure 3b. The hydrophone measurements showed a peak pressure of 85 kPa at 5.4 mm distance from the transducer surface. Our photoacoustic-pulse response was acquired via a USAF resolution test target (R3L3S1P, Thorlabs Inc., Newton, NJ, USA) and amplified by a preamplifier (Olympus 5073PR, Olympus NDT Inc., Waltham, MA, USA) with 39 dB gain. The laser energy measured by a pyroelectric energy meter (PE9-ES-C, Ophir-Spiricon, LLC, North Logan, UT, USA) after spatial filtering was found to be approximately 250 nJ. As seen in Figure 3c, our received photoacoustic signal was then averaged 100 times, and showed a center frequency of 13 MHz with a−6 dB fractional bandwidth of 60%. The SNR was calculated as the 20 $\log_{10}$ ratio of the PA signal amplitude to the standard deviation of noise, which was equal to 38 dB.

Next, the lateral resolution of the OR-PAM system was measured by linear scanning along the edge of a ~2 × 2 mm^2 square block of the USAF resolution-test target. During this test, the block was scanned with a 0.5 μm step size. Figure 3d shows the MAP image of the square edge, with a dashed line showing the 1 mm long scan length. The experiment data of the edge-spread function are shown in Figure 3e. The line-spread function was obtained by taking the first derivative of the fitted edge-spread function; its full-width half-maximum (FWHM) showed a lateral resolution of 8.5 μm. The axial resolution of the system was then estimated by taking the FWHM of a Gaussian envelope applied to a photoacoustic signal from the target. The FWHM was found to be 0.1 μs, which was equal to 150 μm in water, as seen in Figure 3f.

The axial resolution of the PAM system is inversely proportional to the bandwidth of the acoustic receiver and estimated to be 0.88 c/B [27], where B is the −6 dB bandwidth in MHz and c is the ultrasound velocity inside the tissue medium. Using this relation, the axial resolution of the proposed OR-PAM system was expected to be ~167 μm, which aligned well with the experimentally observed value of 150 μm. This axial resolution could further be improved by increasing the TUT's bandwidth using a stronger acoustic absorption material as the backing layer. This would also likely improve the SNR and spatial resolution of the OR-PAM system. Additionally, since no matching layer was used in the current TUT, the transmitted acoustic energy propagated through the tissue was ~17%, considering the acoustic impedance of the $LiNbO_3$ wafer and the tissue was 34 and 1.5 MRayls, respectively. If a transparent matching layer with proper acoustic impedance was added, such as a two-matching-layer design using glass slide and parylene coating, we could achieve transmission coefficient as high as ~45%, as the acoustic impedance mismatch between the piezoelectric material and the tissue would be reduced. This would increase our acoustic transmission and receiving sensitivities, and further result in an improved SNR.

3.2. Phantom- and Biological-Tissue-Imaging Experiments

Next, our OR-PAM system was validated by imaging a 12 μm diameter dense carbon-fiber network (that simulated capillary blood vessels) embedded in an agarose phantom gel. Step size was set at 2 μm to cover an area of 0.5 × 0.5 mm^2. The photoacoustic signal was then acquired via the high-speed data-acquisition system and averaged 100 times to generate the image. This MAP image of the carbon fiber can be seen in Figure 4a, where each fiber is clearly distinguishable with sufficient resolution and contrast.

Further, we demonstrated the feasibility of utilizing the OR-PAM for vasculature imaging using chicken embryos. Chicken embryos were used as an animal model to visualize different development phases [28], and OR-PAM could reveal their important vasculature information for clinical relevance [29].

For this study, Day 4 fertile chicken eggs (E4) were obtained from the Poultry Education and Research Center (PERC) at The Pennsylvania State University. These eggs were gently cracked, and the embryos carefully placed on weigh boats under sterile conditions. The embryos were then incubated at 38 °C with 3% CO_2 in a humidified incubator. For imaging, the CAM attached to each embryo was removed by cutting around its edges, and then each embryo was quickly and gently transferred to a Petri dish and rinsed with deionized water. Finally, each embryo was placed on top of an agarose-gel phantom bed for imaging. Figure 4b shows a photograph of the CAM: the scanning area is marked by a white box. Scan step size was set at 20 μm to cover a 2 × 2 mm^2 area, and imaging data were averaged 500 times to provide a sufficient SNR. The vasculature image from MAP, seen in Figure 4c, clearly shows the vascular-branch pattern marked in Figure 4b with adequate contrast and resolution.

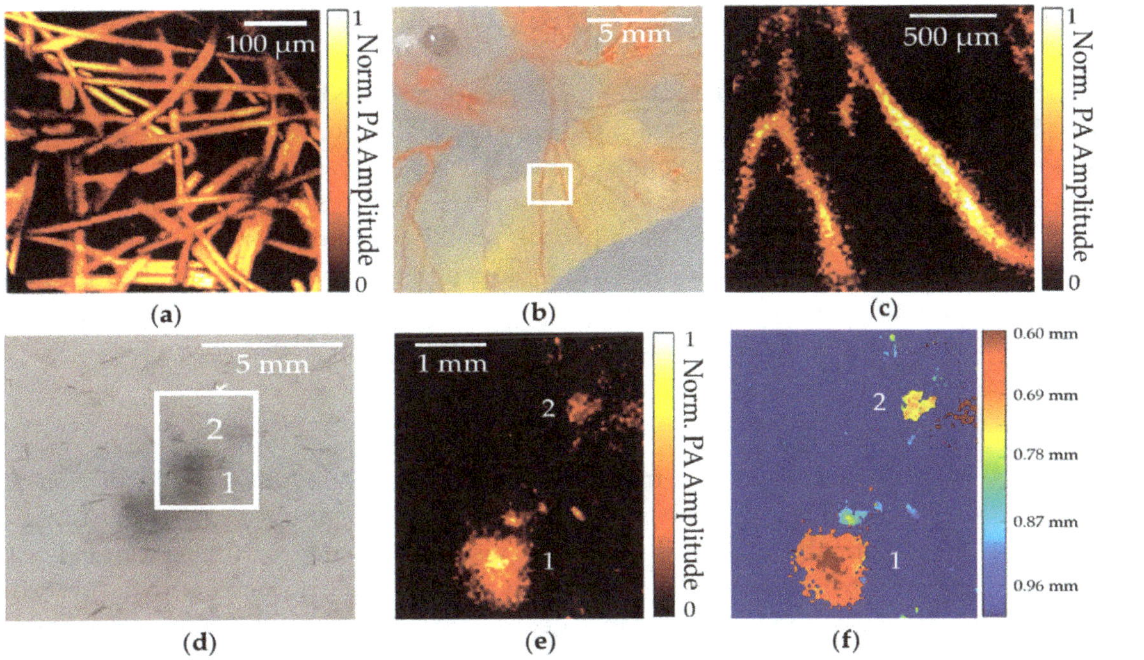

Figure 4. Imaging capabilities of transparent ultrasound-transducer-based OR-PAM system. (**a**) MAP image of carbon-fiber phantom with 0.5 × 0.5 mm^2 area. PA: photoacoustic; (**b**) Photograph of chick-embryo chorioallantoic membrane (CAM) with imaging area marked by blue box; (**c**) MAP image of CAM vasculature inside blue box of (**b**); (**d**) Photograph of melanoma phantom; (**e**) MAP image of melanin particles detected under mouse skin; (**f**) Color-coded depth profiling of melanoma phantom. Color bar represents depth relative to skin surface.

Next, the OR-PAM's application in melanoma imaging was demonstrated by scanning a melanoma phantom. The depth of melanoma invasion under the skin, also known as Breslow's depth, is one of the three most important prognostic factors in melanoma detection, and it reveals important details about how tumor cells invade [30]. To demonstrate the feasibility of TUT-based OR-PAM wearable imaging of melanoma patients without the need for thick gel coupling, we conducted the following melanoma-tissue experiment.

Approximately 2 mg of melanin particles (M8631, Sigma Aldrich, St. Louis, MO, USA; optical absorption coefficient ~1100 cm^{-1} at 532 nm [31]) was mixed with 100 mg of 1.5% agarose phantom gel and placed under a piece of mouse skin at different depths. The scan area was set as 3.5 × 4.5 mm^2 to cover two melanoma spots under the skin, as shown by the white box region in Figure 4d (animal protocols were approved by the Institutional Animal Care and Use Committee, Pennsylvania State University, University Park, State College, PA, USA).

Pulse energy after the spatial filter was set at ~600 nJ to yield an optical fluence of ~14.7 mJ/cm^2, which was below the American National Standards Institute (ANSI) safety skin maximum permissible exposure (MPE) limit of 20 mJ/cm^2 at 532 nm [32]. A-lines were averaged 300 times to generate the MAP image, as seen in Figure 4e. The image was then color-coded with a distance relative to the skin surface, which showed clear melanoma boundaries and depth information, as seen in Figure 4f. The feasibility of the high-contrast melanoma imaging demonstrated here could benefit clinical point-of-care depth detection and the monitoring of melanoma cells using wearable TUT-based OR-PAM.

The main limitations of our first-generation TUT-based OR-PAM system were scan speed (100 × 100 steps took 50 min) and SNR. Scan speed could be improved by using state-of-the-art scanning methods, such as galvo-mirror-based scanning of the optical beam like that employed in conventional OR-PAM systems. This could achieve a scanning speed of 1000 × 1000 steps in 100 s [7]. The SNR could be improved by further investigating novel high-acoustic absorption backing and proper impedance-matching layers. Using a better backing layer and the described two-matching-layer design, we could improve bandwidth by 60% [22,33] and transmission coefficient by ~160%.

Furthermore, fabricating the TUT with a higher-frequency $LiNbO_3$ wafer would further increase bandwidth [34] and lead to an improvement in the spatial resolution of the OR-PAM system. During the scanning, blood diffusion from certain areas of these *ex ovo* samples resulted in low-contrast vascular images: vascular contrast is expected to improve when imaging living subjects *in vivo*. Despite these limitations, the novel TUT-based OR-PAM approach presented here showed promising results that could lead to the miniaturization of OR-PAM for emerging wearable and high-throughput imaging applications. Additionally, the total cost of the proposed TUT is less than 50 USD, well below that of current OR-PAM setups that require additional optical components and instruments.

4. Conclusions

A novel OR-PAM system based on a transparent $LiNbO_3$ ultrasound transducer was developed, characterized, and validated using both inanimate and biological subjects. The transducer was ITO-coated with 80% optical transmission in the visible and near-infrared optical-wavelength regions, and had a center frequency of 13 MHz with a fractional photoacoustic bandwidth of 60%. The resultant transparency of the $LiNbO_3$ transducer facilitated a shared pathway for both light and acoustic-wave propagation.

Our approach also removed the need for additional optical components (such as acoustic-optic prisms) and large-coupling media used in conventional OR-PAM systems. Instead, the OR-PAM presented in this work has a much smaller, lighter imaging head—the TUT itself—with minimal acoustic coupling. Imaging experiments demonstrated an SNR of 38 dB, and a lateral and axial resolution of 8.5 and 150 μm, respectively.

The OR-PAM's feasibility of vascular imaging was demonstrated using Day 4 CAM and melanoma depth profiling using melanoma-tissue phantoms. In the future, the proposed TUT could be integrated in conventional optical-microscopy techniques to allow multimodal microscopy that is capable of both ultrasound stimulation and sensing. Eventually, the TUT technology could be further scaled to develop miniaturized photoacoustic endomicroscopy and microendoscopy devices for space-constrained point-of-care clinical applications, e.g., prostate and pancreas needle biopsies [35–37].

Author Contributions: Conceptualization, H.C., A.D., and S.-R.K.; software, H.C., S.A., and A.D.; investigation, S.-R.K.; biological resources, L.A., H.J., R.R., and Y.W.; data curation, H.C., A.D., and S.A.; writing—original-draft preparation, H.C. and S.A.; experiment design, H.C., S.A., A.D., and S.-R.K.; hardware, H.C., A.D., C.W., and M.O.; supervision, S.-R.K.; project administration, S.-R.K.; funding acquisition, Y.W. and S.-R.K.

Acknowledgments: We acknowledge Eugene Gerber for his kind support in the machining of parts.

References

1. Lan, B.; Liu, W.; Wang, Y.C.; Shi, J.; Li, Y.; Xu, S.; Sheng, H.; Zhou, Q.; Zou, J.; Hoffmann, U.; et al. High-speed widefield photoacoustic microscopy of small-animal hemodynamics. *Biomed. Opt. Express* **2018**, *9*, 4689–4701. [CrossRef] [PubMed]
2. Yao, J.; Wang, L.; Yang, J.M.; Maslov, K.I.; Wong, T.T.; Li, L.; Huang, C.H.; Zou, J.; Wang, L.V. High-speed label-free functional photoacoustic microscopy of mouse brain in action. *Nat. Methods* **2015**, *12*, 407. [CrossRef] [PubMed]
3. Wang, L.; Maslov, K.; Wang, L.V. Single-cell label-free photoacoustic flowoxigraphy *in vivo*. *Proc. Natl. Acad. Sci. USA* **2013**, *110*, 5759–5764. [CrossRef] [PubMed]

4. Zhang, W.; Li, Y.; Nguyen, V.P.; Huang, Z.; Liu, Z.; Wang, X.; Paulus, Y.M. High-resolution, *in vivo* multimodal photoacoustic microscopy, optical coherence tomography, and fluorescence microscopy imaging of rabbit retinal neovascularization. *Light Sci. Appl.* **2018**, *7*, 103. [CrossRef] [PubMed]
5. Cao, R.; Li, J.; Ning, B.; Sun, N.; Wang, T.; Zuo, Z.; Hu, S. Functional and oxygen-metabolic photoacoustic microscopy of the awake mouse brain. *Neuroimage* **2017**, *150*, 77–87. [CrossRef] [PubMed]
6. Maslov, K.; Zhang, H.F.; Hu, S.; Wang, L.V. Optical-resolution photoacoustic microscopy for *in vivo* imaging of single capillaries. *Opt. Lett.* **2008**, *33*, 929–931. [CrossRef]
7. Kim, J.Y.; Lee, C.; Park, K.; Han, S.; Kim, C. High-speed and high-SNR photoacoustic microscopy based on a galvanometer mirror in non-conducting liquid. *Sci. Rep.* **2016**, *6*, 34803. [CrossRef]
8. Wong, T.T.; Zhang, R.; Zhang, C.; Hsu, H.C.; Maslov, K.I.; Wang, L.; Shi, J.; Chen, R.; Shung, K.K.; Zhou, Q.; et al. Label-free automated three-dimensional imaging of whole organs by microtomy-assisted photoacoustic microscopy. *Nat. Commun.* **2017**, *8*, 1386. [CrossRef]
9. Chen, Q.; Guo, H.; Jin, T.; Qi, W.; Xie, H.; Xi, L. Ultracompact high-resolution photoacoustic microscopy. *Opt. Lett.* **2018**, *43*, 1615–1618. [CrossRef]
10. Rebling, J.; Estrada, H.; Gottschalk, S.; Sela, G.; Zwack, M.; Wissmeyer, G.; Ntziachristos, V.; Razansky, D. Dual-wavelength hybrid optoacoustic-ultrasound biomicroscopy for functional imaging of large-scale cerebral vascular networks. *J. Biophotonics* **2018**, *11*, e201800057. [CrossRef]
11. Dangi, A.; Agrawal, S.; Tiwari, S.; Jadhav, S.; Cheng, C.; Datta, G.R.; Trolier-McKinstry, S.; Pratap, R.; Kothapalli, S.R. Ring PMUT array based miniaturized photoacoustic endoscopy device. In Proceedings of the Photons Plus Ultrasound: Imaging and Sensing 2019, International Society for Optics and Photonics, San Francisco, CA, USA, 27 February 2019; Volume 10878, p. 1087811.
12. Dangi, A.; Agrawal, S.; Datta, G.R.; Srinivasan, V.; Kothapalli, S.R. Towards a Low-Cost and Portable Photoacoustic Microscope for Point-of-Care and Wearable Applications. *IEEE Sens. J.* **2019**. [CrossRef]
13. Ansari, R.; Zhang, E.Z.; Desjardins, A.E.; Beard, P.C. All-optical forward-viewing photoacoustic probe for high-resolution 3D endoscopy. *Light Sci. Appl.* **2018**, *7*, 75. [CrossRef] [PubMed]
14. Li, H.; Dong, B.; Zhang, X.; Shu, X.; Chen, X.; Hai, R.; Czaplewski, D.A.; Zhang, H.F.; Sun, C. Disposable ultrasound-sensing chronic cranial window by soft nanoimprinting lithography. *Nat. Commun.* **2019**, *10*, 1–9. [CrossRef] [PubMed]
15. Dong, B.; Sun, C.; Zhang, H.F. Optical detection of ultrasound in photoacoustic imaging. *IEEE Trans. Biomed. Eng.* **2016**, *64*, 4–15. [CrossRef] [PubMed]
16. Gougheri, H.S.; Dangi, A.; Kothapalli, S.R.; Kiani, M. A Comprehensive Study of Ultrasound Transducer Characteristics in Microscopic Ultrasound Neuromodulation. *IEEE Trans. Biomed. Circuits Syst.* **2019**, *13*, 835–847. [CrossRef]
17. Tufail, Y.; Matyushov, A.; Baldwin, N.; Tauchmann, M.L.; Georges, J.; Yoshihiro, A.; Tillery, S.I.H.; Tyler, W.J. Transcranial pulsed ultrasound stimulates intact brain circuits. *Neuron* **2010**, *66*, 681–694. [CrossRef]
18. Zhang, X.; Wu, X.; Adelegan, O.J.; Yamaner, F.Y.; Oralkan, Ö. Backward-mode photoacoustic imaging using illumination through a CMUT with improved transparency. *IEEE Trans. Ultrason. Ferroelectr. Freq. Control* **2017**, *65*, 85–94. [CrossRef]
19. Li, Z.; Ilkhechi, A.K.; Zemp, R. Transparent capacitive micromachined ultrasonic transducers (CMUTs) for photoacoustic applications. *Opt. Express* **2019**, *27*, 13204–13218. [CrossRef]
20. Dangi, A.; Agrawal, S.; Kothapalli, S.R. Lithium niobate-based transparent ultrasound transducers for photoacoustic imaging. *Opt. Lett.* **2019**, *44*, 5326–5329. [CrossRef]
21. Baba, A.; Searfass, C.T.; Tittmann, B.R. High temperature ultrasonic transducer up to 1000 C using lithium niobate single crystal. *Appl. Phys. Lett.* **2010**, *97*, 232901.
22. Fei, C.; Chiu, C.T.; Chen, X.; Chen, Z.; Ma, J.; Zhu, B.; Shung, K.K.; Zhou, Q. Ultrahigh frequency (100 MHz–300 MHz) ultrasonic transducers for optical resolution medical imagining. *Sci. Rep.* **2016**, *6*, 28360. [CrossRef] [PubMed]
23. Liu, W.; Shcherbakova, D.M.; Kurupassery, N.; Li, Y.; Zhou, Q.; Verkhusha, V.V.; Yao, J. Quad-mode functional and molecular photoacoustic microscopy. *Sci. Rep.* **2018**, *8*, 11123. [CrossRef] [PubMed]
24. Zhou, Q.; Cha, J.H.; Huang, Y.; Zhang, R.; Cao, W.; Shung, K.K. Alumina/epoxy nanocomposite matching layers for high-frequency ultrasound transducer application. *IEEE Trans. Ultrason. Ferroelectr. Freq. Control* **2009**, *56*, 213–219. [PubMed]

25. Shung, K.K.; Zippuro, M. Ultrasonic transducers and arrays. *IEEE Eng. Med. Biol. Mag.* **1996**, *15*, 20–30. [CrossRef]
26. Chen, Q.; Wang, Q.M. The effective electromechanical coupling coefficient of piezoelectric thin-film resonators. *Appl. Phys. Lett.* **2005**, *86*, 022904. [CrossRef]
27. Zhang, C.; Maslov, K.I.; Yao, J.; Wang, L.V. *In vivo* photoacoustic microscopy with 7.6-μm axial resolution using a commercial 125-MHz ultrasonic transducer. *J. Biomed. Opt.* **2012**, *17*, 116016. [CrossRef]
28. Dorrell, M.I.; Marcacci, M.; Bravo, S.; Kurz, T.; Tremblay, J.; Rusing, J.C. *Ex ovo* model for directly visualizing chick embryo development. *Am. Boil. Teach.* **2012**, *74*, 628–634.
29. Laufer, J.G.; Zhang, E.Z.; Treeby, B.E.; Cox, B.T.; Beard, P.C.; Johnson, P.; Pedley, B. *In vivo* preclinical photoacoustic imaging of tumor vasculature development and therapy. *J. Biomed. Opt.* **2012**, *44817*, 056016. [CrossRef]
30. Balch, C.M.; Soong, S.J.; Gershenwald, J.E.; Thompson, J.F.; Reintgen, D.S.; Cascinelli, N.; Urist, M.; McMasters, K.M.; Ross, M.I.; Kirkwood, J.M.; et al. Prognostic factors analysis of 17,600 melanoma of 14patients: Validation of the American Joint Committee on Cancer melanoma staging system. *J. Clin. Oncol.* **2001**, *19*, 3622–3634. [CrossRef]
31. Ansari, M.A.; Mohajerani, E. Mechanisms of laser-tissue interaction: Optical properties of tissue. *J. Lasers Med. Sci.* **2011**, *2*, 119.
32. American National Standards Institute. *American National Standard for Safe Use of Lasers*; Laser Institute of America: New York, NY, USA, 2007.
33. Szabo, T.L.; Lewin, P.A. Piezoelectric materials for imaging. *J. Ultrasound Med.* **2007**, *26*, 283–288. [CrossRef] [PubMed]
34. Shung, K.K.; Cannata, J.; Zhou, M.Q.; Lee, J. High Frequency Ultrasound: A New Frontier for Ultrasound. In Proceedings of the 2009 Annual International Conference of the IEEE Engineering in Medicine and Biology Society, Hilton Minneapolis, Minnesota, 2–6 September 2009; pp. 1953–1955.
35. Kothapalli, S.R.; Sonn, G.A.; Choe, J.W.; Nikoozadeh, A.; Bhuyan, A.; Park, K.K.; Cristman, P.; Fan, R.; Moini, A.; Lee, B.C.; et al. Simultaneous transrectal ultrasound and photoacoustic human prostate imaging. *Sci. Trans. Med.* **2019**, *11*, 507. [CrossRef] [PubMed]
36. Huang, S.; Qin, Y.; Chen, Y.; Pan, J.; Xu, C.; Wu, D.; Chao, W.Y.; Wei, J.T.; Tomlins, S.A.; Wang, X.; et al. Interstitial assessment of aggressive prostate cancer by physio-chemical photoacoustics: An *ex vivo* study with intact human prostates. *Med. Phys.* **2018**, *45*, 9. [CrossRef] [PubMed]
37. Tummers, W.S.; Miller, S.E.; Teraphongphom, N.T.; Gomez, A.; Steinberg, I.; Huland, D.M.; Hong, S.; Kothapalli, S.R.; Hasan, A.; Ertsey, R.; et al. Intraoperative pancreatic cancer detection using tumor-specific multimodality molecular imaging. *Ann. Surg. Oncol.* **2018**, *25*, 1880–1888. [CrossRef] [PubMed]

12

Towards Clinical Translation of LED-Based Photoacoustic Imaging

Yunhao Zhu [1,2,†], Ting Feng [3,4,†], Qian Cheng [4], Xueding Wang [2], Sidan Du [1], Naoto Sato [5], Jie Yuan [1,2,*] and Mithun Kuniyil Ajith Singh [6,*]

1 Department of Electronic Science and Engineering, Nanjing University, Nanjing 210023, China; yunhaoz@umich.edu (Y.Z.); coff128@nju.edu.cn (S.D.)
2 Department of Biomedical Engineering, University of Michigan, Ann Arbor, MI 48109, USA; xdwang@umich.edu
3 Department of Electronic and Optical Engineering, Nanjing University of Science and Technology, Nanjing 210094, China; fengting@njust.edu.cn
4 Institution of Acoustics, Tongji University, Shanghai 200092, China; Q.cheng@tongji.edu.cn
5 Research and Development Division, CYBERDYNE INC, Tsukuba 3050818, Japan; sato_naoto@cyberdyne.jp
6 Research and Business Development Division, CYBERDYNE INC, 3013 Rotterdam, The Netherlands
* Correspondence: yuanjie@nju.edu.cn (J.Y.); mithun_ajith@cyberdyne.jp (M.K.A.S.)
† These authors contributed equally.

Abstract: Photoacoustic imaging, with the capability to provide simultaneous structural, functional, and molecular information, is one of the fastest growing biomedical imaging modalities of recent times. As a hybrid modality, it not only provides greater penetration depth than the purely optical imaging techniques, but also provides optical contrast of molecular components in the living tissue. Conventionally, photoacoustic imaging systems utilize bulky and expensive class IV lasers, which is one of the key factors hindering the clinical translation of this promising modality. Use of LEDs which are portable and affordable offers a unique opportunity to accelerate the clinical translation of photoacoustics. In this paper, we first review the development history of LED as an illumination source in biomedical photoacoustic imaging. Key developments in this area, from point-source measurements to development of high-power LED arrays, are briefly discussed. Finally, we thoroughly review multiple phantom, ex-vivo, animal in-vivo, human in-vivo, and clinical pilot studies and demonstrate the unprecedented preclinical and clinical potential of LED-based photoacoustic imaging.

Keywords: photoacoustic; LED; clinic; optical imaging

1. Introduction

Photoacoustic imaging (PAI) holds strong potential in providing structural, functional and molecular information on tissue, with scalable resolution and imaging depth [1]. Since the optical scattering is high in biological tissue, ballistic optical microscopic techniques cannot provide any useful information beyond a depth of 1 mm. PAI overcomes this difficulty since it involves acoustic detection and sound scattering in tissue is orders of magnitude lower than that of light. In PAI, short-pulsed light is irradiated on the tissue, and endogenous optical absorbers in the tissue absorb light resulting in a temperature rise [2]. This transient temperature rise results in thermoelastic expansion and produces light-induced ultrasound (US) waves, which then can be detected by US detectors placed on the skin surface for reconstructing an optical absorption map with acoustic resolution [3]. In a clinical context, PAI is easy to combine with US imaging and is capable of providing anatomical, functional, molecular, and metabolic information by utilizing the signature optical absorption contrast of the vasculature, hemodynamics, oxygen metabolism, biomarkers, and gene expression. Utilizing the useful information provided by PAI, a plethora of clinical applications have been explored in vascular biology [4–7], oncology [8,9], neurology [2,10,11], ophthalmology [12,13], dermatology [14,15], gastroenterology [16–20], osteology [21–24], and cardiology [25,26].

In laser-based PAI, where the tissue of interest is illuminated by a pulsed laser beam, the optical energy used usually ranges from tens to hundreds of mJ per pulse, with a typical pulse duration of 5–10 ns. Most of the commercial and research lab-made PAI systems utilize Q-switched Nd:YAG pumped OPO (optical parametric oscillator), Ti: Sapphire or dye laser systems. However, because of their high cost, larger footprint and strict requirement for eye-safety goggles and laser-safe rooms, these laser sources are not suitable for a clinical environment. Furthermore, the repetition rate of most high-power laser sources is relatively low (~10 Hz), which limits the imaging speed, especially when the signal-to-noise ratio (SNR) is not sufficient and frame averaging is a necessity. In recent years, laser diodes (LD) and light emitting diodes (LEDs) have been heavily explored to be used as an illumination source in PAI, resulting in portable, affordable and clinically translatable PAI systems [6,7,27–37]. LD offers a higher pulse repetition rate (PRR) (typical 2–4 KHz), average power around 6 W, and optical energy of around 0.56–2.5 mJ per pulse, but is only available at wavelengths greater than 750 nm [38,39]. Additionally, for an LD-based PAI system, laser-safe rooms and goggles are requirements, just as in the case of conventional laser sources. On the other hand, LEDs, which are available in a wide wavelength range (e.g., 470, 520, 620, 660, 690, 750, 820, 850, 940 and 980 nm) provide lower optical energy in the range of μJ per pulse, but at a higher repetition rate (~16 KHz) offering the possibility to average more frames without compromising on temporal resolution. Compared to fixed pulse widths in lasers, the optical pulse width of an LED/LD source can be tuned based on the required spatial resolution and imaging depth [39,40].

The pulse width of LED/LD sources is tens of nanoseconds, whereas that of solid-state lasers could be less than ten nanoseconds. The temporal pulse width imposes a limit to the spatial resolution of the imaging system. For example, the 35-ns pulse width of the 850-nm LED corresponds to a spatial resolution of 52.5 μm (=35 ns × 1500 μm/μs). The LD usually offers more energy than LEDs. An LD light source's (Quantel, Bozeman, MT) pulse width, for example, can be tuned from 30 ns to 200 ns, with the pulse energy correspondingly changing from 1–4 mJ. As a limitation, the LED array can only reach up to 0.200 mJ per pulse (highest reported optical output for 850 nm LED arrays). LD, even though it can offer higher pulse energy, is the same as class-IV lasers in terms of optical coherence and subsequent eye/skin safety issues. Owing to its portability, affordability, imaging speed and safety aspects, LED-based PAI holds potential in real-time functional and structural characterization of tissue in various superficial and sub-surface imaging applications and also to accelerate the clinical translation of PAI. Typically used laser, LD and LED performance are listed in Table 1.

Table 1. Comparison of pulsed laser, laser diodes and LED [6,7,27–40].

	Energy (mJ)	PRR (Hz)	Pulse Width (ns)	Cost *	Advantages	Disadvantages
Laser	5 ~120	~10	<10	$70–200 K	Powerful, ~5 cm penetration depth, tunable wavelength	Bulky size, eye protection and laser safe rooms needed
LD	0.5–2.5	~1 K–6 K	30–200	~$10–25 K	Integration in a handheld probe feasible, high PRR	Limited penetration depth, eye protection and laser safe rooms needed, wavelength tuning not possible
LED	0.2	~200–16 K	30–100	$10–15 K	Integration in a handheld probe feasible, high PRR, no need for laser-safe rooms or eye-safety goggles	Limited penetration depth, wavelength tuning not possible

* Cost includes the driving electronics and may vary based on different features, number of wavelengths etc. Integration to a US probe may also involve extra development cost.

In this paper, we review the progress of LED-based PAI technology and its potential preclinical and clinical applications.

2. Fundamental Development of LED-Based PAI Technology

PAI has already demonstrated its unparalleled potential in multiple preclinical and clinical applications and is quite mature in a research setting. At this point, this technology is facing an exciting transition from bench to bedside and LD- and LED-based systems are being explored heavily because of their portability, affordability, and ease of use in a clinical setting. LDs operating in pulsed mode have been investigated by different research groups for multiple point-of-care applications [36–38]. However, typical commercial pulsed LDs are available only in the near-infrared wavelength range, and combining multiple wavelengths in a handheld setting is a cumbersome process [41,42]. On the other hand, the LEDs could be fabricated to operate in a 400 nm to 1000 nm wavelength range (not continuously) with reasonable optical energy by developing arrays of multiple elements and overdriving them [43]. Within this wavelength range, PAI could provide high contrast for melanin, hemoglobin, and fat to an extent, making LEDs one of the ideal illumination sources for multispectral PAI of tissue up to a depth of 1–1.5 cm.

An LED is a semiconductor device based on a p–n junction diode. A p-n junction diode is a two-terminal semiconductor device, which allows the electric current in only one direction and blocks the electric current in the opposite or reverse direction. If the diode is forward biased by applying a voltage, it allows the electric current flow. A small increase in voltage results in a significant change in current flow. Holes (from the P-type material) and electrons (from the N-type material) flowing across the junction promote strong electron–hole radiative recombination, resulting in the emission of a large number of photons [44]. Typically, LEDs are designed for continuous wave (CW) operation, but it is also feasible to drive them with pulsed current. In the pulsed mode, output energy of LEDs is dependent on the peak current, and this can be far higher than the CW rated current, especially if the duty cycle is kept low (<0.1%) to avoid any thermal damage. Since LEDs, when overdriven in a pulsed mode, can generate significantly higher optical output than in conventional CW operation, these types of overdriven pulsed-mode LEDs are often referred to as high-power LEDs. However, operating an LED at excessively high drive currents may lead to faster ageing due to heat generation, and this can even cause immediate failure of the LEDs. The quantum efficiency of the device will also drop with increasing current [45]. Considering this, it is important to design and develop efficient, safe electronic drivers and heat sinks to use LEDs in high-power mode.

About a decade ago, Hansen first proposed the use of LEDs working at a 627-nm wavelength as an inexpensive and compact excitation source for biomedical PAI [46]. In this proof-of-concept work, he demonstrated the feasibility of using LEDs as a light source in PAI for the first time. The basic idea of creating pulsed high-power LED is that, when the low-power LED is overdriven, they can deliver optical output that is far higher than their normal specifications in CW-operation [47–50]. The LED they used was Luxeon LXHL_PD09 which has been measured to yield approximately 250 mW of light output when supplied with 1 A DC current. A derivative of the MOSFET-based circuit presented by Alton and Raji was employed as a driver for generating pulsed current [51]. When the LED was supplied with 60-ns current pulses with peak value of 40 A, it was able to provide pulse energy of 400 nJ per pulse with pulse width of 60 ns, and light focusing was performed to generate the radiant energy required for generating a photoacoustic (PA) response. Also, 50,000 A-line signals were averaged to detect PA response from a non-realistic phantom. Based on the PRR of the proposed LED (200 Hz), this system requires 250 s to acquire an image, which was not good enough for imaging tissue in real-time. Owing to the advances in solid-state device technology and efforts of different research groups in the last decade, there were significant improvements in the performance of LEDs (improvement of pulse energy, PRR, etc.), which consequently resulted in the step-by-step development and commercialization of an LED-based PAI system that is comparable to a laser-based machine.

In 2013, Allen et al. proposed the use of high-power LEDs (CBT−120 from Luminus) working at 400-nm to 65-nm wavelengths as an illumination source in biomedical PAI [43]. In this work, the pulse energy of the LED is increased to 22 μJ per pulse with a pulse width of 500 ns, by overdriving the LED elements by 10 times their rated current. The driver they used was made based on MOSFET, which is described in work of Chaney et al. [51]. As a result of increase in light energy, with the same PRR of 200 Hz, they were able to significantly reduce the frame averaging (by 1000 times), which is commendable.

In 2016, Allen et al. further improved their system performance by using high-power LED (SST−90 from Luminus) elements working at 400-nm to 650-nm wavelengths, driven by a commercial electronic driver (PCO−7120, Directed Energy, Inc., Loveland, CO, USA), which provided 9 μJ per pulse, with a pulse duration of 200 ns, a peak current of 50 A and a PRR of 500 Hz when overdriving LEDs by 20 times their nominal current [33]. They confirmed that the duty cycle was 0.01%, still below the 1% which has been previously reported as safe (no noticeable damage to the device) [45]. In this work, they first imaged a realistic tissue-mimicking phantom by averaging 5000 image frames and using a wide field illumination strategy. The best imaging depth they achieved was 15 mm in 1% intralipid (Figure 1).

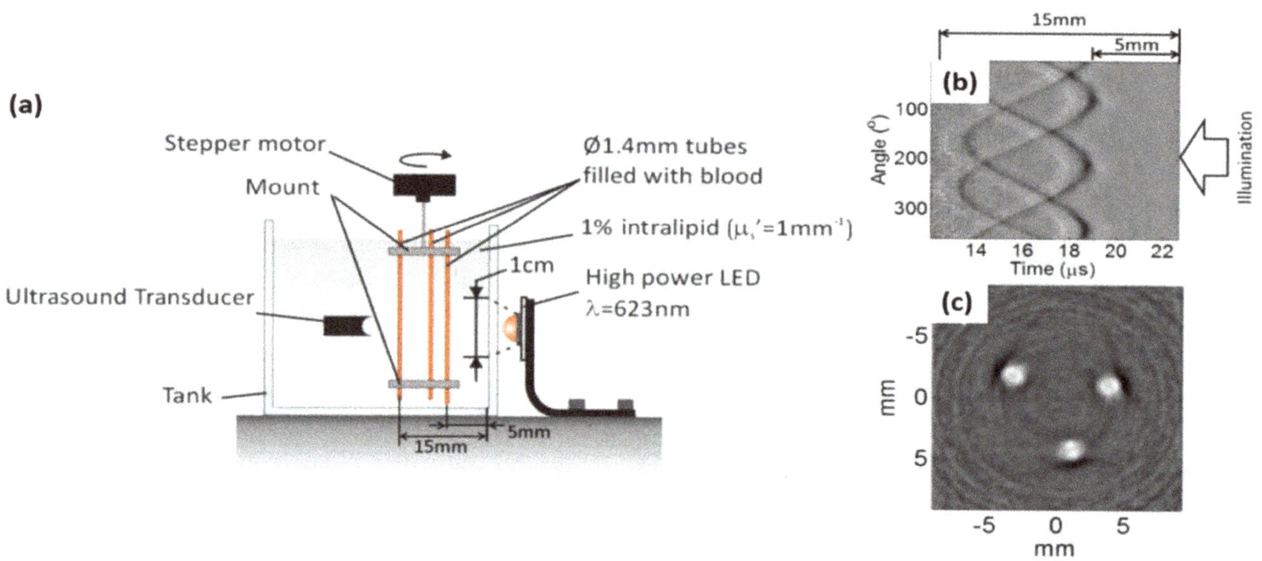

Figure 1. (**a**) PAI setup. (**b**) Time-resolved PA signals of three 1.4 mm tubes filled with human blood (35% haematocrit) and immersed in 1% Intralipid (μs′ = 1 mm^{-1}). (**c**) Reconstructed PA image. Energy = 9 μJ, averaging image frames = 5000. Reprinted from Ref. [33].

The pioneering works mentioned above laid the foundation for LED-based PAI, especially demonstrating the feasibility of using visible light for PAI, which is not possible using lasers or LDs. Oxygen saturation imaging is one of the most important applications of PAI, and it is of paramount importance to have illumination wavelengths suitable for this. Considering the absorption peak for deoxy-hemoglobin (690 nm) and oxy-hemoglobin (850 nm), it was critical to develop LEDs in these wavelength ranges too. Considering this, there has been significant efforts from different researchers in this direction, which are detailed below.

In 2016 and 2017, Agano et al. for the first time proposed the use of high-power LED arrays working at 850 nm with optical energy of 200 μJ per pulse and with a pulse duration of ~70–100 ns. They optimized the SNR by increasing the optical output, by developing highly noise-efficient front end electronics with multiple stages of amplification (~106 dB), and also by matching the US transducer's frequency characteristics with LED light pulse width [34,35,52]. To increase the optical output, they developed LED arrays and further optimized them using hybrid techniques. The single LED element provided output energy of 0.024 μJ per pulse, with a pulse duration of 70 ns and 1 A DC-current.

By developing LED elements with double stack structure, arranging them in an array, and applying 20 times the rated current, they were able to achieve 200 μJ per pulse at a wavelength of 850 nm. The repetition rate of this first commercial LED-based PAI system (AcousticX) was 4 KHz. In 2018, Zhu et al. improved the PRR of LEDs to 16 KHz and used the same system for demonstrating its dynamic structural and functional imaging capabilities [6]. The performance of the mentioned LED-based PAI technology is summarized in Table 2.

Table 2. Summary of the Fundamental development of LED-based PAI technology.

Year	Authors	Pulse Width (ns)	Peak Current (A)	Pulse Energy (mJ)	Repetition Rate (Hz)	Wavelength (nm)
2011	Hansen et al. [46]	60	40	0.0004	200	627
2013	Allen et al. [43]	500	200	0.0022	200	623
2016	Allen et al. [33]	200	50	0.0009	500	623
2016–2017	Agano et al. [34,35,52]	70 *	15–20	0.15–0.2 **	4000	850
2018	Zhu et al. [6]	70 *	20	0.2 **	4000–16,000	850

* Pulse width is tunable from 35–150 ns and above measurements are with 70 ns; ** value is measured from the arrays of the LED.

The AcousticX system was thoroughly characterized for its imaging depth, spatial resolution, frame rate, and oxygen saturation imaging accuracy in multiple studies. When using a 9-MHz US probe and 850-nm LED arrays, Xia et al. reported mean axial and lateral resolutions of 220 μm and 460 μm respectively, which was similar for both US and PA imaging. They also reported an imaging depth of 2.8 cm at an interleaved US and PA frame rate of 30 Hz. Imaging depth was further improved to 3.8 cm after averaging more frames, resulting in a final frame rate of 1.5 Hz. In another study, Hariri et al. reported mean axial and lateral resolution of 268 μm and 570 μm respectively, when using a combination of a 7-MHz US probe and 850-nm LED arrays. They also obtained an imaging depth of 3.2 cm (frame rate = 15 Hz) in their phantom study. In this molecular imaging study, they also measured the sensitivity of the system in detecting commonly used molecular contrast agents. The limits of detection for ICG, MB, and DiR were reported to be 9 μM, 0.75 mM, and 68 μM, respectively. Oxygen saturation imaging is one of the most important applications of PAI. Using a two-wavelength (750/850 nm) approach, Kalloor Joseph et al. evaluated the potential of AcousticX in oxygen saturation imaging using phantom and in-vivo small animal imaging experiments. Based on 28 human-blood-based in-vitro measurements, a standard error of 8.4% was observed between actual oxygen saturation values and the oxygen saturation image formed by the system. In the same work, they showed repeatability and reproducibility of oxygen saturation imaging using an in-vivo mouse oxygen breathing challenge experiment.

From the beginning of 2017, there has been a tremendous push in this area and multiple studies using LED-based PAI were reported. In the next section, we will review the potential preclinical and clinical applications demonstrated using AcousticX, the commercially available LED-based PA and US imaging system.

3. Preclinical and Clinical Applications of LED-Based PAI

Several preclinical and clinical studies utilizing LED-based PAI are reviewed in this section to provide a perspective for future clinical translation.

3.1. Phantom and Ex-Vivo Studies

3.1.1. Guidance on Minimally Invasive Procedures with Peripheral Tissue Targets

Precise and efficient device guidance is critical for minimally invasive vascular access procedures. US imaging is commonly used in clinics for this purpose, but the visualization of medical needles and tissue targets are often challenging [53]. PAI with high contrast for metallic needles and vasculature holds strong potential for guiding these needle-based vascular access procedures. However, the bulky and expensive solid-state laser that is required for tissue illumination is hindering the transition of PAI from bench to clinic, for this point-of-care application [54–56]. In 2018, Xia et al. used AcousticX and demonstrated the potential of LED-based PAI and US imaging in guiding minimally invasive procedures [32]. Their results demonstrated that LED-based PAI enabled needle visualization with SNRs that were 1.2 to 2.2 times higher than those obtained with US imaging, over insertion angles of 26 to 51 degrees. In the reported phantom study, an imaging depth close to 4 cm was achieved as shown in Figure 2a–c. In this work, they also demonstrated that LED-based PAI can visualize the superficial vasculature of the finger and wrist of a human volunteer in real time, along with conventional pulse-echo US. Based on these promising results, it can be concluded that LED-based PAI combined with US imaging holds potential in guiding minimally invasive procedures with peripheral tissue targets.

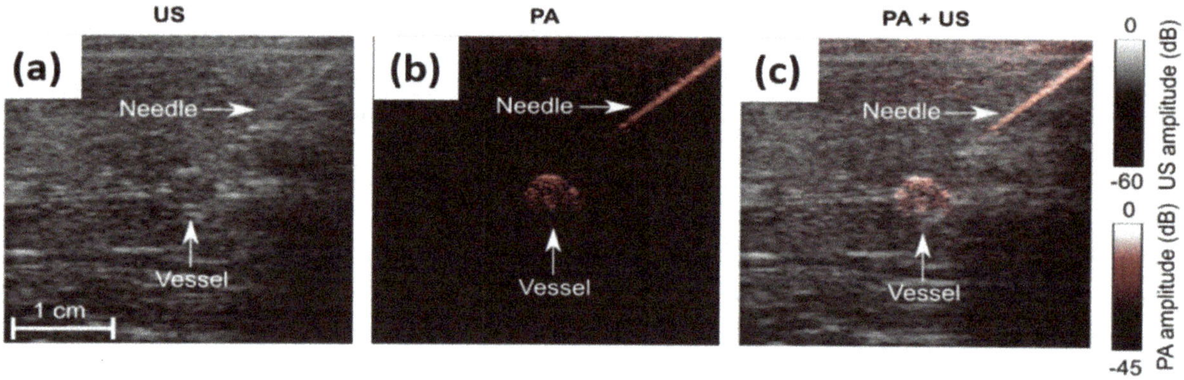

Figure 2. (**a**) US, (**b**) PA and (**c**) US-PA overlay images showing a medical needle inserted towards a vessel-mimicking phantom embedded in chicken tissue, respectively. Here, the uppermost 5 mm, which contained the US gel, is not shown. Reprinted from Ref. [32].

3.1.2. Imaging of Human Placental Vasculature

Accurate guidance is important not only for vascular access procedures, but also for minimally invasive fetal surgeries, for example, for the procedure performed to treat twin-to-twin transfusion syndrome (TTTS) [57]. TTTS is caused by imbalanced blood flow between twin vascular connections (anastomoses) in the placenta. If not treated in time, it will bring high morbidity and risk of death [58]. In current clinical practice of the TTTS procedure, in-vivo imaging of the placenta is performed using white-light fetal endoscopy and external B-mode US imaging. Both these methods do not provide sufficient contrast to visualize small anastomotic vessels below the surface of the chorionic placenta [59]. In 2018, Maneas et al. employed the LED-based PA imaging for wide field imaging of the human placental vasculature ex vivo, taking advantage of high optical absorption contrast offered by oxy- and deoxy-hemoglobin [60,61]. Previous studies have shown that PA signals from placental vessels can be detected using external clinical US probes [62,63]. Here, they used an LED-based PAI system (AcousticX) to image chorionic (fetal) superficial and subsurface vasculature in normal and TTTS-treated human placentas [64]. The LED-based PAI system based on a clinical US probe enabled fast interleaved 2D PA and US imaging (Figure 3). This work gives direct confirmation that volumetric LED-based PAI of the human placenta can generate detailed 3D maps of surface and subsurface vasculature up to a depth of around 7 mm. The authors also foresee that interventional PA imaging for visualizing the chorionic surface and superficial placental blood vessels with high spatial resolution may be valuable for minimally invasive fetal treatments.

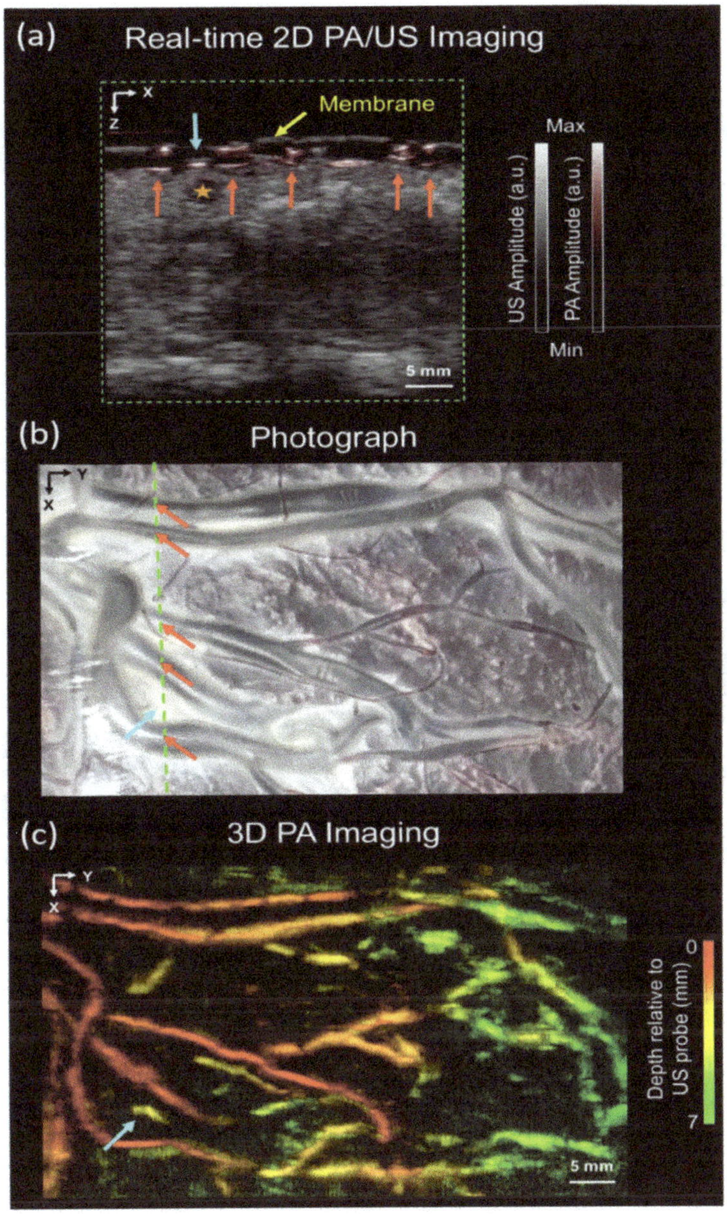

Figure 3. Wide-field PA-US images of the chorionic placental vasculature in an untreated part of a TTTS photocoagulated placenta. (**a**) 2D PA and US overlay image, acquired from a region corresponding to the green line in (**b**), which is a photograph of the imaged placenta. (**c**) 3D PA image displayed as a maximum intensity projection (MIP) of the reconstructed image volume. Reprinted from Ref. [64].

3.1.3. Imaging of Intraocular Tumors

PA imaging has shown great potential in diagnosis and characterization of cancer, especially in applications like head and neck tumor imaging [65–70]. As a head and neck cancer, intraocular tumors are relatively rare, but life-threatening [70,71]. Xu et al. have demonstrated the ability of laser-based PA imaging to characterize intraocular tumors through molecular composition and structural heterogeneity [72]. Zhu et al. recently explored the feasibility of using LED-based PAI to image intraocular tumors in a complete human eyeball. Figure 4a,b shows 2D US and PA images of the eyeball of a choroidal melanoma tumor, respectively. US is shown in grayscale and PA is shown in pseudo-color. Figure 4c is the PA/US overlay image, offering complementary information. PA results show that LED-based PA imaging has sufficient penetration depth to cover the entire tumor volume. Figure 4d shows a 3D PA image of the eyeball. In this work, single-wavelength LED arrays were used to visualize vasculature. LED arrays with multiple wavelengths can be potentially used to observe individual molecular components in the future. These results reveal the potential of LED-based PAI in the broad area of cancer diagnosis and staging.

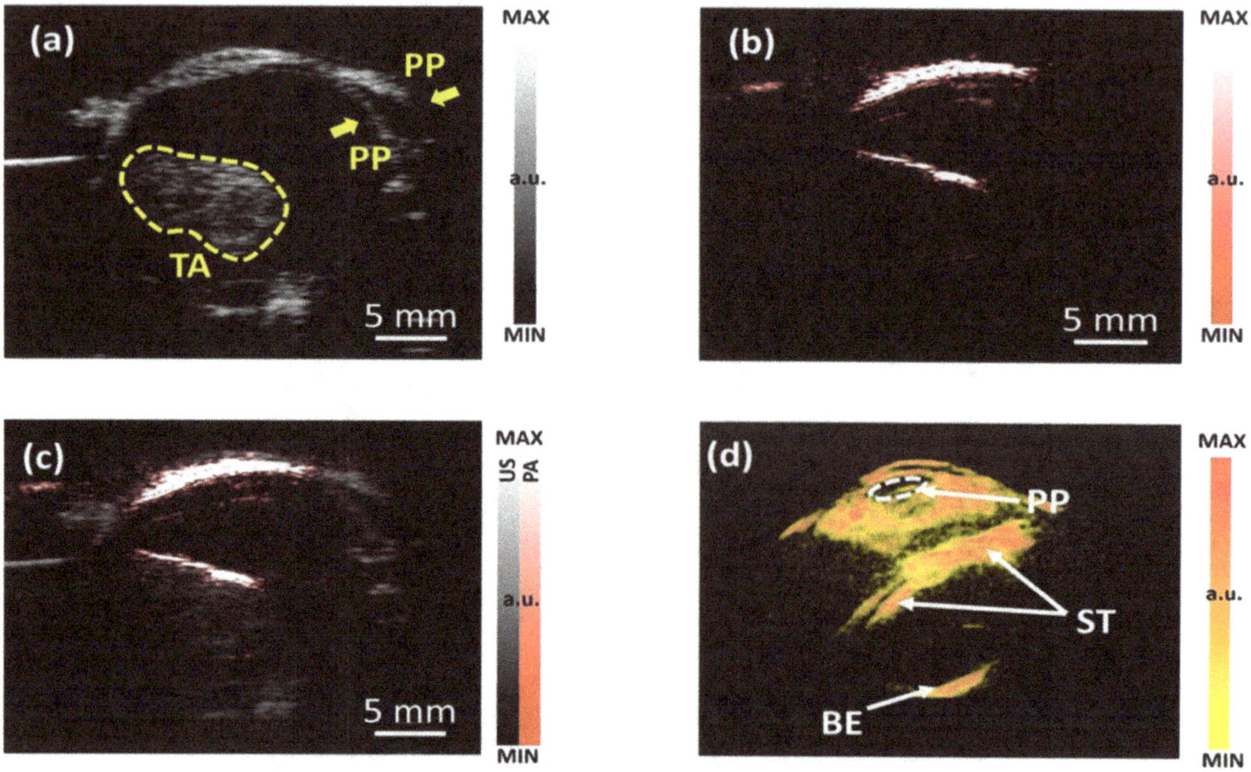

Figure 4. (**a**) 2D B-scan US image and (**b**) PA image of an ocular globe ex vivo with a tumor inside (confirmed in clinic). (**c**) PA and US combined image. (**d**) Perspective view of a 3D PA image of ocular globe with a choroidal melanoma tumor. PP-pupil. TA-tumor area. ST-the surface of the tumor. BE-the back of the eye. Reprinted from Ref. [6].

3.2. In-Vivo Preclinical Small Animal Imaging Studies

3.2.1. Non-Invasive Monitoring of Angiogenesis

Vascularization of engineered constructs is required to integrate an implant within the host blood supply. The ability to non-invasively monitor neovascularization of an implanted construct is ultimately critical for translation. Laser speckle contrast analysis (LASCA), a widely used imaging technique within regenerative medicine, has high spatial resolution, but offers limited imaging depth and is only sensitive to perfused blood vessels [73–75]. In 2019, Zhu et al. used LED-based PA and US imaging to potentially solve this challenge in regenerative medicine [7]. They used an LED-based PA-US dual-mode system to image and monitor angiogenesis for 7 days in fibrin-based scaffolds, which were subcutaneously implanted in mice. Scaffolds, with or without basic fibroblast growth factor (bFGF), were imaged on days 0 (i.e., post implantation), 1, 3, and 7 with both LASCA and PA-US imaging systems (Figure 5). Quantified perfusion measured by LASCA and PA imaging was compared with histologically determined blood vessel density on day 7. Vessel density corroborated changes in perfusion measured by both LASCA and PA. PAI enabled delineation of differences in neovascularization in the upper and the lower regions of the scaffold. Overall, this study has demonstrated that PAI could be a noninvasive and highly sensitive method for monitoring deep-seated vascularization in regenerative applications.

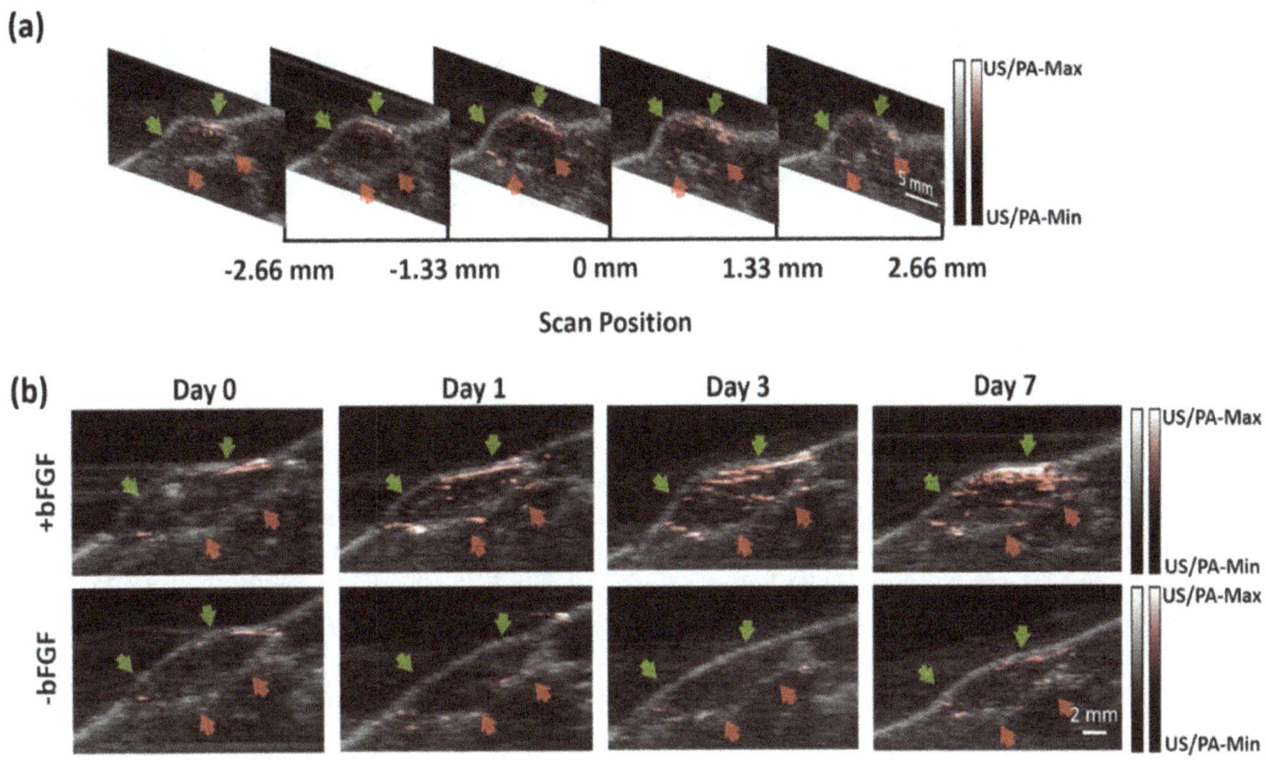

Figure 5. Longitudinal LED-based PA-US imaging of two subcutaneous implants. Green and red arrows indicate the upper and lower edges of the scaffold, as determined through the B-mode US. (**a**) A series of two-dimensional US-PA images from a +bFGF scaffold on day 7 at different scan positions. Note that only images within the range of −2.5 to 2.5 mm are used for MIP image. (**b**) A series of longitudinal MIP US-PA images of +bFGF and −bFGF scaffolds from the same mouse. PA intensity represented in red has the greatest difference on day 7. Reprinted from Ref. [7].

3.2.2. Noninvasive Imaging of Pressure Ulcers

Hariri et al. used PAI as a noninvasive method for detecting early tissue damage that cannot be visually observed. They used a mouse model of pressure ulcers by implanting subdermal magnets in the dorsal flank and periodically applying an external magnet to the healed implant site. The magnet-induced pressure was applied in cycles, and the extent of ulceration was dictated by the number of cycles. They evaluated these ulcers with LED-based PAI. Figure 6 shows baseline (top) and stage I ulcers (bottom) via US, PA, and US/PA overlay images obtained using LED excitation. The insets in Figure 6B–C are photographs of mice without and with pressure ulcers, respectively. They used a LED-based PAI system to detect early stage (stage I) pressure ulcers and observed a 2.5-fold increase in PA signal. Importantly, they confirmed the capacity of this technique to detect dysregulated skin even before stage I ulcers have erupted. They also observed significant changes in PA intensity during healing, suggesting that this approach can monitor therapy. These findings were confirmed with histology (not shown here). These results suggest that this PA-based approach might have clinical value for monitoring skin diseases, including pressure ulcers.

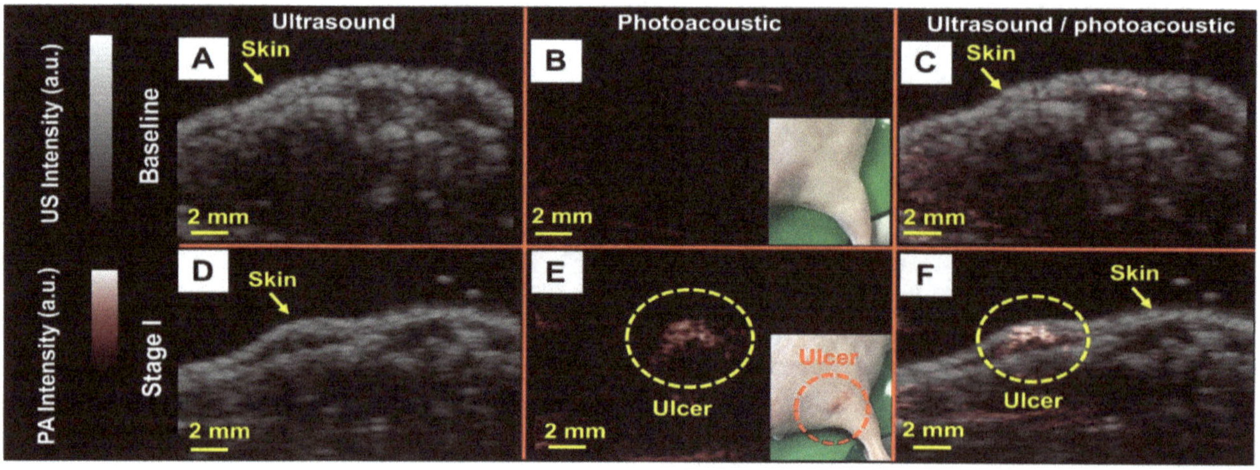

Figure 6. LED-based PA evaluation of pressure ulcers at stage I. (**A**) B-mode US image at baseline conditions when no pressure has been applied. (**B**) B-mode PA image at baseline at the same position as panel A. Minor PA signal is observed from the epidermis. The photographic inset shows the mouse in absence of ulcer. (**C**) B-mode PA/US overlay at baseline conditions. (**D**) B-mode US image at stage I. (**E**) B-mode PA image at stage I at the same position as panel D. We observed a 2.5-fold increase in PA intensity compared to baseline. The photographic inset shows the stage I ulcer. (**F**) B-mode PA/US overlay at stage I. The image depth is 1 cm and the scale bars are 2 mm. Reprinted with permission from Ref. [76].

3.2.3. Oxygen Saturation Imaging in Rheumatoid Arthritis Diagnosis

Multiwavelength LED-based PAI is a useful tool for functionally characterizing tissue in different clinical applications, for example, to obtain oxygen saturation. Hypoxia in the joints are biomarkers of Rheumatoid Arthritis (RA). The ability to accurately estimate the oxygen concentration makes multiwavelength PAI a potential tool for early detection of RA. Joseph et al. used in vivo animal study to find the capability of measuring the oxygen saturation using this system [77]. First, ex-vivo PA oxygen saturation imaging using human blood was validated against oximeter readings and further verified with in-vivo animal studies. The PA oxygen saturation estimation correlates with oximeter readings, which is confirmed with in-vivo studies. In the case of oxygen saturation, an approximately 5-mm imaging depth was achieved. This imaging depth is considered sufficient for RA imaging of the finger joint.

Results from the blood oxygen saturation imaging are shown in Figure 7. Figure 7a–c shows an oxygen saturation map of two tubes, one with normal blood (oxygen concentration approximately 65%) and another with blood having 18%, 43% and 87% oxygen concentration respectively. This correlates with the estimated oxygen saturation generated by the imaging system. Further, in-vivo imaging of the thigh muscle of the mouse is shown in Figure 7d–f. In the case of the mouse breathing normal air, an average oxygen concentration of 61.1% was observed and with 100% oxygen it was 105.3% using the system. This shows that the system can provide a fairly accurate estimate of oxygen saturation with in-vivo imaging. Through their results, they have shown that early stage rheumatoid arthritis changes such as synovial angiogenesis and hypoxia can be imaged using the LED-based PA imaging system. The results give a direct confirmation that multispectral LED-based PA holds potential in early detection and staging of RA in animal studies.

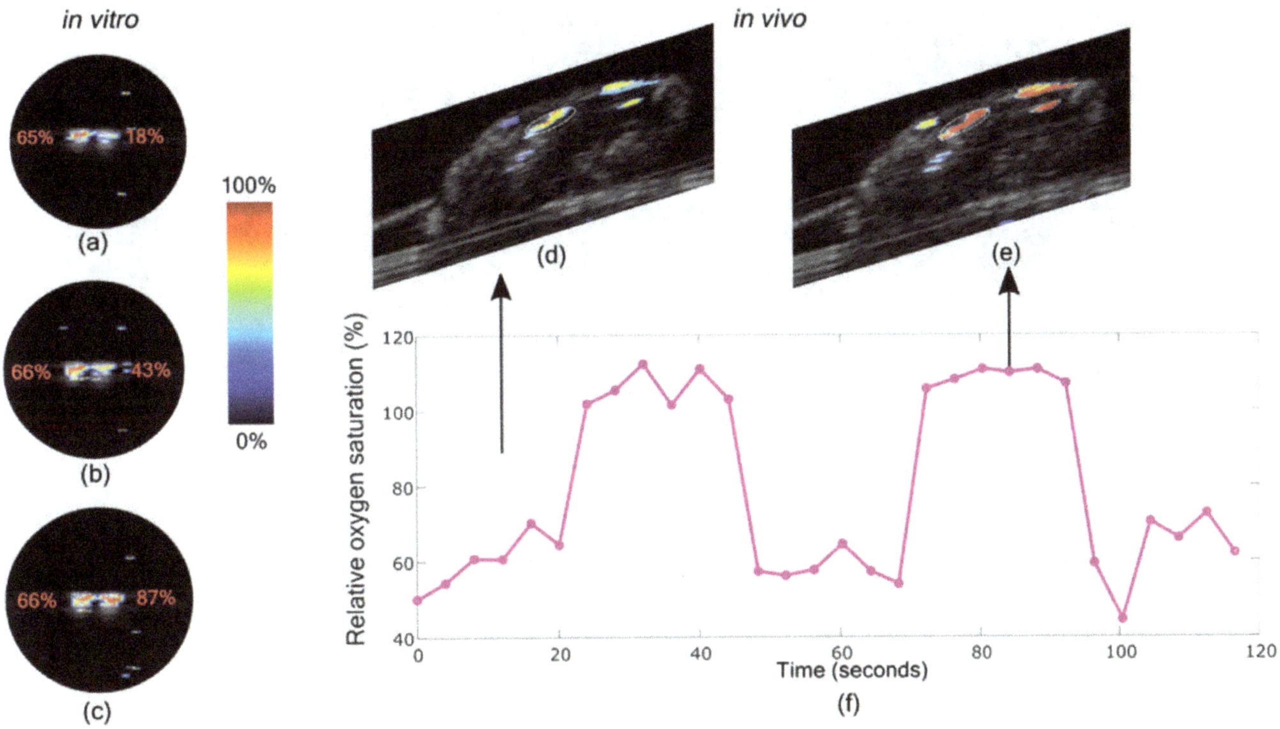

Figure 7. (**a–c**) The in-vitro study oxygen saturation map, with three different oxygen concentrations in the tube on the right, keeping oxygen unchanged in the left tube. The oxygen concentrations values in left and right tube: (**a**) 65% and 18%, (**b**) 66% and 43%, (**c**) 66% and 87%, (**d**) PA and (**e**) US imaging of mouse knee. In-vivo oxygen saturation images of mouse thigh muscle during high and low cycles of oxygen concentration. (**f**) Average oxygen saturation in the region of interested plotted over time. Reprinted from Ref. [77].

3.2.4. Molecular Imaging: Detection and Monitoring of Reactive Oxygen and Nitrogen Species

Reactive oxygen and nitrogen substances (RONS) regulate important functions in living systems. Endogenous RONS contribute to signal transduction, smooth muscle relaxation, and blood pressure regulation [66,67]. RONS disorders can cause diseases, such as cancer, and RONS detection can be used to diagnose and treat infections and various diseases [68–70].

In 2019, Hariri et al. reported on molecular imaging of RONS using near-infrared absorbing small molecules (CyBA) and an LED-based PA imaging system [29]. They evaluated CyBA's ability to measure inflammation in mice. Figure 8a–d shows the US/PA images from the injection location of CyBA and zymosan at 0, 10, 20, and 60 min, respectively (Figure 8). These figures show an increasing trend in PA signals due to the diffused probe (CyBA) at the region of interest (ROI), marked using a yellow circle. Figure 8e represents the quantitative analysis of CyBA's in-vivo PA imaging assessment. These results indicated a gradual increase in PA intensity, and a ~3.2-fold increase was quantified 90 min after CyBA injection. It also shows the flat PA intensity trend of separated zymosan and the dye.

As we know, the LED output energy is about 1000-fold lower than that of conventional Nd:YAG lasers. However, it turns out to be a positive factor here: the higher power generated by Nd:YAG lasers bleach dyes, but not the light from LEDs. Therefore, their work not only revealed the sensitivity of PA in detecting RONS, but also emphasized the practicality of LED-based PAI in the clinic for molecular imaging applications involving dyes. In this work, they demonstrated that advantages of LED as an illumination source may help to accelerate the clinical translation of PAI. It is foreseen that LED-based PAI and reported probes can be used for clinical monitoring of RONS, especially for keloid diagnosis and for drug toxicity studies [78].

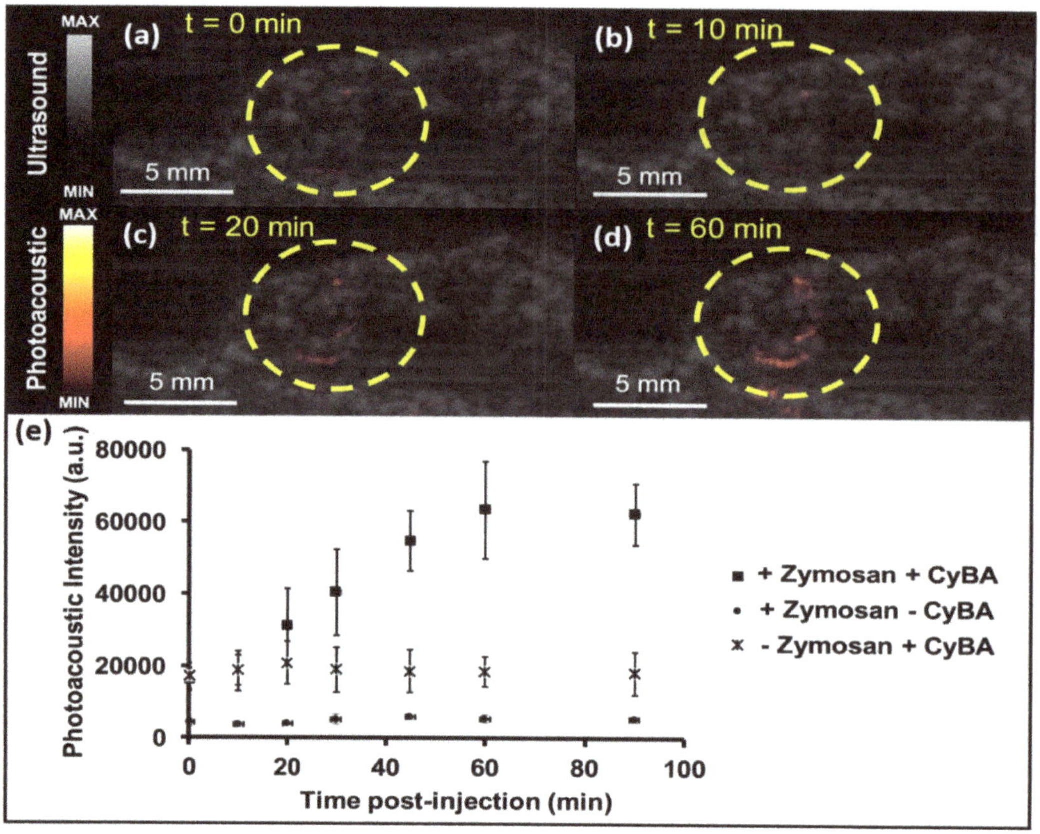

Figure 8. In-vivo PA evaluation of CyBA. US-PA image at (**a**) baseline, (**b**) 10, (**c**) 20, and (**d**) 60 min after CyBA injection. (**e**) Quantitative analysis of PA intensity as a function of time post-injection of CyBA. Reprinted from Ref. [29].

3.2.5. Imaging of Tumor Vasculature Using Contrast Enhancement

Contrast enhancement is prevalently used in vasculature imaging. Xavierselvan et al. tested the LED-based PAI system for its ability to image the vasculature in the tumor using contrast enhancement [79]. For their study, they used subcutaneous head and neck tumor (FaDu) xenografts in nude mice. When the tumor size reached about 100 mm^3, the tumors were imaged using the AcousticX system. The image shows heterogenous vascular density in the tumor which demonstrates the ability of the LED-based PAI system to obtain vascular information from tissues that are more than 1 cm deep.

Through their study, they found LED-based PAI was a more affordable option for various research groups to avail the opportunity of utilizing the technology to understand nanoparticle or drug uptake non-invasively at high resolution. Figure 9 demonstrates the capability of the LED-based PAI system in imaging a naphthalocyanine (NC) dye, which has strong absorption in the NIR region (~absorption peak at 860 nm). Before and after 100 μL of NC dye was injected intratumorally into the FaDu tumor interstitium, the distribution of dye inside the tumor was imaged respectively. The NC dye has distributed into almost all parts of the tumor, but a strong PA signal was received from the top of tumor, which is potentially due to these areas receiving stronger light energy.

3.2.6. Imaging of Molecular-Labelled Cells

Hariri et al. have previously used PA imaging for stem cell imaging [80,81]. In a recent work [27], they used labeled cells to understand the in-vivo molecular imaging performance of AcousticX. They used DiR, which is an effective contrast agent for cellular imaging. The cells used here were human mesenchymal stem cells (HMSCs; Lonza, PT−2501, NJ, USA).

Figure 10 shows PA images before and after injection of DiR, DiR + HMSC, and HMSC, respectively. The needle generates a strong PA signal and simultaneous US acquisition, offering detailed structural information along with the functional details from DiR-labeled cells. A strong PA signal in the presence of DiR is visible in Figure 10D. A signal increase is also visible when HMSC is labelled using DiR, as shown in Figure 10H. Unlabeled HMSCs were also injected as control but there was no increase in PA signal. This study showed the potential of LED-based PA in cellular imaging.

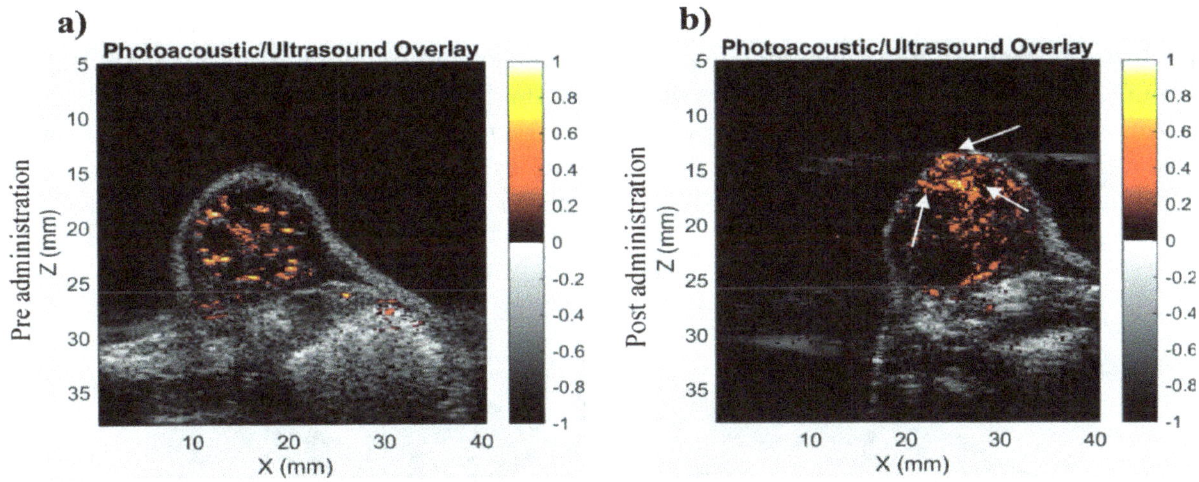

Figure 9. Contrast enhancement in LED-based PAI using exogeneous contrast agents. Combined overlay of PA and US image of subcutaneous FaDu tumor in mice before (**a**) and after (**b**) the NC dye administration. PA images were acquired using 850 nm LED light source (areas with greater contrast is shown with white arrows). Reprinted with permission from Ref. [79].

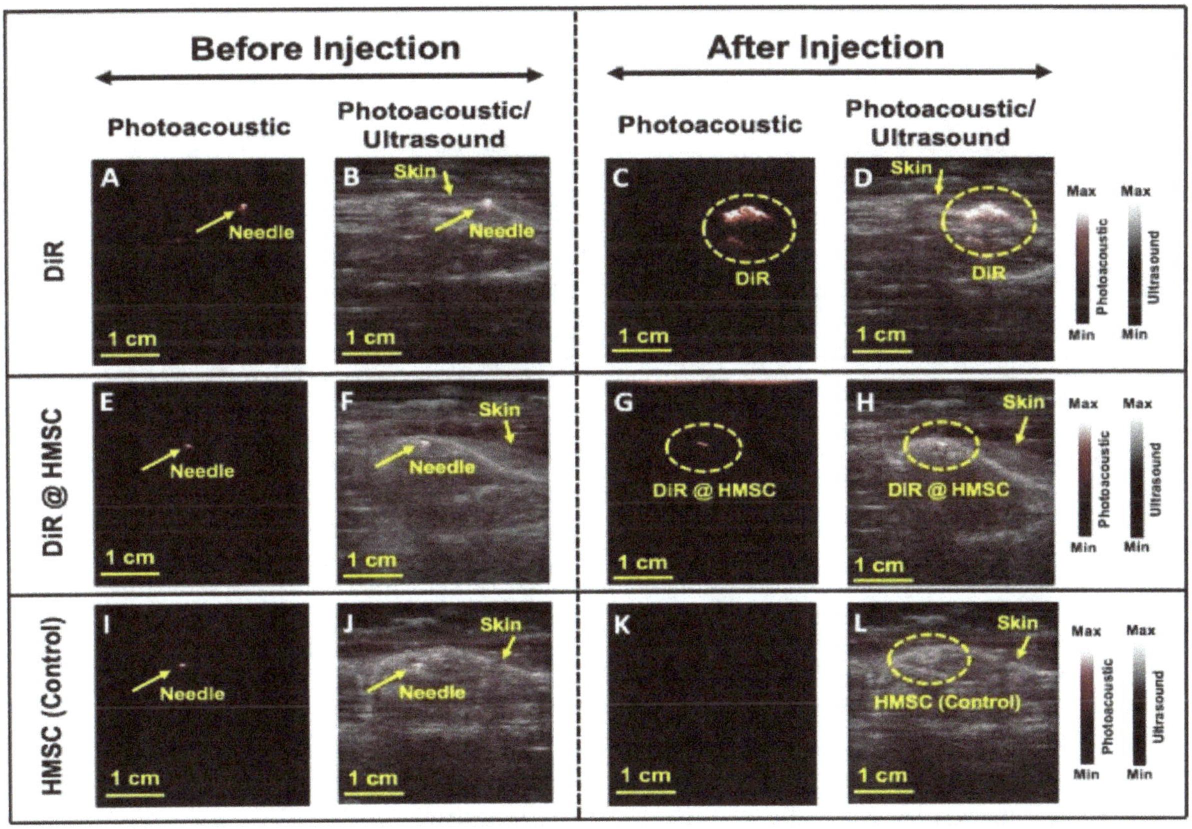

Figure 10. Images were separated in three groups: injecting DiR (**A–D**), DiR + HMSC (**E–H**), and HMSC (**I–L**). Each group contains PA and overlaid PA-US images before and after injection. Needles marked in images are subcutaneously injected on spinal cord area before DiR injection. The needle has a strong PA signal. Reprinted from Ref. [27].

3.3. *In-Vivo Human Volunteer Studies*

3.3.1. Imaging of Peripheral Microvasculature and Function

Hypoxia is an important biomarker that reflects the occurrence and development of many diseases, such as cancer [82]. Multispectral PA imaging has been demonstrated to detect the relative hemoglobin oxygen saturation and hypoxia in biological samples in vivo in a non-invasive manner by detecting the spectral differences between oxygenated hemoglobin and deoxyhemoglobin [83–85]. Figure 11a shows LED-based PA and US B-scan images of a human finger along the sagittal section, which is from our recent work [6]. To show the arterial pulsation (shown by the arrow), four frames of the movie are shown. In this work, we also explored the feasibility of LED-based PA imaging to measure blood oxygen content on human finger blood vessels using a pair of two-wavelength LED bars (850 nm and 690 nm), as shown in Figure 11b [6].

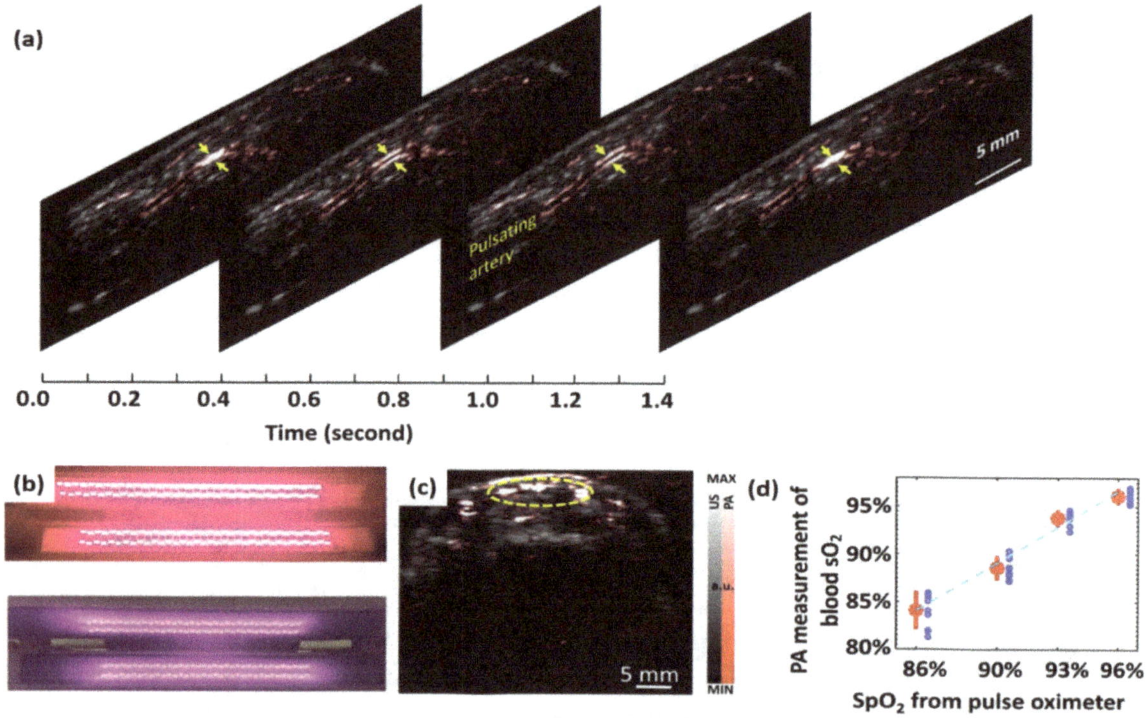

Figure 11. (**a**) Four frames from a PA imaging video (index finger, longitudinal section) presenting the pulsation of an artery marked by the arrows. (**b**) Photo of a pair of dual-wavelength LED bars that emits 690-nm and 850-nm light alternatively. (**c**) PA-US combined image showing a cross-section of the vasculature in a human finger. (**d**) Correlation between the LED-PAI-based blood sO2 in the finger and the SpO2 readouts from a pulse oximeter. Reprinted from Ref. [6].

Functional PA imaging of blood oxygenation saturation in blood vessels was performed on the index fingers of volunteers. Figure 11c is an example of a PA 2D image resolving blood vessels in an axial view of a finger, which is overlaid on a US image in grayscale. In order to quantify the functional information of PA imaging results, the oxygenation saturation levels of pixels in the ROI are averaged, as shown by the yellow dotted circle. The quantitative PA measurement of blood oxygenation saturation in the finger is then correlated with the reading of a pulse oximeter, which is the gold standard. As shown in Figure 11d, the blood oxygenation measured by LED-PAI and the reading of the pulse oximeter have a good correlation (R-squared ~ 0.98).

3.3.2. Simultaneous Imaging of Veins and Lymphatic Vessels

Using dual-wavelength LED arrays working at 820/940-nm wavelengths, Kuniyil Ajith Singh et al. demonstrated that LED-based PAI could differentiate veins and lymphatic vessels (after injecting ICG) in human volunteers [86]. Utilizing a simple image division algorithm (assuming that ICG will not absorb 940-nm light), they showed that LED-based PAI can clearly differentiate veins and lymphatic vessels in real time, as shown in Figure 12. This multispectral PA/US approach holds strong potential in guiding procedures like lymphaticovenous anastomosis, where it is crucial to differentiate venous blood and lymphatic vessels.

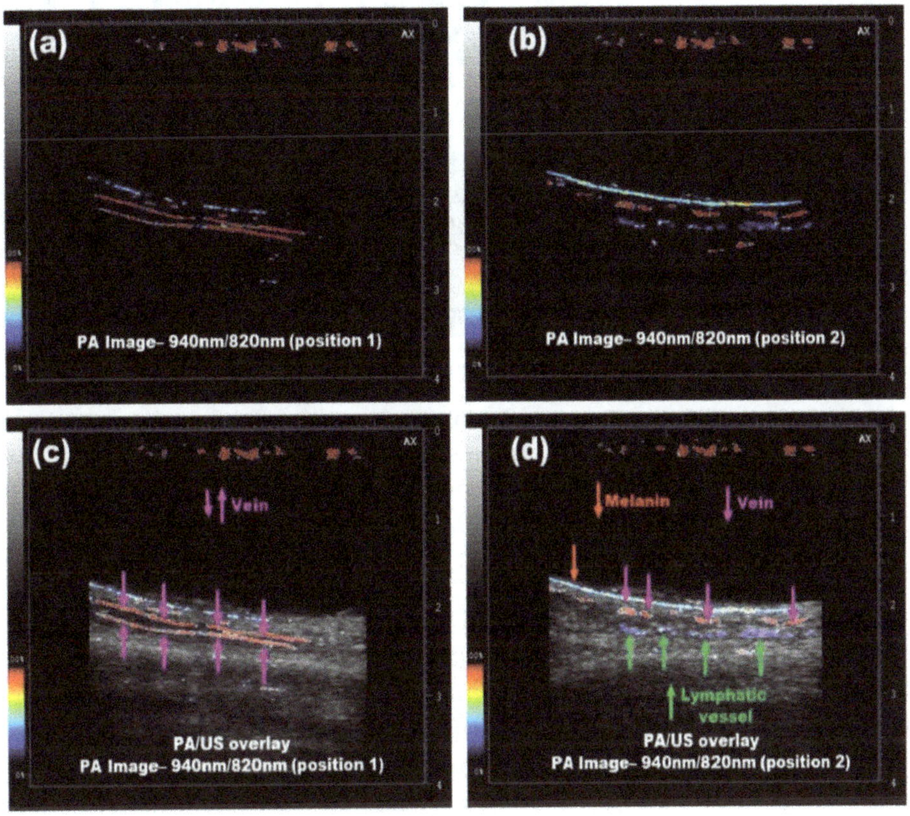

Figure 12. Real-time imaging of lymphatic vessels and veins simultaneously using LED-based PAI. (**a**) PA image: 940 nm/820 nm image generated when the probe was aligned to a vein (position 1); (**b**) PA image: 940 nm/820 nm image generated when the probe was aligned to a lymphatic vessel (position 2); (**c**) 940 nm/820 nm PA image overlaid on US image when the probe was in position 1; and (**d**) 940 nm/820 nm PA image overlaid on US image when the probe was aligned to position 2. Reprinted from Ref. [86].

3.3.3. Full View Tomography of Finger Joints

It is well known that 2D PA and US imaging using linear arrays suffers from limited-view artifacts. Additionally, due to the directivity limitations of US transducers, there is a high probability of loss of information. One way to overcome this limitation is to scan around the object of interest and generate full-view 3D tomographic images with higher spatial resolution and no limited view problems. However, most of the commercially available and lab-made 3D PA/US tomography systems utilize pulsed lasers, which are expensive, bulky and not suitable for a point-of-care setting. Joseph et al. recently demonstrated the possibility to generate full view LED-based 3D PA and US tomographic images of human finger joints (Figure 13) [87,88]. This proof-of-concept study gives a direct confirmation that inexpensive and portable LEDs along with commercially available linear array US probes can generate high-quality 3D tomographic images with rich information suitable for multiple point-of-care clinical applications. In another promising study, Agrawal et al. developed a multispectral molecular LED-based 3D PA tomography system and demonstrated the potential in unmixing and separating three optical absorbers (melanin, methylene blue and ICG) embedded inside a tissue mimicking phantom [89].

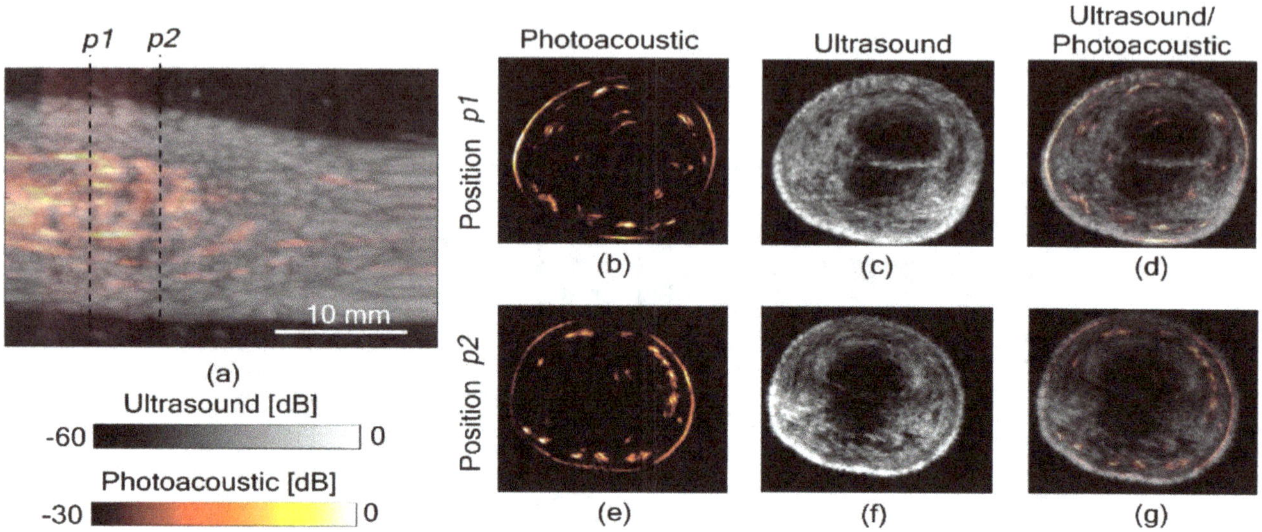

Figure 13. In-vivo finger joint tomographic imaging using multi-angle spatial compounding. (**a**) Overlaid LED-based PA and US MIP image showing finger joint from a linear scan. (**b**) PA, (**c**) US and (**d**) combined tomographic images of the finger joint (p1). (**e**) PA, (**f**) US and (**g**) combined tomographic images 5 mm in front of the joint (p2), respectively. Reprinted from [87].

3.4. Clinical Pilot Studies

3.4.1. Imaging of Inflammatory Arthritis

Since PAI can detect hyper-vascularization and hypoxia, two key early markers of rheumatoid arthritis, it has been explored extensively in multiple preclinical and early clinical pilot studies [90–94]. Relatively small joints are usually first affected by inflammatory arthritis, and PAI in combination with conventional US imaging holds strong potential in this area. Early results from animal models and human subjects clearly indicate that PAI is expected to be translated soon to clinics as an affordable point-of-care tool for early detection of inflammatory diseases [95–99]. Janggun et al. explored the feasibility of using an LED-based PA system to detect inflammation of soft tissues surrounding joints, and the ability to distinguish arthritic joints from normal ones by assessing enhanced blood signal in synovial tissue [31].

Figure 14 shows representative US Doppler and PA images of the three groups compared in this study, including clinically active arthritis joints, subclinical active arthritis joints, and normal healthy joints. Figure 14a shows a case of a clinically active case of arthritis, with hyperemia seen at the same location in both Doppler and PA images. Figure 14b shows a case of subclinical active arthritis, in which hyperemia is only visible in the PA image of the patient's metacarpophalangeal (MCP) joint, but not in the US Doppler image. The normal subjects also underwent US Doppler scans as the patient volunteers, followed by scanning of same location of joints using LED-based PA imaging. When compared with the results of arthritic joints, no significant hyperemia was found in the synovium area of normal subjects, which has also been confirmed by US Doppler imaging. Figure 14c shows the normal situation; no hyperemia was seen in the US Doppler or PA image. Finally, Figure 14d,e shows the statistical results indicating there is significant difference between different groups, confirmed using a two-tailed *p*-test. This clinical pilot study gives a direct confirmation that LED-based PAI offers higher sensitivity to angiogenic microvasculature than US doppler imaging, the current gold standard.

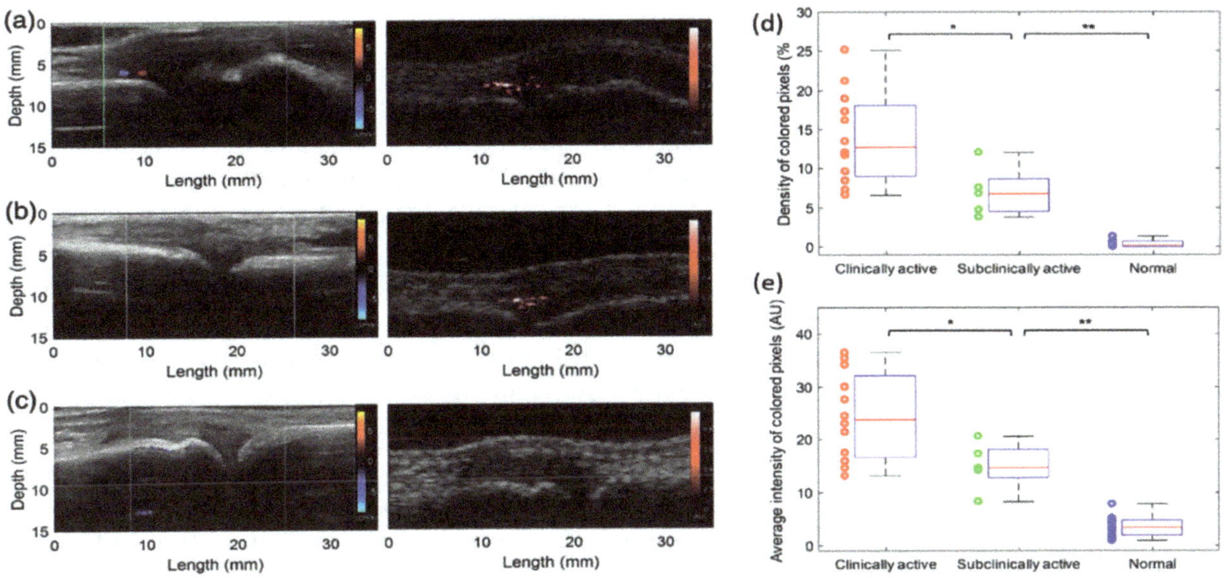

Figure 14. US Doppler (left) and PA (right) images acquired from LED-based system from three groups: (**a**) clinically active arthritis joints, (**b**) subclinical active arthritis joints, and (**c**) normal healthy joints). (**d**) The quantified results showing the density of colored pixels and (**e**) the average intensity of colored pixels in PA images of the three groups. * $p < 0.05$, ** $p < 0.005$. Reprinted from Ref. [31].

3.4.2. Diagnosis and Treatment Monitoring of Port Wine Stain

Port wine stain (PWS) is a benign capillary vascular malformation, with significant social and emotional impact. In a recent clinical pilot study, Cheng et al. demonstrated that LED-based PAI can be used as a point-of-care tool for clinical evaluation and treatment monitoring of PWS disease [100]. We foresee that LED-PAI will a have profound impact in this application, in which vascular contrast with depth information (~1 cm) is key for good diagnosis.

PWS is categorized as a benign capillary vascular malformation, which is difficult to cure. In general, PWS appears on the face, but it can affect other areas of the body too. The affected skin surface may thicken slightly and develop an irregular, pebbled surface in adulthood. PWS's cosmetic appearance causes substantial mental stress for the patients. In the study by Cheng et al., 22 patients were enrolled and separated into two groups based on their age (group 1: 3–6 years, group 2: above 6 years). The representative PA/US images (PWS region and normal region with clear difference in vascular contrast) are shown in Figure 15, along with the masked photograph of patient. The significant difference between the two different age groups also corresponds well with the given knowledge of PWS disease. Based on this result, it is clear that PAI as an imaging tool holds good potential in evaluation of PWS. Through this clinical pilot study, they demonstrated for the first time that LED-based PAI can be used as a point-of-care tool for clinical evaluation and PDT-treatment monitoring of PWS disease.

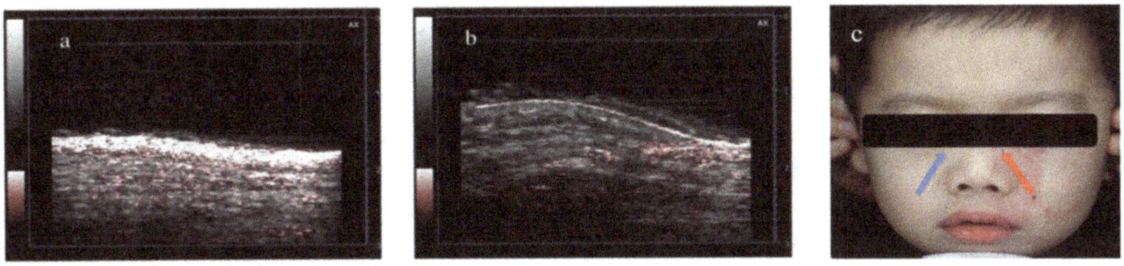

Figure 15. Typical PA/US overlay image of (**a**) PWS region (ROI) and (**b**) control region (HR). (**c**) Photograph of a PWS patient with imaging assisting marks. Reprinted with permission from Ref. [101].

4. Discussion

In this paper, we first reviewed the historical development of LED-based PAI, starting from the first report on single-point measurements to latest clinical pilot studies using high-power LED arrays. In the span of 10 years, there has been significant growth in this field, especially with the improvement of pulse energy (nJ to hundreds of μJ) and PRR (200 Hz to 16,000 Hz) of LEDs and also the advancements in low-noise data acquisition electronics. All these developments have resulted in commercialization of the technology, and it is worth mentioning that LED-PAI is now capable of functional imaging (oxygenation and blood flow imaging) of superficial and sub-surface tissue (more than 1 cm) at frame rates unachievable for laser-based systems (500 Hz). Even though LED-based PAI cannot be used for applications requiring larger imaging depth (for example, a full breast), it holds potential in several superficial imaging applications, specifically in rheumatology and dermatology.

Compared to solid-state lasers, the energy level of LED is two orders lower. However, the PRR of LED is much higher than that of a laser, which then can largely benefit the imaging quality by averaging more frames. Besides the emission energy level, another major difference between the pulsed LEDs and the solid-state lasers is the temporal pulse width. The pulse width of LED is tens of nanoseconds, whereas that of the solid-state lasers could be less than ten nanoseconds. The temporal pulse width imposes a limit on the spatial resolution of the imaging system. For example, the 70-ns pulse width of the 850-nm LED corresponds to a spatial resolution of 105 μm (=70 ns × 1500 μm/μs). This point, however, turns out to benefit the detection efficiency, especially when using bandlimited US probes for detection. The PA signal generated by a solid-state laser with a pulse width of 3.5 ns has a frequency component up to almost 300 MHz, in which anything above ~12 MHz will not be detected using a conventional mid-frequency range US probe. For a typical 5-MHz commercial US probe with 80% detection bandwidth, when using a 3.5-ns laser pulse, PA signal detection efficiency is 40 times less than the attainable efficiency when using an LED array generating 100-ns light pulses [102]. The resolution offered by a typical 5–10-MHz clinical US probe is 200 μm. Therefore, the pulse width of the LEDs can potentially be extended to 100 ns without affecting the spatial resolution (70 ns setting is used in all the studies reported in this paper).

In the second part of this paper, we reviewed some of the preclinical and clinical applications reported using LED-based PAI (in sequence of phantom, ex-vivo, small animal, and human in-vivo studies) as listed in Table 3. It is clear from the results that multispectral LED-based PA and US imaging holds strong potential in multiple applications, for example, guiding minimally invasive procedures, blood oxygen saturation imaging, diagnosis and staging of inflammatory arthritis, peripheral vascular assessment, guidance of surgical procedures like lymphaticovenous anastomosis, etc. In all the studies, an imaging depth of 0.5–1 cm was achieved at 10-Hz US and PA frame rates, which is good enough for multiple clinical applications. However, it is of paramount importance to improve the imaging depth for exploring more clinical applications, especially in the area of breast imaging and cardio-vascular medicine. To solve this issue and accelerate the clinical translation of LED-based PAI, several reconstruction and image processing techniques have been reported recently [103–105]. Use of clinically approved contrast agents (for example, ICG) may also be also useful to enhance the imaging depth.

The LED-based PA imaging system described here (AcousticX) is safe for both skin and eye exposure. Since LED emissions are incoherent, the ANSI safety limits for collimated laser beams do not apply. Instead, the international electrotechnical commission (IEC) 62471 is followed. According to IEC 62471, the exposure limit for skin is based on thermal injury due to the temperature rise in tissue. Assuming that the illumination on the same skin area lasts continuously for 5 s using two 850-nm LED bars working at a 4-KHz pulse repetition rate, the estimated exposure is 4.57×10^3 W·m^{-2}, which is below the thermal hazard limit for skin of 5.98×10^3 W·m^{-2}. For eye safety, two aspects need to be considered, which are retinal thermal hazard exposure limit (weak visual stimulus) and infrared radiation eye safety limit. Assuming a continuous illumination at the front of the eye for 5 s using two 850-nm LED bars working at a 4-KHz pulse repetition rate, the estimated exposures are

2.92×10^3 W·m^{-2}·sr^{-1} for retinal thermal exposure and 4.57×10^3 W·m^{-2} for infrared radiation exposure, both lower than the safety limits for eye of 1.34×10^5 W·m^{-2}·sr^{-1} and 5.38×10^3 W·m^{-2}, respectively.

Table 3. Summary of preclinical and clinical applications of LED-based PAI.

Target	Application		Depth (mm)	Contrast Agent	Wavelength (nm)
Medical needles, Vasculature	Guidance of minimally invasive procedures with peripheral tissue targets [32]	Phantom and ex vivo studies	38	N/A	850
Vasculature	Imaging of human placental vasculature [64]		7	N/A	850
Tumor	Imaging of intraocular tumors [6]		10	N/A	850
Vasculature	Non-invasive monitoring of angiogenesis [7]	Animal in vivo	10	N/A	850
Ulcer	Noninvasive imaging of pressure ulcers [76]		10	N/A	690
Oxygen saturation	Oxygen saturation imaging in Rheumatoid arthritis [77]		5	N/A	750/850
Molecular	Detection and monitoring of reactive oxygen and nitrogen species [29]		10	CyBA	850
Tumor/Contrast agents	Imaging of tumor using contrast enhancement [79]		10	NC	850
Cells/ Contrast agents	Imaging of molecular-labelled cells [27]		10	DiR	850
Vasculature	Imaging of peripheral microvasculature and function [6]	Healthy human in vivo	10	N/A	690/850
Vasculature	Simultaneous imaging of veins and lymphatic vessels [86]		10	ICG	940/820
Finger joints	Full view tomography of finger joints [87]		5	N/A	850
Finger joints	Imaging of inflammatory arthritis [31]	Patient in vivo	5	N/A	850
Skin	Imaging of port wine stain [101]		10	N/A	850

To date, the maximum imaging depth achieved by LED-based PA imaging in an in-vivo setting is 1 cm. Even though this is encouraging considering the low pulse energy, it is important to improve LED optical output for better usefulness in more clinical applications. To an extent, signal averaging helps to improve SNR without effecting frame rate. However, if the magnitudes of the acoustic signals generated by the weak illumination are significantly below the noise-equivalent pressure level of the US probe, averaging will not effectively improve SNR. In terms of translational potential, addition of PA imaging to a clinical US system will have relatively easier clinical acceptance. Considering the acoustic bandwidth limitation of conventional pulse-echo US probes, we believe that the lower pulse width (70 ns is the setting used in all the applications reported in this paper) of LEDs is not a bottleneck. We foresee work on two aspects to improve the imaging depth: (1) use of nanostack technology to squeeze more light out of LED elements, with multiple p-n junctions embedded in the epitaxial layer, increasing the region's light generation and thereby leading to a higher optical output, and (2) improving the driving electronics to increase the PRR further, consequently resulting in the possibility to average more frames and improve SNR without losing temporal resolution. LED might compete with LD with market share during clinical translation, but will not have much overlap with Nd: YAG OPO-based PAI system which focus on deep-tissue applications. However, LED-PAI may be a suitable option for point-of-care applications like guidance of peripheral vascular access procedures, rheumatoid arthritis screening, PWS diagnosis and treatment monitoring, etc.

Looking into the future, it is foreseen that advances in high-power LED technology, mainly driven by the lighting industry, and significant developments in machine/deep learning and signal processing algorithms will increase the use of LEDs in the context of PAI. LED arrays in different shapes could be also developed to find different applications, for example, developing ring-shape LEDs for breast 3D imaging and coupling light into optical fibers for minimally invasive and endoscopic procedures.

Worth mentioning here, if sufficient focusing can be achieved, LEDs will be the ideal candidate for acoustic-resolution PA microscopy (PAM). There have also been some recent reports in this direction. In 2017, Dai et al. presented a PAM system based on miniature LEDs working at a 405-nm source, which showed the capability of in-vivo mapping of vasculature networks in biological tissue [106,107]. They used a high-power LED (power~1.2 W) working at 405 nm wavelength, and a pulse width of 200 ns. The repetition rate was extended to 40 KHz towards meeting the high demand of scanning speed in a PAM setting. They acquired a complete PAM image in vivo in about 1 h, which is an encouraging result for the first LED-based PAM proof-of-concept study, but this temporal resolution is not good enough for clinical studies. On the other hand, for optical resolution PAM, the use of LEDs is likely to be challenging, as it would be difficult to achieve the necessary micron-scale diffraction-limited spot sizes. It would be also interesting to develop new low-frequency US probes (2–3 MHz) with ultra-high bandwidth and sensitivity to achieve higher imaging depth without compromising spatial resolution.

5. Conclusions

The use of LEDs as an illumination source introduces some limitations. First, the LEDs cannot be spectrally tuned, which eliminates the possibility of PA spectroscopic applications in which multiple chromophores are involved. Second, the pulse width of the LED is low when compared to a laser (30–100 ns), which affects the stress confinement satisfaction and can impact the efficiency of acoustic wave generation. Third, LEDs have low optical output power—this can limit penetration depth at higher frame rates. However, LED-based PAI systems offers several advantages, including a significant reduction in cost, smaller footprint, no requirement of laser calibration and monitoring, and no need for optical goggles or light-tight shields. Thus, LED-based systems are not only suitable for point-of-care non-invasive applications complementing US imaging, but also ideal for personalized or wearable PA equipment, and we foresee that this technology could additionally have broad utility in a number of therapeutic drug monitoring applications.

With wide optical wavelength range, flexible pulse-width setting, small footprint, low cost, and energy efficiency, LED-based PAI holds strong potential in functional and molecular preclinical and clinical imaging. We foresee that the addition of LED-based PAI to conventional US imaging in a clinical scanner will have a huge impact in point-of-care diagnostic imaging and also accelerate the clinical translation of PAI.

Author Contributions: Conceptualization, M.K.A.S. and J.Y.; methodology, N.S.; software, N.S.; investigation, Y.Z., T.F. and Q.C.; resources, Q.C. and X.W.; data curation, Y.Z. and T.F.; writing—original draft preparation, Y.Z. and T.F.; writing—review and editing, Y.Z., T.F., M.K.A.S. and J.Y.; supervision, S.D. All authors have read and agreed to the published version of the manuscript.

References

1. Wang, L.V.; Hu, S. Photoacoustic tomography: in vivo imaging from organelles to organs. *Science* **2012**, *335 6075*, 1458–1462. [CrossRef]
2. Wang, X.; Pang, Y.; Ku, G.; Xie, X.; Stoica, G.; Wang, L.V. Noninvasive laser-induced photoacoustic tomography for structural and functional in vivo imaging of the brain. *Nat. Biotechnol.* **2003**, *21*, 803–806. [CrossRef] [PubMed]
3. Beard, P. Biomedical photoacoustic imaging. *Interface Focus* **2011**, *1*, 602–631. [CrossRef]
4. Oladipupo, S.; Hu, S.; Kovalski, J.; Yao, J.; Santeford, A.; Sohn, R.E.; Shohet, R.; Maslov, K.; Wang, L.V.; Arbeit, J.M. VEGF is essential for hypoxia-inducible factor-mediated neovascularization but dispensable for endothelial sprouting. *Proc. Natl. Acad. Sci. USA* **2011**, *108*, 13264–13269. [CrossRef] [PubMed]

5. Oladipupo, S.S.; Hu, S.; Santeford, A.C.; Yao, J.; Kovalski, J.R.; Shohet, R.V.; Maslov, K.; Wang, L.V.; Arbeit, J.M. Conditional HIF-1 induction produces multistage neovascularization with stage-specific sensitivity to VEGFR inhibitors and myeloid cell independence. *Blood J. Am. Soc. Hematol.* **2011**, *11*, 4142–4153. [CrossRef] [PubMed]
6. Zhu, Y.; Xu, G.; Yuan, J.; Jo, J.; Gandikota, G.; Demirci, H.; Agano, T.; Sato, N.; Shigeta, Y.; Wang, X. Light emitting diodes based photoacoustic imaging and potential clinical applications. *Sci. Rep.* **2018**, *8*, 1–12. [CrossRef]
7. Zhu, Y.; Lu, X.; Dong, X.; Yuan, J.; Fabiilli, M.L.; Wang, X. LED-Based Photoacoustic Imaging for Monitoring Angiogenesis in Fibrin Scaffolds. *Tissue Eng. Part C Methods* **2019**, *25*, 523–531. [CrossRef]
8. Erpelding, T.N.; Kim, C.; Pramanik, M.; Jankovic, L.; Maslov, K.; Guo, Z.; Margenthaler, J.A.; Pashley, M.D.; Wang, L.V. Sentinel lymph nodes in the rat: noninvasive photoacoustic and US imaging with a clinical US system. *Radiology* **2010**, *256*, 102–110. [CrossRef]
9. Kim, C.; Cho, E.C.; Chen, J.; Song, K.H.; Au, L.; Favazza, C.; Zhang, Q.; Cobley, C.M.; Gao, F.; Xia, Y. In vivo molecular photoacoustic tomography of melanomas targeted by bioconjugated gold nanocages. *ACS Nano* **2010**, *4*, 4559–4564. [CrossRef]
10. Hu, S.; Wang, L. Neurovascular photoacoustic tomography. *Front. Neuroenerg.* 2010. [CrossRef]
11. Hu, S.; Yan, P.; Maslov, K.; Lee, J.-M.; Wang, L.V. Intravital imaging of amyloid plaques in a transgenic mouse model using optical-resolution photoacoustic microscopy. *Opt. Lett.* **2009**, *34*, 3899–3901. [CrossRef] [PubMed]
12. Hu, S.; Rao, B.; Maslov, K.; Wang, L.V. Label-free photoacoustic ophthalmic angiography. *Opt. Lett.* **2010**, *35*, 1–3. [CrossRef] [PubMed]
13. Jiao, S.; Jiang, M.; Hu, J.; Fawzi, A.; Zhou, Q.; Shung, K.K.; Puliafito, C.A.; Zhang, H.F. Photoacoustic ophthalmoscopy for in vivo retinal imaging. *Opt. Express* **2010**, *18*, 3967–3972. [CrossRef] [PubMed]
14. Zhang, E.Z.; Povazay, B.; Laufer, J.; Alex, A.; Hofer, B.; Pedley, B.; Glittenberg, C.; Treeby, B.; Cox, B.; Beard, P. Multimodal photoacoustic and optical coherence tomography scanner using an all optical detection scheme for 3D morphological skin imaging. *Biomed. Opt. Express* **2011**, *2*, 2202–2215. [CrossRef]
15. Favazza, C.P.; Wang, L.V.; Jassim, O.W.; Cornelius, L.A. In vivo photoacoustic microscopy of human cutaneous microvasculature and a nevus. *BIOMEDO* **2011**, *16*, 016015. [CrossRef]
16. Yang, J.-M.; Favazza, C.; Chen, R.; Yao, J.; Cai, X.; Maslov, K.; Zhou, Q.; Shung, K.K.; Wang, L.V. Toward dual-wavelength functional photoacoustic endoscopy: Laser and peripheral optical systems development. In Proceedings of the Photons Plus Ultrasound: Imaging and Sensing , San Francisco, CA, USA, 9 February 2012; p. 822316.
17. Yang, J.-M.; Maslov, K.; Yang, H.-C.; Zhou, Q.; Shung, K.K.; Wang, L.V. Photoacoustic endoscopy. *Opt. Lett.* **2009**, *34*, 1591–1593. [CrossRef]
18. Zhu, Y.; Johnson, L.A.; Huang, Z.; Rubin, J.M.; Yuan, J.; Lei, H.; Ni, J.; Wang, X.; Higgins, P.D.; Xu, G. Identifying intestinal fibrosis and inflammation by spectroscopic photoacoustic imaging: an animal study in vivo. *Biomed. Opt. Express* **2018**, *9*, 1590–1600. [CrossRef]
19. Zhu, Y.; Johnson, L.A.; Rubin, J.M.; Appelman, H.; Ni, L.; Yuan, J.; Wang, X.; Higgins, P.D.; Xu, G. Strain-photoacoustic imaging as a potential tool for characterizing intestinal fibrosis. *Gastroenterology* **2019**, *157*, 1196–1198. [CrossRef]
20. Zhu, Y.; Johnson, L.; Rubin, J.; Wang, X.; Higgins, P.; Xu, G. Characterization of intestinal fibrosis and inflammation with transcutaneous spectroscopic PA imaging (Conference Presentation). *Photons Plus Ultrasound Imaging Sens.* **2018**, 10494. [CrossRef]
21. Feng, T.; Perosky, J.E.; Kozloff, K.M.; Xu, G.; Cheng, Q.; Du, S.; Yuan, J.; Deng, C.X.; Wang, X. Characterization of bone microstructure using photoacoustic spectrum analysis. *Opt. Express* **2015**, *23*, 25217–25224. [CrossRef] [PubMed]
22. Kaiplavil, S.; Mandelis, A.; Wang, X.; Feng, T. Photothermal tomography for the functional and structural evaluation, and early mineral loss monitoring in bones. *Biomed. Opt. Express* **2014**, *5*, 2488–2502. [CrossRef] [PubMed]

23. Feng, T.; Kozloff, K.M.; Tian, C.; Perosky, J.E.; Hsiao, Y.-S.; Du, S.; Yuan, J.; Deng, C.X.; Wang, X. Bone assessment via thermal photo-acoustic measurements. *Opt. Lett.* **2015**, *40*, 1721–1724. [CrossRef] [PubMed]
24. Wang, X.; Feng, T.; Cao, M.; Perosky, J.E.; Kozloff, K.; Cheng, Q.; Yuan, J. Photoacoustic measurement of bone health: A study for clinical feasibility. In Proceedings of the 2016 IEEE International Ultrasonics Symposium (IUS), Tours, France, 18–21 September 2016.
25. Jansen, K.; Van Der Steen, A.F.; van Beusekom, H.M.; Oosterhuis, J.W.; van Soest, G. Intravascular photoacoustic imaging of human coronary atherosclerosis. *Opt. Lett.* **2011**, *36*, 597–599. [CrossRef]
26. Wang, B.; Yantsen, E.; Larson, T.; Karpiouk, A.B.; Sethuraman, S.; Su, J.L.; Sokolov, K.; Emelianov, S.Y. Plasmonic intravascular photoacoustic imaging for detection of macrophages in atherosclerotic plaques. *Nano Lett.* **2009**, *9*, 2212–2217. [CrossRef]
27. Hariri, A.; Lemaster, J.; Wang, J.; Jeevarathinam, A.S.; Chao, D.L.; Jokerst, J.V. The characterization of an economic and portable LED-based photoacoustic imaging system to facilitate molecular imaging. *Photoacoustics* **2018**, *9*, 10–20. [CrossRef]
28. Hariri, A.; Jeevarathinam, A.S.; Zhao, E.; Jokerst, J.V. Molecular imaging of oxidative stress sensing using LED-based photoacoustic imaging (Conference Presentation). *Photons Plus Ultrasound Imaging Sens.* **2019**, 10878. [CrossRef]
29. Hariri, A.; Zhao, E.; Jeevarathinam, A.S.; Lemaster, J.; Zhang, J.; Jokerst, J.V. Molecular imaging of oxidative stress using an LED-based photoacoustic imaging system. *Sci. Rep.* **2019**, *9*, 1–10. [CrossRef]
30. Xia, W.; Maneas, E.; Huynh, N.T.; Singh, M.K.A.; Brown, N.M.; Ourselin, S.; Gilbert-Kawai, E.; West, S.J.; Desjardins, A.E. Imaging of human peripheral blood vessels during cuff occlusion with a compact LED-based photoacoustic and ultrasound system. *Photons Plus Ultrasound Imaging Sens.* **2019**, 10878. [CrossRef]
31. Jo, J.; Xu, G.; Zhu, Y.; Burton, M.; Sarazin, J.; Schiopu, E.; Gandikota, G.; Wang, X. Detecting joint inflammation by an LED-based photoacoustic imaging system: a feasibility study. *BIOMEDO* **2018**, *23*, 110501. [CrossRef]
32. Xia, W.; Kuniyil Ajith Singh, M.; Maneas, E.; Sato, N.; Shigeta, Y.; Agano, T.; Ourselin, S.; J West, S.; E Desjardins, A. Handheld real-time LED-based photoacoustic and ultrasound imaging system for accurate visualization of clinical metal needles and superficial vasculature to guide minimally invasive procedures. *Sensors* **2018**, *18*, 1394. [CrossRef] [PubMed]
33. Allen, T.J.; Beard, P.C. High power visible light emitting diodes as pulsed excitation sources for biomedical photoacoustics. *Biomed. Opt. Express* **2016**, *7*, 1260–1270. [CrossRef] [PubMed]
34. Agano, T.; Sato, N.; Nakatsuka, H.; Kitagawa, K.; Hanaoka, T.; Morisono, K.; Shigeta, Y. Attempts to increase penetration of photoacoustic system using LED array light source. *Photons Plus Ultrasound Imaging Sens.* **2015**, 9323. [CrossRef]
35. Agano, T.; Sato, N.; Nakatsuka, H.; Kitagawa, K.; Hanaoka, T.; Morisono, K.; Shigeta, Y. Comparative experiments of photoacoustic system using laser light source and LED array light source. *Photons Plus Ultrasound Imaging Sens.* **2015**, 9323. [CrossRef]
36. Allen, T.J.; Beard, P.C. Pulsed near-infrared laser diode excitation system for biomedical photoacoustic imaging. *Opt. Lett.* **2006**, *31*, 3462–3464. [CrossRef]
37. Kolkman, R.G.; Steenbergen, W.; van Leeuwen, T.G. In vivo photoacoustic imaging of blood vessels with a pulsed laser diode. *Lasers Med. Sci.* **2006**, *21*, 134–139. [CrossRef]
38. Daoudi, K.; Van Den Berg, P.; Rabot, O.; Kohl, A.; Tisserand, S.; Brands, P.; Steenbergen, W. Handheld probe integrating laser diode and ultrasound transducer array for ultrasound/photoacoustic dual modality imaging. *Opt. Express* **2014**, *22*, 26365–26374. [CrossRef]
39. Kalva, S.K.; Upputuri, P.K.; Pramanik, M. High-speed, low-cost, pulsed-laser-diode-based second-generation desktop photoacoustic tomography system. *Opt. Lett.* **2019**, *44*, 81–84. [CrossRef]
40. Agano, T.; Singh, M.K.A.; Nagaoka, R.; Awazu, K. Effect of light pulse width on frequency characteristics of photoacoustic signal—An experimental study using a pulse-width tunable LED-based photoacoustic imaging system. *Int. J. Eng. Technol.* **2018**, *7*, 4300–4303.
41. Upputuri, P.K.; Pramanik, M. Pulsed laser diode based optoacoustic imaging of biological tissues. *Biomed. Phys. Eng. Express* **2015**, *1*, 045010. [CrossRef]
42. Wang, T.; Nandy, S.; Salehi, H.S.; Kumavor, P.D.; Zhu, Q. A low-cost photoacoustic microscopy system with a laser diode excitation. *Biomed. Opt. Express* **2014**, *5*, 3053–3058. [CrossRef]

43. Allen, T.J.; Beard, P.C. Light emitting diodes as an excitation source for biomedical photoacoustics. *Photons Plus Ultrasound Imaging Sens.* **2013**, 8581. [CrossRef]
44. Allen, T.J. High-Power Light Emitting Diodes; An Alternative Excitation Source for Photoacoustic Tomography. In *LED-Based Photoacoustic Imaging*; Springer: Berlin/Heidelberg, Germany, 2020; pp. 23–43.
45. Willert, C.; Stasicki, B.; Klinner, J.; Moessner, S. Pulsed operation of high-power light emitting diodes for imaging flow velocimetry. *Meas. Sci. Technol.* **2010**, *21*, 075402. [CrossRef]
46. Hansen, R.S. Using high-power light emitting diodes for photoacoustic imaging. *Ultrason. Imaging Tomogr. Ther.* **2011**, *7968*. [CrossRef]
47. Ikuta, T.; Shimizu, R. The dynamic response of magnetic domain walls to applied fields in yttrium orthoferrite, observed by a stroboscopic technique. *J. Phys. D Appl. Phys.* **1974**, *7*, 726. [CrossRef]
48. McFarlane, W. An inexpensive nanosecond light pulser for use in photomultiplier system testing. *Rev. Sci. Instrum.* **1974**, *45*, 286–289. [CrossRef]
49. Araki, T.; Misawa, H. Light emitting diode-based nanosecond ultraviolet light source for fluorescence lifetime measurements. *Rev. Sci. Instrum.* **1995**, *66*, 5469–5472. [CrossRef]
50. Araki, T.; Fujisawa, Y.; Hashimoto, M. An ultraviolet nanosecond light pulse generator using a light emitting diode for test of photodetectors. *Rev. Sci. Instrum.* **1997**, *68*, 1365–1368. [CrossRef]
51. Chaney, A.; Sundararajan, R. Simple MOSFET-based high-voltage nanosecond pulse circuit. *IEEE Trans. Plasma Sci.* **2004**, *32*, 1919–1924. [CrossRef]
52. Agano, T.; Sato, N. Photoacoustic Imaging System using LED light source. In Proceedings of the 2016 Conference on Lasers and Electro-Optics (CLEO), San Jose, CA, USA, 5–10 June 2016; pp. 1–2.
53. Narouze, S.N. *Atlas of Ultrasound-Guided Procedures in Interventional Pain Management*; Springer: Berlin/Heidelberg, Germany, 2018.
54. Wang, L.V.; Yao, J. A practical guide to photoacoustic tomography in the life sciences. *Nat. Methods* **2016**, *13*, 627. [CrossRef]
55. Kim, C.; Erpelding, T.N.; Maslov, K.I.; Jankovic, L.; Akers, W.J.; Song, L.; Achilefu, S.; Margenthaler, J.A.; Pashley, M.D.; Wang, L.V. Handheld array-based photoacoustic probe for guiding needle biopsy of sentinel lymph nodes. *BIOMEDO* **2010**, *15*, 046010. [CrossRef]
56. Su, J.L.; Karpiouk, A.B.; Wang, B.; Emelianov, S.Y. Photoacoustic imaging of clinical metal needles in tissue. *BIOMEDO* **2010**, *15*, 021309. [CrossRef] [PubMed]
57. Pratt, R.; Deprest, J.; Vercauteren, T.; Ourselin, S.; David, A.L. Computer-assisted surgical planning and intraoperative guidance in fetal surgery: a systematic review. *Prenat. Diagn.* **2015**, *35*, 1159–1166. [CrossRef] [PubMed]
58. Lewi, L.; Deprest, J.; Hecher, K. The vascular anastomoses in monochorionic twin pregnancies and their clinical consequences. *Am. J. Obstet. Gynecol.* **2013**, *208*, 19–30. [CrossRef] [PubMed]
59. Guiot, C.; Gaglioti, P.; Oberto, M.; Piccoli, E.; Rosato, R.; Todros, T. Is three-dimensional power Doppler ultrasound useful in the assessment of placental perfusion in normal and growth-restricted pregnancies? *Ultrasound Obstet. Gynecol.* **2008**, *31*, 171–176. [CrossRef] [PubMed]
60. Ntziachristos, V.; Razansky, D. Molecular imaging by means of multispectral optoacoustic tomography (MSOT). *Chem. Rev.* **2010**, *110*, 2783–2794. [CrossRef]
61. Maneas, E.; Xia, W.; Singh, M.K.A.; Sato, N.; Agano, T.; Ourselin, S.; West, S.J.; David, A.L.; Vercauteren, T.; Desjardins, A.E. Human placental vasculature imaging using an LED-based photoacoustic/ultrasound imaging system. In Proceedings of the Photons Plus Ultrasound: Imaging and Sensing 2018, San Francisco, CA, USA, 19 February 2018.
62. Xia, W.; Maneas, E.; Nikitichev, D.I.; Mosse, C.A.; Dos Santos, G.S.; Vercauteren, T.; David, A.L.; Deprest, J.; Ourselin, S.; Beard, P.C. Interventional photoacoustic imaging of the human placenta with ultrasonic tracking for minimally invasive fetal surgeries. In *International Conference on Medical Image Computing and Computer-Assisted Intervention*; Springer: Berlin/Heidelberg, Germany, 2015.
63. Xia, W.; Nikitichev, D.I.; Mari, J.M.; West, S.J.; Pratt, R.; David, A.L.; Ourselin, S.; Beard, P.C.; Desjardins, A.E. Performance characteristics of an interventional multispectral photoacoustic imaging system for guiding minimally invasive procedures. *BIOMEDO* **2015**, *20*, 086005. [CrossRef]

64. Maneas, E.; Aughwane, R.; Huynh, N.; Xia, W.; Ansari, R.; Kuniyil Ajith Singh, M.; Hutchinson, J.C.; Sebire, N.J.; Arthurs, O.J.; Deprest, J. Photoacoustic imaging of the human placental vasculature. *J. Biophotonics* **2019**, e201900167. [CrossRef]
65. Mallidi, S.; Larson, T.; Tam, J.; Joshi, P.P.; Karpiouk, A.; Sokolov, K.; Emelianov, S. Multiwavelength photoacoustic imaging and plasmon resonance coupling of gold nanoparticles for selective detection of cancer. *Nano Lett.* **2009**, *9*, 2825–2831. [CrossRef]
66. Krishna, V.; Singh, A.; Sharma, P.; Iwakuma, N.; Wang, Q.; Zhang, Q.; Knapik, J.; Jiang, H.; Grobmyer, S.R.; Koopman, B. Polyhydroxy fullerenes for non-invasive cancer imaging and therapy. *Small* **2010**, *6*, 2236–2241. [CrossRef]
67. Kircher, M.F.; De La Zerda, A.; Jokerst, J.V.; Zavaleta, C.L.; Kempen, P.J.; Mittra, E.; Pitter, K.; Huang, R.; Campos, C.; Habte, F. A brain tumor molecular imaging strategy using a new triple-modality MRI-photoacoustic-Raman nanoparticle. *Nat. Med.* **2012**, *18*, 829. [CrossRef] [PubMed]
68. Li, M.-L.; Oh, J.-T.; Xie, X.; Ku, G.; Wang, W.; Li, C.; Lungu, G.; Stoica, G.; Wang, L.V. Simultaneous molecular and hypoxia imaging of brain tumors in vivo using spectroscopic photoacoustic tomography. *Proc. IEEE* **2008**, *96*, 481–489.
69. Levi, J.; Kothapalli, S.-R.; Bohndiek, S.; Yoon, J.-K.; Dragulescu-Andrasi, A.; Nielsen, C.; Tisma, A.; Bodapati, S.; Gowrishankar, G.; Yan, X. Molecular photoacoustic imaging of follicular thyroid carcinoma. *Clin. Cancer Res.* **2013**, *19*, 1494–1502. [CrossRef] [PubMed]
70. Oyama, T.; Tomori, A.; Hotta, K.; Morita, S.; Kominato, K.; Tanaka, M.; Miyata, Y. Endoscopic submucosal dissection of early esophageal cancer. *Clin. Gastroenterol. Hepatol.* **2005**, *3*, S67–S70. [CrossRef]
71. Polednak, A.P.; Flannery, J.T. Brain, other central nervous system, and eye cancer. *Cancer* **1995**, *75*, 330–337. [CrossRef]
72. Xu, G.; Xue, Y.; Özkurt, Z.G.; Slimani, N.; Hu, Z.; Wang, X.; Xia, K.; Ma, T.; Zhou, Q.; Demirci, H. Photoacoustic imaging features of intraocular tumors: Retinoblastoma and uveal melanoma. *PLoS ONE* **2017**, *12*, e0170752. [CrossRef]
73. Draijer, M.; Hondebrink, E.; van Leeuwen, T.; Steenbergen, W. Review of laser speckle contrast techniques for visualizing tissue perfusion. *Lasers Med. Sci.* **2009**, *24*, 639. [CrossRef]
74. Briers, J.D. Laser speckle contrast imaging for measuring blood flow. *Opt. Appl.* **2007**, *37*, 139–152.
75. Dunn, A.K. Laser speckle contrast imaging of cerebral blood flow. *Ann. Biomed. Eng.* **2012**, *40*, 367–377. [CrossRef]
76. Hariri, A.; Chen, F.; Moore, C.; Jokerst, J.V. Noninvasive staging of pressure ulcers using photoacoustic imaging. *Wound Repair Regen.* **2019**, *27*, 488–496. [CrossRef]
77. Joseph, F.K.; Xavierselvan, M.; Singh, M.K.A.; Mallidi, S.; van der Laken, C.; van de Loo, F.; Steenbergen, W. LED-based photoacoustic imaging for early detection of joint inflammation in rodents: Towards achieving 3Rs in rheumatoid arthritis research. *Photons Plus Ultrasound Imaging Sens.* **2020**, 11240. [CrossRef]
78. Shuhendler, A.J.; Pu, K.; Cui, L.; Uetrecht, J.P.; Rao, J. Real-time imaging of oxidative and nitrosative stress in the liver of live animals for drug-toxicity testing. *Nat. Biotechnol.* **2014**, *32*, 373. [CrossRef] [PubMed]
79. Xavierselvan, M.; Mallidi, S. LED-Based Functional Photoacoustics—Portable and Affordable Solution for Preclinical Cancer Imaging. In *LED-Based Photoacoustic Imaging: From Bench to Bedside*; Singh, M.K.A., Ed.; Springer Singapore: Singapore, 2020; pp. 303–319.
80. Jokerst, J.V.; Thangaraj, M.; Kempen, P.J.; Sinclair, R.; Gambhir, S.S. Photoacoustic imaging of mesenchymal stem cells in living mice via silica-coated gold nanorods. *ACS Nano* **2012**, *6*, 5920–5930. [CrossRef] [PubMed]
81. Nam, S.Y.; Ricles, L.M.; Suggs, L.J.; Emelianov, S.Y. In vivo ultrasound and photoacoustic monitoring of mesenchymal stem cells labeled with gold nanotracers. *PLoS ONE* **2012**, *7*, e37267. [CrossRef]
82. Bristow, R.G.; Hill, R.P. Hypoxia and metabolism: Hypoxia, DNA repair and genetic instability. *Nat. Rev. Cancer* **2008**, *8*, 180–192. [CrossRef]
83. Wang, X.; Xie, X.; Ku, G.; Wang, L.V.; Stoica, G. Noninvasive imaging of hemoglobin concentration and oxygenation in the rat brain using high-resolution photoacoustic tomography. *BIOMEDO* **2006**, *11*, 024015. [CrossRef]
84. Yang, S.; Xing, D.; Zhou, Q.; Xiang, L.; Lao, Y. Functional imaging of cerebrovascular activities in small animals using high-resolution photoacoustic tomography. *Med. Phys.* **2007**, *34*, 3294–3301. [CrossRef]
85. Kim, C.; Favazza, C.; Wang, L.V. In vivo photoacoustic tomography of chemicals: high-resolution functional and molecular optical imaging at new depths. *Chem. Rev.* **2010**, *110*, 2756–2782. [CrossRef]

86. Singh, M.K.A.; Agano, T.; Sato, N.; Shigeta, Y.; Uemura, T. Real-time in vivo imaging of human lymphatic system using an LED-based photoacoustic/ultrasound imaging system. In Proceedings of the Photons Plus Ultrasound: Imaging and Sensing 2018, San Francisco, CA, USA, 19 February 2018.
87. Joseph, F.K.; Boink, Y.; Dantuma, M.; Singh, M.K.A.; Manohar, S.; Steenbergen, W. Tomographic imaging with an ultrasound andLED-based photoacoustic system. *Biomed. Opt. Express* **2020**, *11*, 2152–2165. [CrossRef]
88. Francis, K.J.; Boink, Y.E.; Dantuma, M.; Singh, M.K.A.; Manohar, S.; Steenbergen, W. Light Emitting Diodes Based Photoacoustic and Ultrasound Tomography: Imaging Aspects and Applications. In *LED-Based Photoacoustic Imaging*; Springer: Berlin/Heidelberg, Germany, 2020; pp. 245–266.
89. Agrawal, S.; Fadden, C.; Dangi, A.; Yang, X.; Albahrani, H.; Frings, N.; Heidari Zadi, S.; Kothapalli, S.-R. Light-Emitting-Diode-Based Multispectral Photoacoustic Computed Tomography System. *Sensors* **2019**, *19*, 4861. [CrossRef]
90. Wang, X.; Chamberland, D.L.; Carson, P.L.; Fowlkes, J.B.; Bude, R.O.; Jamadar, D.A.; Roessler, B.J. Imaging of joints with laser-based photoacoustic tomography: An animal study. *Med. Phys.* **2006**, *33*, 2691–2697. [CrossRef] [PubMed]
91. Zhang, H.F.; Maslov, K.; Sivaramakrishnan, M.; Stoica, G.; Wang, L.V. Imaging of hemoglobin oxygen saturation variations in single vessels in vivo using photoacoustic microscopy. *Appl. Phys. Lett.* **2007**, *90*, 053901. [CrossRef]
92. Sun, Y.; Sobel, E.; Jiang, H. Quantitative three-dimensional photoacoustic tomography of the finger joints: an in vivo study. *J. Biomed. Opt.* **2009**, *14*, 064002. [CrossRef] [PubMed]
93. Xu, G.; Rajian, J.R.; Girish, G.; Kaplan, M.J.; Fowlkes, J.B.; Carson, P.L.; Wang, X. Photoacoustic and ultrasound dual-modality imaging of human peripheral joints. *J. Biomed. Opt.* **2013**, *18*, 10502. [CrossRef] [PubMed]
94. Van Es, P.; Biswas, S.K.; Moens, H.J.B.; Steenbergen, W.; Manohar, S. Initial results of finger imaging using photoacoustic computed tomography. *J. Biomed. Opt.* **2014**, *19*, 060501. [CrossRef] [PubMed]
95. Sun, Y.; Sobel, E.S.; Jiang, H. First assessment of three-dimensional quantitative photoacoustic tomography for in vivo detection of osteoarthritis in the finger joints. *Med. Phys.* **2011**, *38*, 4009–4017. [CrossRef]
96. Rajian, J.R.; Girish, G.; Wang, X. Photoacoustic tomography to identify inflammatory arthritis. *J. Biomed. Opt.* **2012**, *17*, 96011–96013. [CrossRef]
97. Rajian, J.R.; Shao, X.; Chamberland, D.L.; Wang, X. Characterization and treatment monitoring of inflammatory arthritis by photoacoustic imaging: a study on adjuvant-induced arthritis rat model. *Biomed. Opt. Express* **2013**, *4*, 900–908. [CrossRef]
98. Beziere, N.; von Schacky, C.; Kosanke, Y.; Kimm, M.; Nunes, A.; Licha, K.; Aichler, M.; Walch, A.; Rummeny, E.J.; Ntziachristos, V.; et al. Optoacoustic imaging and staging of inflammation in a murine model of arthritis. *Arthritis Rheumatol.* **2014**, *66*, 2071–2078. [CrossRef] [PubMed]
99. Jo, J.; Xu, G.; Cao, M.; Marquardt, A.; Francis, S.; Gandikota, G.; Wang, X. A Functional Study of Human Inflammatory Arthritis Using Photoacoustic Imaging. *Sci. Rep.* **2017**, *7*, 15026. [CrossRef]
100. Zhang, H.; Pan, J.; Wen, L.; Shen, S.; Zhang, Y.; Wang, P.; Cheng, Q.; Wang, X.; Wang, X. A novel light emitting diodes based photoacoustic evaluation method for port wine stain and its clinical trial (Conference Presentation). *Photons Plus Ultrasound Imaging Sens.* **2019**, 10878. [CrossRef]
101. Cheng, Q.; Qian, M.; Wang, X.; Zhang, H.; Wang, P.; Wen, L.; Pan, J.; Gao, Y.; Wu, S.; Zhang, M. Diagnosis and Treatment Monitoring of Port-Wine Stain Using LED-Based Photoacoustics: Theoretical Aspects and First In-Human Clinical Pilot Study. In *LED-Based Photoacoustic Imaging: From Bench to Bedside*; Springer: Berlin/Heidelberg, Germany, 2020; pp. 351–377.
102. Agano, T.; Sato, N.; Awazu, K. LED-based photoacoustic imaging system: Why it achieves the same signal to noise ratio as solid-state-laser-based system: A review. *Photons Plus Ultrasound Imaging Sens.* **2020**, 11240. [CrossRef]
103. Anas, E.M.A.; Zhang, H.K.; Kang, J.; Boctor, E. Enabling fast and high quality LED photoacoustic imaging: a recurrent neural networks based approach. *Biomed. Opt. Express* **2018**, *9*, 3852–3866. [CrossRef] [PubMed]
104. Mozaffarzadeh, M.; Hariri, A.; Moore, C.; Jokerst, J.V. The double-stage delay-multiply-and-sum image reconstruction method improves imaging quality in a led-based photoacoustic array scanner. *Photoacoustics* **2018**, *12*, 22–29. [CrossRef]
105. Singh, M.K.A.; Sivasubramanian, K.; Sato, N.; Ichihashi, F.; Sankai, Y.; Xing, L. Deep learning-enhanced LED-based photoacoustic imaging. *Photons Plus Ultrasound Imaging Sens.* **2020**, 11240. [CrossRef]

106. Dai, X.; Yang, H.; Jiang, H. In vivo photoacoustic imaging of vasculature with a low-cost miniature light emitting diode excitation. *Opt. Lett.* **2017**, *42*, 1456–1459. [CrossRef]
107. Dai, X.; Yang, H.; Jiang, H. Low-cost high-power light emitting diodes for photoacoustic imaging. In Proceedings of the Photons Plus Ultrasound: Imaging and Sensing 2017, San Francisco, CA, USA, 29 January–1 February 2017; p. 100644.

13

Multiangle Long-Axis Lateral Illumination Photoacoustic Imaging Using Linear Array Transducer

João H. Uliana [1], Diego R. T. Sampaio [1], Guilherme S. P. Fernandes [1], María S. Brassesco [2], Marcello H. Nogueira-Barbosa [3], Antonio A. O. Carneiro [1] and Theo Z. Pavan [1,*]

1 Department of Physics, FFCLRP, University of São Paulo, Ribeirão Preto 14040-901, SP, Brazil; joaouliana@usp.br (J.H.U.); diegothomaz@gmail.com (D.R.T.S.); guilherme.santos.fernandes@usp.br (G.S.P.F.); adilton@usp.br (A.A.O.C.)

2 Department of Biology, FFCLRP, University of São Paulo, Ribeirão Preto 14040-901, SP, Brazil; solbrassesco@usp.br

3 Department of Medical Images, Hematology and Clinical Oncology, Ribeirão Preto Medical School, University of São Paulo, Ribeirão Preto 14040-901, SP, Brazil; marcello@fmrp.usp.br

* Correspondence: theozp@usp.br

Abstract: Photoacoustic imaging (PAI) combines optical contrast with ultrasound spatial resolution and can be obtained up to a depth of a few centimeters. Hand-held PAI systems using linear array usually operate in reflection mode using a dark-field illumination scheme, where the optical fiber output is attached to both sides of the elevation plane (short-axis) of the transducer. More recently, bright-field strategies where the optical illumination is coaxial with acoustic detection have been proposed to overcome some limitations of the standard dark-field approach. In this paper, a novel multiangle long-axis lateral illumination is proposed. Monte Carlo simulations were conducted to evaluate light delivery for three different illumination schemes: bright-field, standard dark-field, and long-axis lateral illumination. Long-axis lateral illumination showed remarkable improvement in light delivery for targets with a width smaller than the transducer lateral dimension. A prototype was developed to experimentally demonstrate the feasibility of the proposed approach. In this device, the fiber bundle terminal ends are attached to both sides of the transducer's long-axis and the illumination angle of each fiber bundle can be independently controlled. The final PA image is obtained by the coherent sum of subframes acquired using different angles. The prototype was experimentally evaluated by taking images from a phantom, a mouse abdomen, forearm, and index finger of a volunteer. The system provided light delivery enhancement taking advantage of the geometry of the target, achieving sufficient signal-to-noise ratio at clinically relevant depths.

Keywords: photoacoustic imaging; illumination scheme; in vivo; mouse; Monte Carlo; linear array

---

1. Introduction

Photoacoustic imaging (PAI) is a technique based on the photoacoustic (PA) effect, which consists of pressure waves generation due to the absorption of light [1–5]. Currently, laser-based PAI systems use short-duration laser pulses (i.e., ~10^{-9} s) ensuring thermal and stress confinement. As pulsed-light propagates within the target material, its absorption increases the local temperature, causing a thermal-elastic expansion [6] and generating a pressure wave. Thus, PAI encodes the optical absorption information into pressure waves, therefore combining optical contrast with ultrasound spatial resolution [4].

PAI can provide physiological and anatomical information of tissues by accessing their optical, thermal, and mechanical proprieties [5,7]. Since PA signal magnitude is temperature-dependent,

PAI has been used, for example, to map temperature variation within tissues during hyperthermia procedures [8–11]. Moreover, PA magnitude is proportional to the optical absorption of a chromophore; therefore, multi-wavelength PAI is capable of identifying structures with different optical absorption profiles [12,13]. In this context, a typical application of multispectral PAI is to estimate blood oxygen saturation (sO_2) from the relative concentrations of oxyhemoglobin (HbO_2) and deoxyhemoglobin (Hb) [14–19]. In addition, exogenous contrast agents, for example, nanoparticles and organic dyes, can be accessed to obtain molecular PAI and for drug delivery studies [20]. PAI is frequently combined with clinical ultrasound arrays. This approach allows simultaneously displaying conventional ultrasound images of different modalities (e.g., B-mode and Doppler) with PAI. Different preclinical and clinical, e.g., breast cancer [21] and joint arthritis [22,23], applications of PAI integrated with ultrasound scanners are under investigation.

Hand-held PAI systems usually operate in reflection mode (also known as epi-mode), where illumination and PA wave detection are arranged on the same side [24–28]. For linear array transducers, it is common to illuminate the tissue using a rectangular optical fiber output, which is attached to both sides of the elevation plane (short-axis) of the transducer, see Figure 1a (here this strategy will be referred to as standard dark-field illumination, following the terminology used in [29–32]). For this dark-field illumination scheme, when the transducer face is in contact with the skin, light is delivered obliquely and relies on light scattering within the target to illuminate the whole field-of-view (FOV) of the transducer. In addition, light absorption outside the imaging plane generates PA waves that can reach the ultrasound transducer. These signals are a source of clutter, which is also an important limiting factor to obtain PA images at deeper regions [33–35]. Different studies have investigated, for this standard dark-field illumination scheme, light delivery optimization to enhance PA image contrast and signal-to-noise ratio (SNR) by varying the distance between the fiber output and the transducer and incidence angle between the light beam and the imaging plane [30,33,36–38]. In [39], the authors verified, through Monte Carlo simulations, that the optimal illumination configuration depends on the optical properties of the tissues under investigation. They observed that thickness and optical scattering of skin play a major role for this optimization. Another possible strategy to optimize light delivery is to accommodate an optically transparent spacer between the transducer and target's surface to deliver light directly to the tissue underneath the transducer [25,27,28,32]. Improvements in light delivery could also be achieved by using a concave-shaped light catcher that redirects the light reflected by the skin surface back to the tissue, improving the PA signal magnitude at higher depths [40,41]. The aforementioned studies evaluated laser-based PAI systems. More recently, pulsed light-emitting diodes (LED)-based PAI technique has been proposed as an interesting and cost-efficient option [42,43]. LED-based PAI with linear array usually operates using a similar setup as shown in Figure 1a [42,44]. The study [44] suggested that the high divergence of LED illumination decreases the source direction dependency on PA signal compared to laser.

Since optimal light delivery to the tissue is essential to increase image depth and SNR, custom transducers, new materials, and new strategies have been developed to explore different illumination geometries to improve the quality of the PA image. For example, an ultrasonic transducer fabricated on a glass substrate has an improved transparency allowing the laser beam to propagate through the transducer's material with low absorption, resulting in overlapped optical excitation and acoustic detection [45]. An ultrasound transducer with a hollow central bore [46] or an optically transparent acoustic transducer [47] could be other options to provide reflection mode illumination. However, these approaches require an extensive redesign of the ultrasound probe and cannot be easily integrated into standard clinical scanners. In epi-mode PAI using standard linear array transducers, optical and acoustic fields can be coaxially arranged (see Figure 1b) by redirecting the laser beam using an optical/acoustic coupler [48] or by using a single or double acoustic reflector to redirect the acoustic waves [29,31,49]. Another strategy for coaxial illumination consists of a custom linear array transducer where the optical fiber outputs and piezoelectric elements are linearly and alternately arranged [50]. These studies [29,31,48–50] showed that this illumination strategy improved light delivery when compared with the standard dark-field approach. In the present paper, this strategy will be referred to as bright-field illumination, following the terminology used in [30–32,49].

An alternative illumination approach, not yet investigated in the literature, would consist of attaching the fiber bundle terminal ends to both sides of the transducer's long-axis (from now on we will refer to this technique as long-axis lateral illumination), see Figure 1c. In the present paper, we propose a long-axis lateral illumination scheme as a new epi-mode PAI strategy, where the light is delivered within the imaging plane similarly to the coaxial arrangement. In the first part of the paper, Monte Carlo simulations of photon propagation were used to compare light delivery for different illumination strategies; i.e., standard dark-field, long-axis lateral, and bright-field illumination. A transparent spacer positioned between the transducer and the tissue surface was considered for all cases. Tissues with three different geometries were simulated; i.e., targets larger and smaller than the lateral dimension of the imaging plane simulating the human forearm and index finger, respectively and an intermediate situation simulating the cross section of a mouse torso where the abdomen was smaller than the image width and the lower limbs fitted the transducer FOV. The simulations demonstrate that the lateral illumination strategy can provide remarkably improved fluence distribution for targets smaller than the imaging plane.

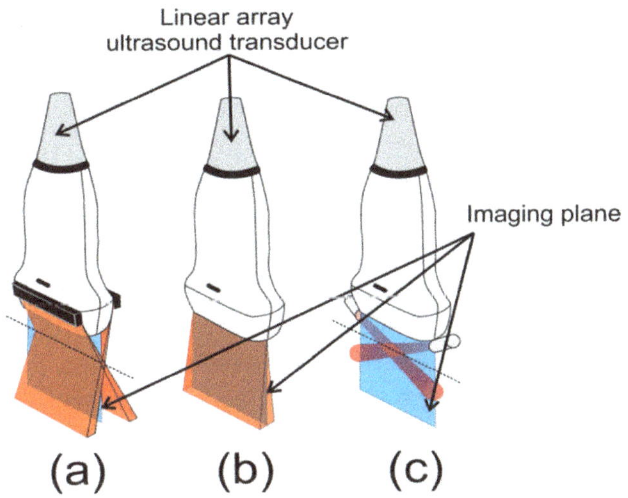

Figure 1. (**a**) Standard dark-field illumination scheme to acquire photoacoustic (PA) image in reflection mode; a rectangular optical fiber terminal illuminates the surface of the target. (**b**) Bright-field illumination where the laser beam and the acoustic field are coaxially aligned. (**c**) Proposed long-axis lateral illumination architecture; the variation of light incidence angle provides wide illumination to the surface of the target.

In the second part of this paper, the development of a simple and easy way to construct a device for long-axis lateral illumination PAI is described. This device employed a nonexpensive commercially available bifurcated optical fiber bundle for light delivery, where no other optical components were required. Since the setup, as shown in Figure 1c, would irradiate only a limited area within FOV, the optical fiber bundle outputs were mounted on movable sockets arranged parallel to the imaging plane to provide multiangle long-axis lateral illumination. The final PA image, covering the full scan area, is then obtained by combining the PA sub-images acquired at different angles. This is a similar strategy as described in [51], where a narrow laser beam scanning approach was proposed for a combined real-time PA-ultrasound imaging system. Then the final PA image was the summation of the sub-images obtained at each laser beam scanning position.

Therefore, this paper presents a novel PAI light delivery where light and sound are coaxially illuminated. Different from other approaches with similar capability [29,31,48,49], the proposed technique does not require an acoustic/optical coupling device. This is an advantage because these coupling modules usually induce important phase distortion to the PA wavefront which can reduce image quality [32]. The light delivery device was prototyped to provide freedom to independently choose the illumination angle, at each side of the transducer, allowing multiangle illumination planning. To show the feasibility of the multiangle long-axis lateral illumination PAI device, images taken from phantom, mouse abdomen, forearm, and index finger of a volunteer were analyzed.

2. Materials and Methods

2.1. Monte Carlo Simulation of Illumination Schemes

The spatial energy deposition may vary depending on the illumination scheme and target shape. To evaluate the performance of the illumination schemes depicted in Figure 1, light transport was simulated using the MCXLAB Matlab toolbox, which is a 3D voxel-based Monte Carlo model [52], for three different target geometries: (i) a cylindrical target shape simulating a situation similar to what was observed for the human index finger (lateral dimension smaller than transducer's width); (ii) geometry similar to the human forearm (lateral dimension larger than transducer's width); (iii) mouse torso as an intermediate case, i.e., part of the target was smaller (mouse abdomen), while the lower limbs of the animal was larger than the transducer's width.

The standard dark-field illumination scheme shown in Figure 1a, based on the setup described in [53], was composed of two optical fiber terminals (38 mm × 1.25 mm) with the same width as the ultrasound linear array used in the experiments of the present paper. Each terminal was positioned so that the light beam incident angle was 20° and the light beams overlapped at the upper surface of the target. For all three illumination schemes, an optically transparent spacer of 19.5 mm (i.e., water) was positioned between the transducer and the target. For the bright-field illumination scheme shown in Figure 1b, the laser beam was coaxial with acoustic detection. In this case, the illumination dimension hitting the target was 38 mm × 5 mm, which is in accordance with [48]. For the long-axis lateral illumination, Figure 1c, the fiber optic bundle terminals were circular in shape with 5 mm diameter. To illuminate the entire transducer FOV, the same multiangle illumination strategy used for the experiments (see next sections for a detailed description) were adopted in the simulations. We verified that at least 5 laser beam incident angles were necessary to ensure a complete illumination. In this case, all simulation parameters were the same as the experimental setup. A total of (5.0×10^6) photons were used to simulate each situation.

The volume dimension for all simulations was 89 mm × 60 mm × 30 mm with a voxel size of 0.25 mm. The volume consisted of two different materials, the background (water) and an inclusion (target) to simulate the tissue. The optical proprieties of the background were: absorption coefficient $\mu_a^{bkg} = 3.5640 \times 10^{-5}$ mm^{-1}, scattering coefficient $\mu_s^{bkg} = 1.0$ mm^{-1}, $g_{bkg} = 1$, and $\eta_{bkg} = 1.37$; where g denotes the anisotropic factor and η denotes the refraction index. For the target, the optical scattering and optical absorption coefficients were chosen for a generic tissue, following the equations [54]:

$$\mu'_s = a(\lambda/500nm)^{-b}, \tag{1}$$

$$\mu_a = BO\mu_a^{HbO_2} + B(1-O)\mu_a^{Hb} + W\mu_a^{water} + F_a\mu_a^{lipid} \tag{2}$$

where μ'_s denotes the reduced scattering coefficient, μ_a denotes the absorption coefficient, B denotes the average blood volume fraction, O is the oxygen saturation of blood, W is the water content, and F_a is the fat content. Selecting a generic tissue composed of 15% of blood at 75% of oxygen saturation, 20% of water, and 10% of fat results in $\mu_a^{tissue} = 0.062$ mm^{-1} at 800 nm. The a and b values were chosen as the mean values estimated for soft tissues ($a = 1.89$ mm^{-1}, $b = 1.286$) [54] resulting in $\mu{\prime}_s^{tissue} = 1.033$ mm^{-1} at 800 nm. The anisotropic factor (g_{tissue}) and the refraction index (η_{tissue}) were 0.95 and 1.37, respectively.

2.2. Device for Multiangle Long-Axis Lateral Illumination

The PA system is composed by an Nd:YAG Laser (Brilliant B, Quantel Laser, Les Ulis, France) and an Optical Parametric Oscillator (MagicPRISM OPO, Opotek, Carlsbad, CA, USA) connected to a trifurcated optical fiber bundle (Oriel Glass Fiber Optic Bundle; numerical aperture 0.56; core diameter: 7.9 mm (common), 5.5 mm (legs); fiber length 36 in; Newport, Irvine, CA, USA). One terminal end of the optical fiber bundle was connected to the sensor of an energy meter (FieldMax II-TOP, Coherent, Santa Clara, CA, USA) providing the measurement of laser fluence in real-time. The other two terminals were used to illuminate the sample. PA and ultrasonic radiofrequency (RF) data were acquired using a commercial ultrasound system (SonixOP, Ultrasonix Medical Corp., Richmond, BC, Canada) connected to a parallel acquisition receiver module (SonixDAQ, Ultrasonix Medical Corp., Richmond, Canada), operating at a sampling frequency of 40 MHz.

The device for multiangle long-axis lateral illumination was developed using a new architecture that differs from most used configurations presented in previous studies [9,23–26,33–38]. The optical fiber bundle terminal ends were attached to movable sockets placed on the lateral sides of the transducer's long-axis (see Figure 1c), so that different focal illumination spots within the transducer FOV could be obtained by varying the incident laser beam angles (see Figures 2 and 3).

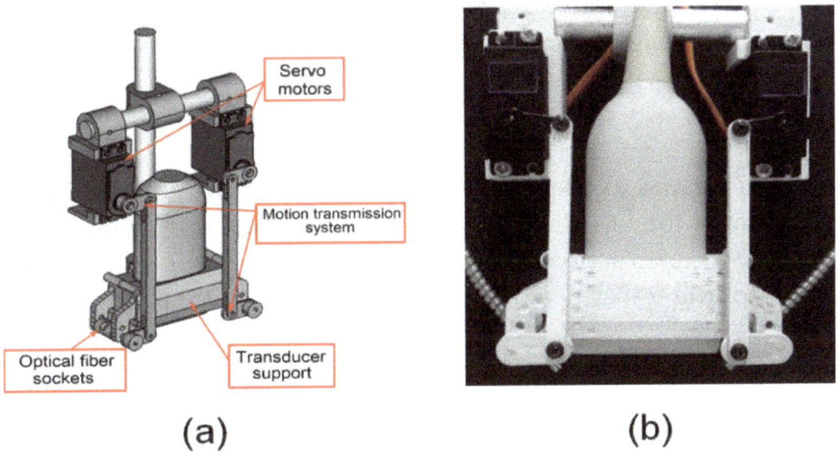

Figure 2. (**a**) Three-dimensional model and (**b**) prototype of the multiangle long-axis lateral illumination device attached to a linear array ultrasound transducer.

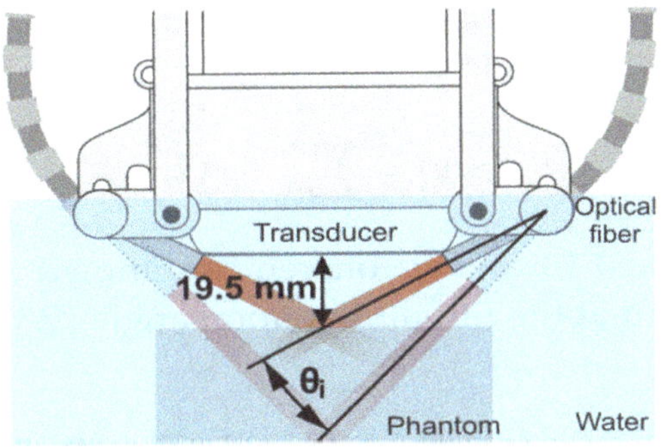

Figure 3. Depiction of the experimental setup used to acquire the multiangle long-axis lateral illumination PA images. The distance of 19.5 mm between the transducer and the phantom surface forces the focal illumination region to be at the phantom surface for $\theta_i = 0°$.

The device consists of three main parts: the ultrasound transducer support, the motion transmission system, and two motors. The support and the motion transmission system were designed using the FreeCAD open-source parametric modeling software, see Figure 2a, and printed with Acrylonitrile Butadiene Styrene (ABS) plastic using a 3D printer (ZMorph 2.0 SX, ZMorph, Wroclaw, Poland), as shown in Figure 2b. The angle of the movable sockets is controlled by the servo motors (MG996R, Tower Pro, Shenzhen, China) connected to the motion transmission systems and controlled by an open-source microcontroller (Arduino UNO, Arduino, Turin, Italy).

A linear L14-5/38 ultrasound transducer (Ultrasonix Medical Corp., Richmond, Canada) with 128 piezoelectric elements and a nominal center frequency of 7.2 MHz, was positioned inside the support, which was then attached to the 3D linear stage (HSC-103, Sigmakoki, Tokyo, Japan). A LabVIEW virtual interface (National Instruments Corp., Austin, TX) was developed to control the position of the device as well as the illumination angles. The timing sequence of the synchronous RF data acquisition and multiangle illumination consists in acquiring a pair of PA and B-mode images for each laser pulse (laser repetition rate is 10 Hz). After K laser pulses (K·100 ms) the illumination angle is incremented, the process is then repeated for n illumination angles. A 3D volume is obtained by moving the transducer along the elevation axis with a 3-axes translational stage.

2.3. Coherently Summing the PA Subframes

The RF data were acquired intercalating the laser pulse with the pulse-echo transmission for obtaining a prebeamformed PA subframe and then a prebeamformed B-mode frame. The PA sub-image and B-mode image were generated with the delay and sum technique. In PA images, the RF signal $s(x_i, t)$ represents the pressure waves generated by the light absorbers and detected by the i-th transducer element. The PA wave time of flight from the absorber position to each element of the array is

$$\delta(x, x_i,\ y) = \sqrt{y^2 + (x - x_i)^2}/c \tag{3}$$

where x and y are the lateral and axial position of the pressure wave source, respectively, while x_i denotes the lateral distance of the i-th element of the array to the central element. The delay and sum technique for PA subframe reconstruction consists in applying a delay $\delta(x, x_i, y)$ to the RF signal $s(x_i, t)$ detected by the elements of the transducer and adding coherently [51]

$$S(x, y) = \sum\nolimits_{x-\alpha}^{x+\alpha} s(x_i, \delta(x, x_i,\ y)) \tag{4}$$

where α is the aperture of receive beamforming, i.e., the number of adjacent elements summed.

The coherent sum of reconstructed PA subframes acquired using each illumination angle, without other processing steps, is equivalent to a reconstructed PA image acquired using a wide illumination due to the linear behavior of the delay and sum operation (Huygens–Fresnel principle) [51]. Thus, PA signals reconstructed using the delay and sum technique can be coherently added to gather the contribution of each illumination angle as:

$$S_C(x, y) = \sum\nolimits_{\theta_0}^{\theta_n} S_{\theta_i}(x, y), \tag{5}$$

where $S_c(x, y)$ is the reconstructed RF signal coherently summed (PA final image), $S_{\theta_i}(x, y)$ is the reconstructed RF signal acquired at the i-th illumination angle (PA subframe), θ_n is the maximum illumination angle.

2.4. Phantom Experiments: Evaluation of Multiangle Long-Axis Lateral Illumination PAI

A cubic phantom with a homogeneous distribution of light absorbers (magnetic nanoparticles) was used to evaluate the multiangle illumination and the PA images. The phantom dimensions were 8.0 cm × 8.0 cm × 3.5 cm, and it was manufactured using a mixture of gelatin (Bloom 250, Gelita, Eberbach, Germany) and agar powder (RM026; Himedia Laboratories-LLC, Kennett Square, USA), diluted at dry-weight concentrations of 4% and 2% of water mass, respectively. Iron oxide nanoparticles (Fe_3O_4) with dimensions ranging from 20 nm to 30 nm (Nanostructured and Amorphous Materials Inc., Houston, TX, USA) in the concentration of 0.1% of water mass were added to act as light absorbers.

Formaldehyde in a weight concentration of 0.5% of gelatin mass was added to increase stiffness and melting temperature. The phantom was manufactured according to the description in [55,56].

To avoid any coupling issues, the experiments were performed using targets immersed in water to guarantee that the gap between the ultrasound transducer and the target was completely filled by an optically transparent coupling medium. However, we believe it would be possible to acquire images using a matching layer. For example, this layer could be ultrasound imaging gel (see, for example, [57]) or a gel pad (see, for example, [58]). This is a topic of ongoing research and should appear in future publications.

The phantom was immersed in a water tank with its surface 19.5 mm from the transducer face. For this condition, the focal illumination region was at the phantom surface for $\theta_i = 0^{\circ}$, considered as the smallest possible angle (see Figure 3). Then, for each illumination angle, two PA subframes were acquired and the angle was varied n times in steps of $\Delta\theta$ until the n-th angle was achieved

$$\theta_n = \theta_{min} + n\Delta\theta. \tag{6}$$

The device moved across the elevation axis to obtain a volume (Table 1), resulting in a total of 360 frames. The PA images were acquired at 720 nm with an average fluence of 15 mJ/cm^2 at the phantom surface. This wavelength was selected for the phantom experiment because one of the energy peaks of the laser is observed at 720 nm; in addition, iron oxide nanoparticles present higher optical absorption at lower wavelengths within the near infrared spectrum region [59]. For the in vivo experiments, 800 nm was selected because it is the isosbestic point of blood [60].

Table 1. Multiangle illumination and acquisition parameters.

Parameters	Phantom	Finger and Forearm	Balb/C Mouse
Angle step	2°	4°	4°
Elevation step	2 mm	2 mm	2 mm
Image axial	45 mm	35 mm	35 mm
Image lateral	38 mm	38 mm	38 mm
Number of angle steps (n)	9	4	4
Number of elevation steps	19	9	5
Number of frames per angle (K)	2	2	2
Wavelength	720 nm	800 nm	800 nm

The phantom was assumed to have a homogeneous distribution of light absorbers; the optical attenuation coefficient was calculated measuring the fluence of transmitted light through the layers of the phantom with different thickness. The estimated light attenuation of the phantom was $\mu^{att}_{phantom} = (0.133 \pm 0.011)$ mm^{-1}. Therefore, an analysis of the light delivery was performed by evaluating the PA signal as a function of axial and lateral directions of an averaged PA image taken over the elevation axis. Since the magnetic nanoparticles at low concentration, which is the case of the present experiment, mainly absorb the light energy, optical scattering was considered negligible for this analysis [59].

We defined image depth as the axial distance between the position of a RF signal inside the target and the target surface, therefore not considering the distance between the transducer face and target surface. The average RF signal of the PA subframes at depths and in lateral direction were evaluated using distinct regions of interest (ROI). Based on the number of elements of the transducer (i.e., 128 elements), we defined a central ROI-1 within FOV, which included the five central elements (62–66) and extended from the phantom surface to the maximum depth, with dimensions 1.5 mm × 25.5 mm. Also, peripheral ROIs (ROI-2 and ROI-3) were defined including two sets of five elements positioned at opposite sides of transducer elements: 5–9 (ROI-2) and 119–123 (ROI-3). ROI-2 and ROI-3 had the same dimensions as ROI-1. In addition, the average PA signal magnitude, in the lateral direction from 0 mm to 2 mm of depth, was calculated for all elements (1–128).

Since the phantom had a homogenous distribution of light absorbers, the PA signal amplitude was related to the amount of light delivered. The quantitative analysis of illumination, in the ROI-1 region, as a function of illumination angle was performed using the mean square root of the RF signal amplitude (A_{RMS}) calculated in each PA subframe:

$$A_{RMS}(\theta) = \sqrt{\frac{\sum_{j=x_a}^{x_b} \sum_{i=y_a}^{y_b} \left(S_\theta\left(x_j, y_i\right)\right)^2}{(y_b - y_a)(x_b - x_a)}} \tag{7}$$

where x_a, x_b, y_a, and y_b are the limits of the ROI-1.

The spatial light delivery information, in the central region of the final PA image, was estimated taking the mean axial position of the RF signal ($\overline{y}$) as a function of illumination angle in ROI-1

$$\overline{y}(\theta) = \frac{\sum_{j=x_a}^{x_b} \sum_{i=y_a}^{y_b} \left(\left|S_\theta\left(x_j, y_i\right)\right| y_i\right)}{\sum_{j=x_a}^{x_b} \sum_{i=y_a}^{y_b} \left(\left|S_\theta\left(x_j, y_i\right)\right|\right)} \tag{8}$$

Thus, A_{RMS} provides information about the mean amount of light delivered per illumination angle in the central region of the transducer while $\overline{y}$ provides spatial information about the mean axial position of generated pressure waves.

The final multiangle PA image SNR was calculated taking the envelope-detected image amplitude [61]:

$$\text{SNR} = \sum_i \sum_j \left[S_H\left(x_i, y_j\right) - \overline{S}_{nH}\right] / \sigma_{nH} \tag{9}$$

where S_H is the Hilbert transform modulus of the RF signal ($S_H = |H\{S_C\}|$), $\overline{S}_{nH}$ and σ_{nH} are the average and standard deviation of the background noise in S_H, respectively.

2.5. In Vivo Experiments: Human (Finger and Forearm) and Animal (Balb/C Mouse)

The index finger of the left hand and left anterior forearm of a human volunteer were photoacoustically imaged using multiangle PAI with illumination parameters according to Table 1. Figure 4a shows photographs of the index finger and forearm where the dashed lines indicate the position and orientation of the transducer. The volunteer immersed his hand and forearm in a water tank; the distance between the transducer face and the skin was chosen so that the laser beams were focused at the skin surface when illumination angle was minimum ($\theta_i = 0°$). The experiments were performed using an average fluence of 9.0 mJ/cm^2 at 800 nm, obtaining a total of 90 frames.

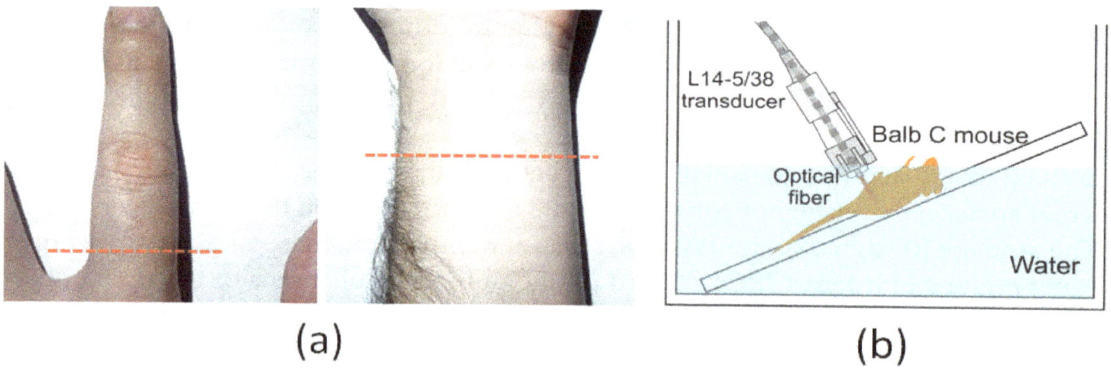

Figure 4. (**a**) Photographs of the index finger and forearm of the volunteer. The dashed lines indicate the position and orientation of the transducer. (**b**) Depiction of the experimental setup used to acquire in vivo PA images of Balb/C mouse.

A male Balb/C mouse, at the age of ten weeks, was anesthetized using vaporized isoflurane (1.0–1.5% isoflurane, Vetflurano, Virbac, São Paulo, Brazil). The animal was positioned in a ramp platform immersed in water with a controlled temperature of 36 °C, as shown in Figure 4b. Using the same wavelength and fluence of the human experiment, PA images of the animal abdomen were acquired.

The experiments involving humans and animals used controlled fluence lower than 20.0 mJ/cm^2, considering the limit for short-pulse lasers at the skin, which is defined by the American National Standards Institute (ANSI). The animal procedures were approved by the Animal Ethical Committee of Ribeirão Preto Medical School, University of São Paulo (process No. 005/2017-1). The experiments with the volunteer were conducted according to the procedure approved by the Research Ethical Committee of Faculty of Philosophy, Science, and Letters of Ribeirão Preto, University of São Paulo (CAAE: 08860819.4.0000.5407).

3. Results and Discussion

3.1. Comparison of Illumination Schemes for Different Target Shapes Using Monte Carlo simulation

Monte Carlo simulations were conducted to analyze the influence of the target shape and illumination scheme on light delivery. Figure 5 shows the normalized fluence maps obtained for all illumination strategies. Figure 5a–c,e–g show the results for the cases where the target is larger and smaller than the image width, respectively. Figure 5i–k show an intermediate situation representing a mouse torso. In this case, the geometry was obtained by segmenting an experimental B-mode image which will be shown in the next sections. Figure 5a,e,i show the results obtained for multiangle long-axis lateral illumination, while in Figure 5b,f,j, the results for the bright-field illumination coaxial with acoustic detection are shown. Finally, Figure 5c,g,k show the results obtained using the standard dark-field illumination scheme. In these images, ROIs were used to compare the light fluence for different spatial locations (white square is ROI-A; black square is ROI-B and magenta square is ROI-C). Figure 5d,h,l show bar graphs comparing the average fluence estimated within ROIs A, B, and C.

In the central region, all illumination schemes presented similar relative fluence at a shallow depth (ROI-A); yet, to some extent it was consistently higher for the bright-field illumination independent of the target shape. For targets with a nonflat surface, the focus region of the two laser beams used in the standard dark-field arrangement can be partially outside of the material and imaging plane as can be seen on the left side of Figure 6. The light delivered outside of the imaging plane contributes less to the PA image generation and can be a clutter source [62]. In this case, both situations, bright-field and long-axis lateral illumination, have the advantage of delivering light inside the imaging plane even when the target's surface is not flat. For this reason, the average fluence within ROIs B and C, located at higher depths, was consistently lower for the standard dark-field illumination scenario. It is important to recall that the light beams used for the standard dark-field were overlapping at the tissue surface. Other studies have shown that light delivery can be increased at higher depths, by using a deeper located illumination focus [30,37,38,53]. However, this strategy can dramatically decrease light delivery at shallow depths. For example, the study [48] showed that by positioning the focus at 13.5 mm depth, the simulated fluence estimated for the standard dark-field optical illumination was considerably lower than what was estimated for the bright-field illumination scheme at depths lower than 10 mm.

For targets smaller than the images' lateral dimension, the long-axis lateral illumination can deliver light to the sides of the target, increasing the penetration of light inside the material, which is depicted at the right side of Figure 6 and can be observed in the Monte Carlo simulation results. Moreover, the long-axis lateral illumination redirects the light to the target while part of the bright-field and standard dark-field illumination schemes do not contribute to PA signal generation. The simulations show that the relative fluence obtained with multiangle long-axis lateral illumination was dramatically improved for the case of a cylindrical geometry with a diameter smaller than the width of the ultrasound probe, which is a similar situation as the human finger as will be described in the next sections. Figure 5h shows that the average fluence for the long-axis lateral illumination scheme, measured within ROI-C, was four times higher than fluence delivered by the bright-field illumination and one order of magnitude higher compared to the dark-field illumination scheme.

For a target that combines parts smaller and parts larger than image width, as the mouse's torso, both long-axis lateral and the bright-field illumination schemes provided a relatively uniform light delivery to the entire target surface. On the other hand, the light delivered by the standard dark-field illumination was considerably higher at the top surface. For this situation, the long-axis lateral illumination provided a little increment of fluence within ROI-C compared to the bright-field illumination scheme.

The next two sections aim to evaluate the feasibility of generating PA images using the long-axis lateral illumination scheme. First, the device and the multiangle imaging strategy are evaluated with a phantom experiment; then the possibility of generating the PA images, in vivo, of targets with similar geometries adopted for the simulations are verified.

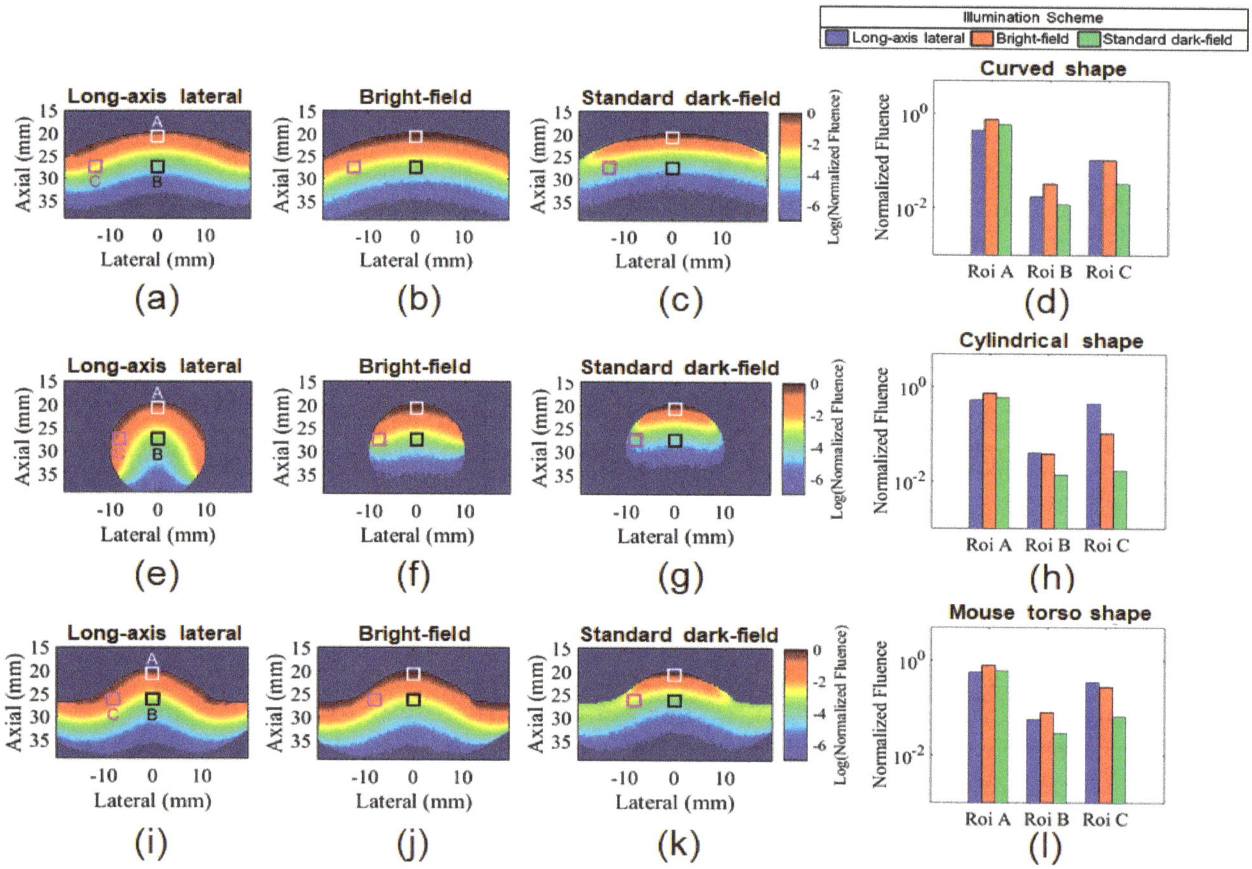

Figure 5. Normalized fluence maps obtained by Monte Carlo simulation for targets larger (**a**–**c**) and smaller (**e**–**g**) than the image width. An intermediate situation representing a mouse torso was also considered (**i**–**k**). All cases were simulated for the bright-field, standard dark-field, and long-axis lateral illumination schemes. Average fluence values were estimated within regions of interest (ROIs) A, B, and C for all cases (**d**,**h**,**l**).

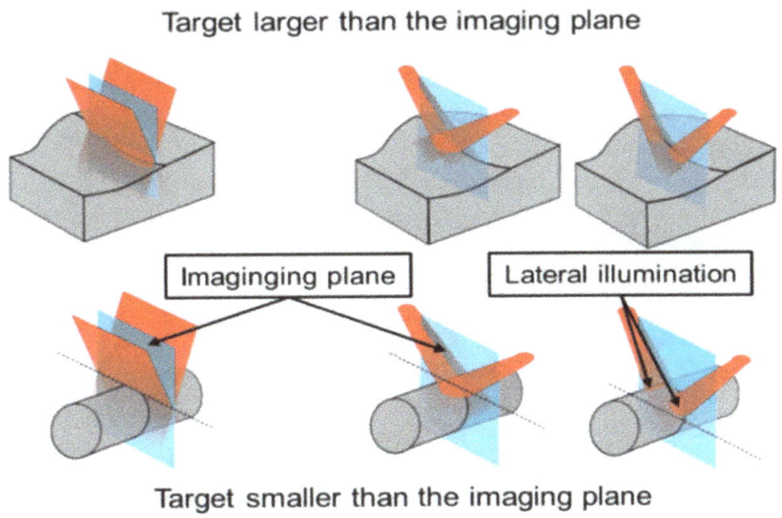

Figure 6. Comparison between the standard dark-field illumination scheme and the multiangle long-axis lateral illumination. For targets larger than the image width with a nonflat surface, the long-axis lateral and the bright-field illumination schemes have the advantage of delivering light within the imaging plane. For targets smaller than the transducer width, the long-axis lateral illumination scheme can deliver light to the sides of the target.

3.2. Analysis of Illumination Angles Contribution to the PA Image of the Phantom

The homogeneous phantom with a flat surface is useful for the characterization of light delivery using different illumination angles. To evaluate the light delivered to the phantom, each PA subframe at θ_i is represented as the average of the 19 PA subframes acquired at different positions of elevation axis (slice) using the same *i*-th illumination angle. The averaged PA subframes in Figure 7 shows the light propagation along depth. The blue arrows indicate the PA signal generated beyond the laser focal region for the illumination angles 0°, 2°, and 4°. This observation can be understood as an advantage of providing illumination from the laterals of the transducer, therefore generating PA signals within FOV for regions not only at the focus. However, the amplitude of the PA signal is a function of the illumination angle, because the laser focus region moves towards higher depth, while the light path increases, reducing the fluence due to light attenuation.

PA signal magnitude increased for depths greater than 10 mm and illumination angles higher than 8°, as it can be seen in Figure 8a. Although illumination along the peripheral areas of the transducer is mostly achieved by just one of the optical fiber outputs, the incident angle of the laser beam in this region decreased relative to the normal surface, delivering light at higher depths, as shown in Figure 8a,b. Moreover, the average PA signal showed the separation of laser beams along the lateral direction; see Figure 8c.

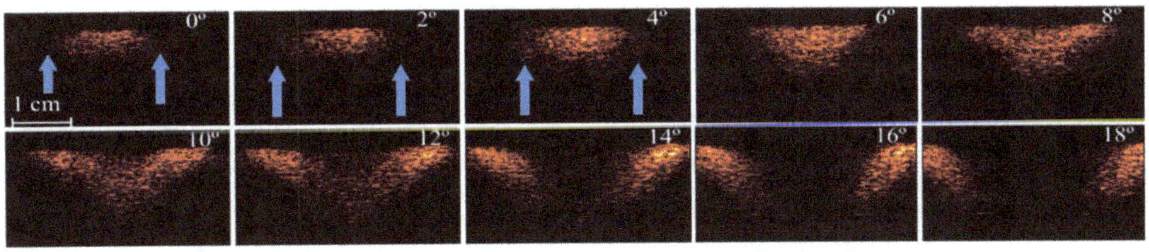

Figure 7. PA subframes of the homogeneous phantom for increasing illumination angles in the range 0°–18°. Each subframe is an average of the phantom's elevational dimension (i.e., 3.8 cm). Blue arrows indicate the generation of PA signals beyond the laser focal region.

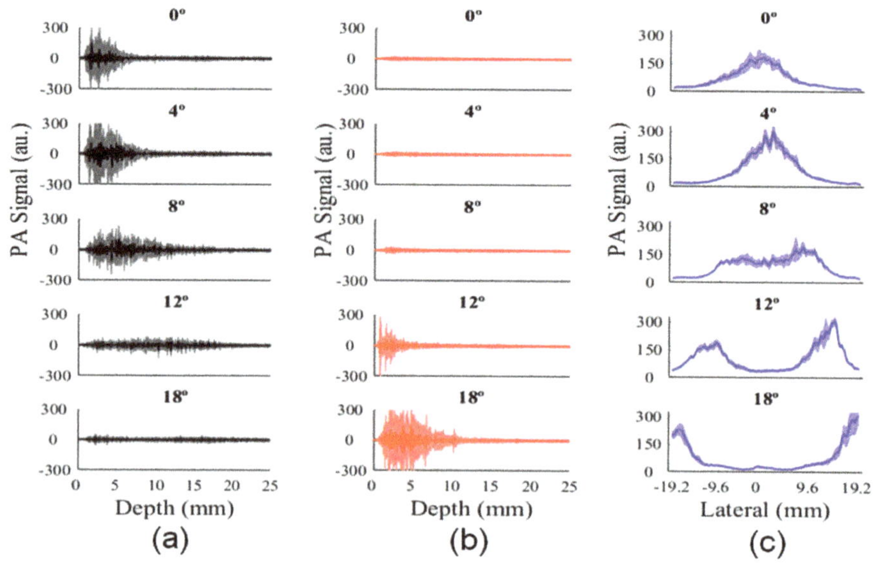

Figure 8. Average PA signal as a function of the illumination angle, along the axial direction at (**a**) central (ROI-1) and (**b**) peripheral ROIs (ROI-2 and ROI-3); (**c**) average PA signal magnitude along lateral direction for depths ranging from 0 mm to 2 mm.

The analysis of the A_{RMS} at the central region revealed a proportional decrease in the amount of light delivered for angles higher than 4°, which is probably related to light attenuation within the phantom (Figure 9a). Besides, a peak of maximum A_{RMS} could be observed for $\theta_i = 4°$, showing that the maximum light delivery to the central area occurred when the laser focus region was completely inside the phantom, where the light was less attenuated (shallow depths). These results show the contribution of illumination using $\theta_i < 4°$ was less significant for the image of the phantom. In addition, the mean depth of the PA signal increased as a function of the illumination angle (Figure 9b), which could be qualitatively inferred from the plots in Figure 8a.

The final PA image was obtained from the summation of the PA subframes at different illumination angles. For example, a PA image of a single image slice of the phantom is shown in Figure 10a. The average PA signal calculated at depths ranging from 0 mm to 25.5 mm for all elements of this PA image showed the contribution of all illumination angles; see Figure 10b. Figure 10c shows SNR as a function of depth demonstrating the multiangle long-axis illumination PA imaging could be used to perform studies at relevant imaging depths.

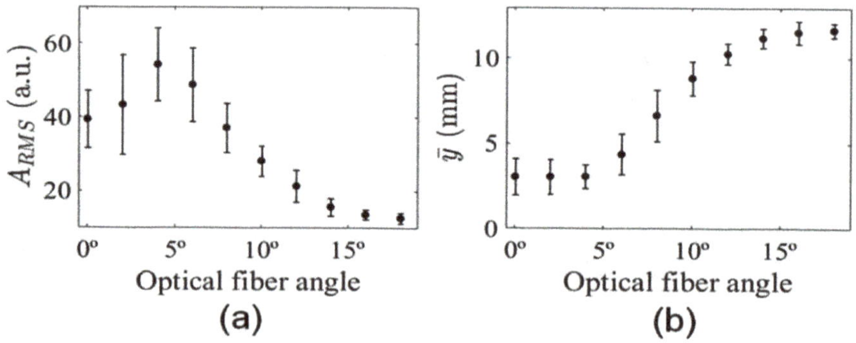

Figure 9. (**a**) Mean square root of PA signal and (**b**) mean depth of PA signal as a function of illumination angle.

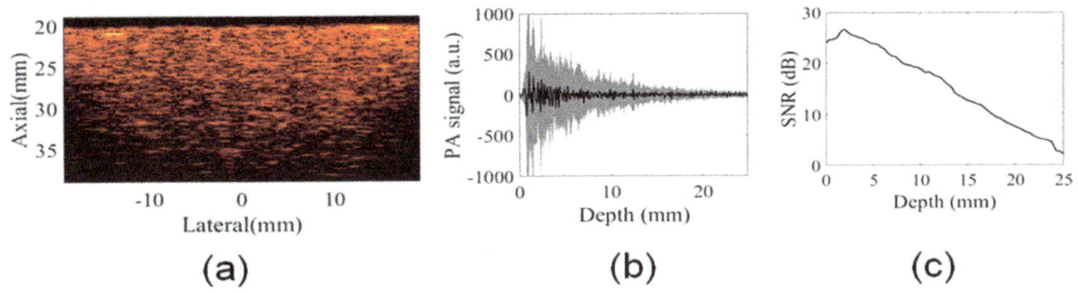

Figure 10. (**a**) Final PA image of a single image slice of the phantom, (**b**) PA signal profile of this PA image shows the contribution of all illumination angles to generate PA signal at depths greater than 10 mm, and (**c**) SNR as a function of image depth.

3.3. *In Vivo PA Images*

Different in vivo experiments were conducted to evaluate the multiangle long-axis lateral illumination PAI. The first in vivo PA images were acquired from a human forearm. In this case, the shape of the surface was larger than the long-axis dimension of the transducer, providing similarities with the flat surface of the phantom and the simulation study. The anatomical structures of the human forearm such as palmaris longus tendon, subcutaneous blood vessels, and epithelial tissue could be identified in the B-mode image as well as in the PA image, as it can be seen in Figure 11a,b. SNR was calculated within two ROIs of 2.4 mm × 1.6 mm in the axial and lateral dimensions, respectively. For the in vivo evaluation, noise ROIs, with the same dimensions, were positioned within 5 mm distance from the structure under analysis. At a tissue depth of 7.3 mm, ROI overlaid the tendon of flexor digitorum superficialis [63] and provided SNR = 14 dB (green rectangle in Figure 11a), while another ROI overlaid a subcutaneous blood vessel and provided SNR = 25 dB at a 2.5 mm tissue depth (cyan rectangle in Figure 11a). Differences in the SNR values between deep and shallow regions were mostly due to light attenuation; the tendon (collagen) also presents an optical absorption coefficient lower than those for melanin or hemoglobin at 800 nm [64], which reduced its SNR on the PA image.

The second acquisition of PA images was obtained from the human index finger, which has a cylindrical-like shape that differs from the forearm or phantom's surface and has a maximum lateral extension of approximately 20 mm. However, the finger cross-section lateral dimension is smaller than the lateral FOV, allowing illumination from laterals to be more efficient. Consequently, the laser focus becomes deeper while the light path within the tissue is shortened, reducing the light attenuation. SNR was analyzed within ROIs of 2.0 mm × 3.0 mm in the axial and lateral dimensions, respectively. Those ROIs were placed over the location of the dorsal and palmar digital arteries at 3.4 mm (cyan rectangle in Figure 11c) and 10.3 mm tissue depths (green rectangle in Figure 11c), resulting in SNR of 22.5 dB and 22 dB, respectively.

Lastly, a challenging combination of both aforementioned surface shapes was observed when acquiring the PA image of the cross-section of the mouse abdomen. The abdomen had a lateral dimension smaller than the lateral length of the transducer, while the lower limbs fit FOV. In this case, illumination angles provided light delivery to the sides of the mouse abdomen and hit the surface of lower limbs obliquely. Furthermore, the mouse skin has an average thickness of 0.5 mm and optical absorption lower than human skin [65], increasing light penetration. In the B-mode image of the mouse, the bladder, femoral artery, and a branch of the abdominal aorta can be identified [66]. PA signals from the femoral artery were evaluated at 1.3 mm (cyan rectangle in Figure 11e) and the aortic branch at 10.5 mm of depth (green rectangle in Figure 11e) presenting SNR = 21.5 dB for the femoral artery and SNR = 17.5 dB for the aortic branch (ROIs of 2.0 mm × 2.8 mm).

For three among the most studied PA targets in biomedical applications, the multiangle long-axis lateral illumination was able to provide PA images with high SNR at a depth of 10.5 mm for target shapes with lateral extension smaller than the lateral length of transducer (mouse and index finger). In the human forearm, a tendon at depth of 7 mm generated PA signal with sufficient SNR for good visualization of the structure. However, it should be mentioned that the in vivo PA images were acquired using a measured laser fluence of 9 mJ/cm^2, which is much lower than the limit for short-pulse laser at the skin. Increasing the laser fluence to values close to the safety limit can improve SNR of PA images at greater depths.

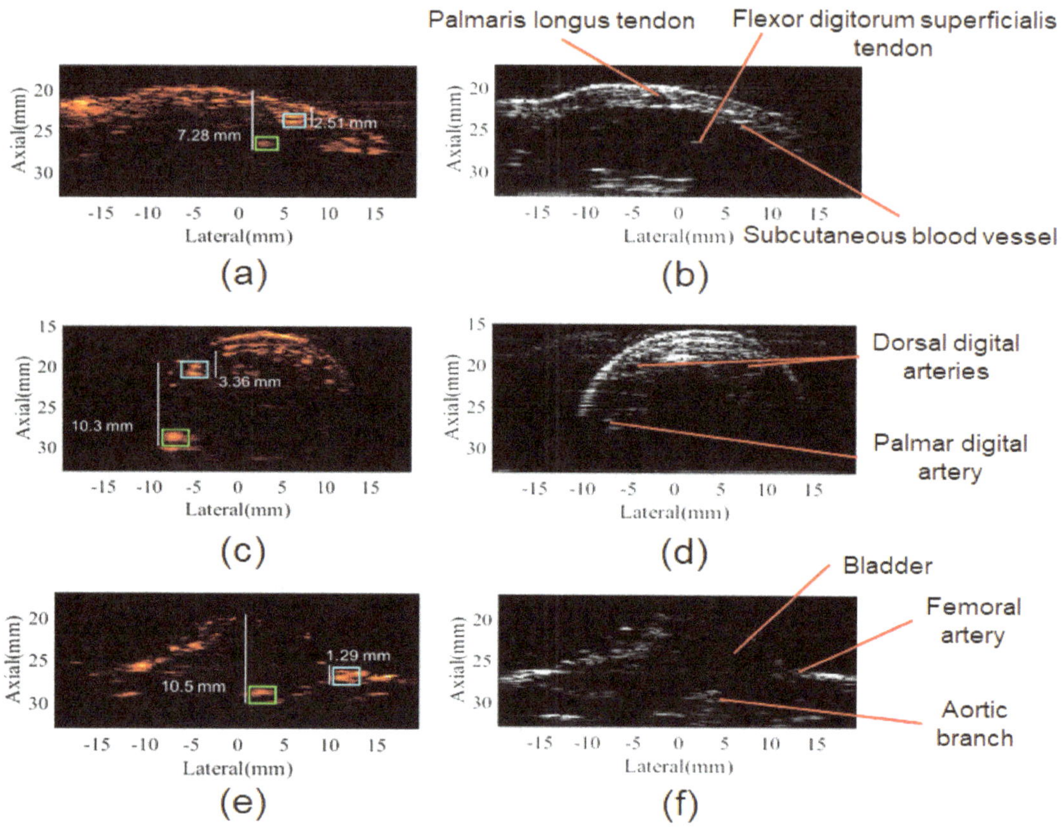

Figure 11. In vivo multiangle long-axis lateral illumination PA and B-mode images. (**a**) PA image and (**b**) B-mode image of the human forearm, anatomical structures such as tendons and subcutaneous blood vessels can be identified; (**c**) PA image and (**d**) B-mode image of the human index finger, the cylindrical shape allows light delivery by the laterals promoting the visualization of the palmar digital artery at depth of 10.3 mm. (**e**) PA image and (**f**) B-mode image of the Balb/Cmouse abdomen, PA signal from an aortic branch at 10.5 mm of depth can be visualized.

Figure S1 shows the subframes acquired at each illumination angle for the in vivo experiments and plots with the corresponding SNR for ROIs positioned at the selected structures (vessels and tendon). The pronounced variation in the SNR values across the subframes acquired at different angles is evident. Clearly, SNR, at each ROI, observed for the final PA image is similar (only slightly higher) to that subframe with the highest SNR where the illumination area comprised the structure of interest. In the case of combining N PA images at the same illumination angle, it is expected that the SNR will be increased by $\sqrt{N}$, which would be higher than SNR obtained with the multiangle approach for a particular ROI. A more concentrated illumination in the proposed approach, when compared to the techniques illustrated in Figure 1a,b, can also help improve SNR at specific locations of the image. This concept has been also explored in other studies [51,53].

Multiangle long-axis lateral illumination could be a useful approach to improve the quality of PA images in preclinical studies with mice, since important anatomic structures are smaller than the FOV. Even for higher frequency linear arrays with a width smaller than the probe used here, murine tumor models still fit in this category [53]. In [53], the authors demonstrated that improving light delivery for this situation can greatly improve PA image quality. Since PA images taken from the human finger joint has shown great potential to evaluate inflammatory arthritis [22,23], it is a possible clinical application where the proposed technique could be beneficial. Future studies will include: (i) evaluating multi-wavelength PA images and fluence correction strategies [57] to monitor blood oxygen saturation and (ii) evaluate the feasibility of using a high divergent source like LED [44] to reduce the number of illumination angles.

Since the pulse repetition frequency of the laser (L_{PRF}) is 10 Hz, the in vivo images of the present study were acquired at a frame rate of 1 frame per second. Each image was composed of two subframes per angle and five different angles were used. The maximum frame rate for this configuration is two frames per second if a single frame was acquired per angle. To acquire the full transducer FOV, a few subframes acquired at different angles are needed; therefore, the frame rate for the proposed technique will be lower than that obtained for the configurations shown in Figure 1a,b. This is a limitation of the proposed approach, especially for the cases where the illumination source operates at low PRF as the laser used in the present study (L_{PRF} = 10 Hz) and monitor fast-changing dynamics is the goal. However, for lasers working at higher repetition rate (L_{PRF} ~ 100 Hz), see, for example, [67]) this limitation can be minimized and the frame rate can be increased. The maximum L_{PRF} supported by the setup depends of the angular velocity of servomotors (ω_s), and the step angle ($\Delta\theta$): $L_{PRF} = \omega_s / \Delta\theta$. The servomotors used in the setup can take 0.2 s to rotate the fibers output from 0° to 60°, resulting in a maximum angular velocity of $\omega_s = 5.2\ rad{\cdot}s^{-1}$ when operating at 5 V. In this case, the setup could acquire PA subframes using = 75 Hz with $\Delta\theta = 4°$ and provide 15 frames per second when five illumination angles are used.

The present paper introduced and evaluated the feasibility of the multiangle long-axis lateral illumination to generate PA images, contributing to the development of new illumination strategies in PAI. An advantage of the setup presented here is that it could be additive to other existing illumination schemes. Light delivery by the laterals of the target could be used together with more conventionally used illumination schemes to improve light delivery to targets with lateral dimension smaller than the transducer's width. The concept of PA images acquired using multiangle illumination can also be applied to setups with similar design as described in [37,38], where the angle of incident light delivered by transducer's short-axis can be controlled.

4. Conclusions

This paper demonstrated the feasibility of using a novel multiangle long-axis lateral illumination PAI. Monte Carlo simulations compared light delivery to tissue for three different illumination schemes: bright-field, standard dark-field, and long-axis lateral illumination. Illumination schemes performance were evaluated for three preclinical and clinically relevant cases for PAI. The shape of the target influenced light delivery for all illumination schemes. Long-axis lateral illumination provided substantial improvement when targets smaller than the lateral width of the transducer were evaluated. The prototype developed to produce multiangle long-axis lateral illumination was evaluated with phantom and in vivo experiments. PA images of good quality were generated from mouse abdomen, forearm, and index finger of a volunteer. Based on the results presented here, a novel PAI system was proposed for preclinical and clinical research. In addition, long-axis lateral illumination could be used together with more conventional illumination schemes to improve light delivery in reflection mode PAI.

Author Contributions: Conceptualization and design, J.H.U. and T.Z.P.; Data curation, J.H.U., D.R.T.S. and G.S.P.F.; Analysis and interpretation of data, J.H.U., D.R.T.S., G.S.P.F., M.S.B., M.H.N.-B. and A.A.O.C. and T.Z.P.; Funding acquisition, A.A.O.C. and T.Z.P.; Investigation, J.H.U and T.Z.P.; Methodology, J.H.U., D.R.T.S., G.S.P.F., M.S.B., M.H.N.-B., A.A.O.C. and T.Z.P.; Project administration, T.Z.P.; Resources, M.S.B., A.A.O.C. and T.Z.P.; Software, J.H.U., D.R.T.S. and G.S.P.F.; Supervision, T.Z.P.; Writing—original draft, J.H.U. and T.Z.P.;

Writing—review & editing, J.H.U., D.R.T.S., G.S.P.F., M.S.B., M.H.N.-B. and A.A.O.C. and T.Z.P. All authors critically read and approved the final version of the manuscript.

References

1. Kresge, C.T.; Leonowicz, M.E.; Roth, W.J.; Vartuli, J.C.; Beck, J.S. Generation of ultrasonic waves from a layered photoacoustic source. *Nature* **1992**, *359*, 710–713. [CrossRef]
2. Kruger, R.A. Photoacoustic ultrasound. *Med. Phys.* **1994**, *21*, 127. [CrossRef] [PubMed]
3. Wang, X.; Xu, Y.; Xu, M.; Yokoo, S.; Fry, E.S.; Wang, L.V. Photoacoustic tomography of biological tissues with high cross-section resolution: Reconstruction and experiment. *Med. Phys.* **2002**, *29*, 2799–2805. [CrossRef] [PubMed]
4. Xu, M.; Wang, L.V. Photoacoustic imaging in biomedicine. *Rev. Sci. Instrum.* **2006**, *77*, 041101. [CrossRef]
5. Beard, P. Biomedical photoacoustic imaging. *Interface Focus* **2011**, *1*, 602–631. [CrossRef]
6. Wang, X.; Pang, Y.; Ku, G.; Xie, X.; Stoica, G.; Wang, L.V. Noninvasive laser-induced photoacoustic tomography for structural and functional in vivo imaging of the brain. *Nat. Biotechnol.* **2003**, *21*, 803–806. [CrossRef]
7. Wang, L.V.; Hu, S. Photoacoustic Tomography: In Vivo Imaging from Organelles to Organs. *Science (80-)* **2012**, *335*, 1458–1462. [CrossRef]
8. Larina, I.V.; Larin, K.V.; Esenaliev, R.O. Real-time optoacoustic monitoring of temperature in tissues. *J. Phys. D Appl. Phys.* **2005**, *38*, 2633–2639. [CrossRef]
9. Shah, J.; Park, S.; Aglyamov, S.R.; Larson, T.; Ma, L.; Sokolov, K.V.; Johnston, K.P.; Milner, T.E.; Emelianov, S.Y. Photoacoustic imaging and temperature measurement for photothermal cancer therapy. *J. Biomed. Opt.* **2008**, *13*, 034024. [CrossRef]
10. Yao, J.; Ke, H.; Tai, S.; Zhou, Y.; Wang, L.V. Absolute photoacoustic thermometry in deep tissue. *Opt. Lett.* **2013**, *38*, 5228–5231. [CrossRef]
11. Ke, H.; Tai, S.; Wang, L.V. Photoacoustic thermography of tissue. *J. Biomed. Opt.* **2014**, *19*, 026003. [CrossRef]
12. Razansky, D.; Vinegoni, C.; Ntziachristos, V. Multispectral photoacoustic imaging of fluorochromes in small animals. *Opt. Lett.* **2007**, *32*, 2891. [CrossRef]
13. Laufer, J.; Zhang, E.; Beard, P. Evaluation of absorbing chromophores used in tissue phantoms for quantitative photoacoustic spectroscopy and imaging. *IEEE J. Sel. Top. Quantum Electron.* **2010**, *16*, 600–607. [CrossRef]
14. Laufer, J.G. Pulsed near-infrared photoacoustic spectroscopy of blood. *Proc. SPIE* **2004**, *5320*, 57–68. [CrossRef]
15. Laufer, J.; Elwell, C.; Delpy, D.; Beard, P. In vitro measurements of absolute blood oxygen saturation using pulsed near-infrared photoacoustic spectroscopy: Accuracy and resolution. *Phys. Med. Biol.* **2005**, *50*, 4409–4428. [CrossRef] [PubMed]
16. Zhang, H.F.; Maslov, K.; Stoica, G.; Wang, L.V. Functional photoacoustic microscopy for high-resolution and noninvasive in vivo imaging. *Nat. Biotechnol.* **2006**, *24*, 848–851. [CrossRef] [PubMed]
17. Zhang, H.F.; Maslov, K.; Sivaramakrishnan, M.; Stoica, G.; Wang, L.V. Imaging of hemoglobin oxygen saturation variations in single vessels in vivo using photoacoustic microscopy. *Appl. Phys. Lett.* **2007**, *90*, 5–7. [CrossRef]
18. Chen, Z.; Yang, S.; Xing, D. In vivo detection of hemoglobin oxygen saturation and carboxyhemoglobin saturation with multiwavelength photoacoustic microscopy. *Opt. Lett.* **2012**, *37*, 3414. [CrossRef]
19. Shao, Q.; Ashkenazi, S. Photoacoustic lifetime imaging for direct *in vivo* tissue oxygen monitoring. *J. Biomed. Opt.* **2015**, *20*, 036004. [CrossRef]
20. Fu, Q.; Zhu, R.; Song, J.; Yang, H.; Chen, X. Photoacoustic Imaging: Contrast Agents and Their Biomedical Applications. *Adv. Mater.* **2019**, *31*, 1–31. [CrossRef]
21. Oraevsky, A.A.; Clingman, B.; Zalev, J.; Stavros, A.T.; Yang, W.T.; Parikh, J.R. Clinical optoacoustic imaging combined with ultrasound for coregistered functional and anatomical mapping of breast tumors. *Photoacoustics* **2018**, *12*, 30–45. [CrossRef] [PubMed]
22. Jo, J.; Xu, G.; Cao, M.; Marquardt, A.; Francis, S.; Gandikota, G.; Wang, X. A Functional Study of Human Inflammatory Arthritis Using Photoacoustic Imaging. *Sci. Rep.* **2017**, *7*, 1–9. [CrossRef] [PubMed]
23. Jo, J.; Tian, C.; Xu, G.; Sarazin, J.; Schiopu, E.; Gandikota, G.; Wang, X. Photoacoustic tomography for human musculoskeletal imaging and inflammatory arthritis detection. *Photoacoustics* **2018**, *12*, 82–89. [CrossRef]

[PubMed]
24. Niederhauser, J.J.; Jaeger, M.; Lemor, R.; Weber, P.; Frenz, M. Combined ultrasound and optoacoustic system for real-time high-contrast vascular imaging in vivo. *IEEE Trans. Med. Imaging* **2005**, *24*, 436–440. [CrossRef]
25. Daoudi, K.; Van Den Berg, P.J.; Rabot, O.; Kohl, A.; Tisserand, S.; Brands, P.; Steenbergen, W. Handheld probe integrating laser diode and ultrasound transducer array for ultrasound/photoacoustic dual modality imaging. *Opt. Express* **2014**, *22*, 26365. [CrossRef]
26. Hai, P.; Zhou, Y.; Zhang, R.; Ma, J.; Li, Y.; Wang, L.V. Label-free high-throughput detection and quantification of circulating melanoma tumor cell clusters. *J. Biomed. Opt.* **2016**, *22*, 1-041004–1-041005-6. [CrossRef]
27. Zhou, Y.; Liang, J.; Wang, L.V. Cuffing-based photoacoustic flowmetry in humans in the optical diffusive regime. *J. Biophotonics* **2016**, *9*, 208–212. [CrossRef]
28. Zhao, L.; Yang, M.; Jiang, Y.; Li, C. Optical fluence compensation for handheld photoacoustic probe: An in vivo human study case. *J. Innov. Opt. Health Sci.* **2017**, *10*, 1740002-1–1740002-18. [CrossRef]
29. Montilla, L.G.; Olafsson, R.; Bauer, D.R.; Witte, R.S. Real-time photoacoustic and ultrasound imaging: A simple solution for clinical ultrasound systems with linear arrays. *Phys. Med. Biol.* **2013**, *58*. [CrossRef]
30. Wang, G.W.G.; Zhao, H.Z.H.; Ren, Q.R.Q.; Li, C.L.C. Simulation of light delivery for photoacoustic breast imaging using the handheld probe. *Chin. Opt. Lett.* **2014**, *12*, 051703–051706. [CrossRef]
31. Lee, Y.J.; Jeong, E.J.; Song, H.W.; Ahn, C.G.; Noh, H.W.; Sim, J.Y.; Song, D.H.; Jeon, M.Y.; Lee, S.; Kim, H.; et al. Photoacoustic imaging probe for detecting lymph nodes and spreading of cancer at various depths. *J. Biomed. Opt.* **2017**, *22*, 091513. [CrossRef] [PubMed]
32. Bai, Y.; Cong, B.; Gong, X.; Song, L.; Liu, C. Compact and low-cost handheld quasibright-field linear-array probe design in photoacoustic computed tomography. *J. Biomed. Opt.* **2018**, *23*, 1. [CrossRef] [PubMed]
33. Held, G.; Preisser, S.; Akarçay, H.G.; Peeters, S.; Frenz, M.; Jaeger, M. Effect of irradiation distance on image contrast in epi-optoacoustic imaging of human volunteers. *Biomed. Opt. Express* **2014**, *5*, 3765. [CrossRef] [PubMed]
34. Frenz, M.; Jaeger, M. Optimization of tissue irradiation in optoacoustic imaging using a linear transducer: Theory and experiments. In Proceedings of the Photons Plus Ultrasound: Imaging and Sensing 2008: The Ninth Conference on Biomedical Thermoacoustics, Optoacoustics, and Acousto-optics, San Jose, CA, USA, 19–24 January 2008.
35. Preisser, S.; Held, G.; Akarçay, H.G.; Jaeger, M.; Frenz, M. Study of clutter origin in in-vivo epi-optoacoustic imaging of human forearms. *J. Opt.* **2016**, *18*, 094003. [CrossRef]
36. Haisch, C.; Eilert-Zell, K.; Vogel, M.M.; Menzenbach, P.; Niessner, R. Combined optoacoustic/ultrasound system for tomographic absorption measurements: Possibilities and limitations. *Anal. Bioanal. Chem.* **2010**, *397*, 1503–1510. [CrossRef]
37. Sivasubramanian, K.; Periyasamy, V.; Wen, K.K.; Pramanik, M. Optimizing light delivery through fiber bundle in photoacoustic imaging with clinical ultrasound system: Monte Carlo simulation and experimental validation. *J. Biomed. Opt.* **2016**, *22*, 041008. [CrossRef]
38. Sangha, G.S.; Hale, N.J.; Goergen, C.J. Adjustable photoacoustic tomography probe improves light delivery and image quality. *Photoacoustics* **2018**, *12*, 6–13. [CrossRef] [PubMed]
39. Sowers, T.; Yoon, H.; Emelianov, S. Investigation of light delivery geometries for photoacoustic applications using Monte Carlo simulations with multiple wavelengths, tissue types, and species characteristics. *J. Biomed. Opt.* **2020**, *25*, 1. [CrossRef]
40. Wang, Z.; Ha, S.; Kim, K. A new design of light illumination scheme for deep tissue photoacoustic imaging. *Opt. Express* **2012**, *20*, 22649. [CrossRef]
41. Yu, J.; Schuman, J.S.; Lee, J.K.; Lee, S.G.; Chang, J.H.; Kim, K. A Light Illumination Enhancement Device for Photoacoustic Imaging: In Vivo Animal Study. *IEEE Trans. Ultrason. Ferroelectr. Freq. Control* **2017**, *64*, 1205–1211. [CrossRef]
42. Xia, W.; Kuniyil Ajith Singh, M.; Maneas, E.; Sato, N.; Shigeta, Y.; Agano, T.; Ourselin, S.; JWest, S.; EDesjardins, A. Handheld real-time LED-based photoacoustic and ultrasound imaging system for accurate visualization of clinical metal needles and superficial vasculature to guide minimally invasive procedures. *Sensors* **2018**, *18*, 1394. [CrossRef] [PubMed]

43. Zhu, Y.; Feng, T.; Cheng, Q.; Wang, X.; Du, S.; Sato, N. Towards Clinical Translation of LED-Based Photoacoustic Imaging: A Review. *Sensors* **2020**, *20*, 2484. [CrossRef]
44. Kuriakose, M.; Nguyen, C.D.; Singh, M.K.A.; Mallidi, S. Optimizing irradiation geometry in LED-based photoacoustic imaging with 3d printed flexible and modular light delivery system. *Sensors* **2020**, *20*, 3789. [CrossRef] [PubMed]
45. Zhang, X.; Wu, X.; Adelegan, O.J.; Yamaner, F.Y.; Oralkan, O. Backward-Mode Photoacoustic Imaging Using Illumination Through a CMUT with Improved Transparency. *IEEE Trans. Ultrason. Ferroelectr. Freq. Control* **2018**, *65*, 85–94. [CrossRef] [PubMed]
46. Chen, Q.X.; Davies, A.; Dewhurst, R.J.; Payne, P.A. Photo-acoustic probe for intra-arterial imaging and therapy. *Electron. Lett.* **1993**, *29*, 1632–1633. [CrossRef]
47. Laufer, J.; Zhang, E.; Raivich, G.; Beard, P. Three-dimensional noninvasive imaging of the vasculature in the mouse brain using a high resolution photoacoustic scanner. *Appl. Opt.* **2009**, *48*, 299–306. [CrossRef]
48. Li, M.; Liu, C.; Gong, X.; Zheng, R.; Bai, Y.; Xing, M.; Du, X.; Liu, X.; Zeng, J.; Lin, R.; et al. Linear array-based real-time photoacoustic imaging system with a compact coaxial excitation handheld probe for noninvasive sentinel lymph node mapping. *Biomed. Opt. Express* **2018**, *9*, 1408–1422. [CrossRef]
49. Wang, Y.; Lim, R.S.A.; Zhang, H.; Nyayapathi, N.; Oh, K.W.; Xia, J. Optimizing the light delivery of linear-array-based photoacoustic systems by double acoustic reflectors. *Sci. Rep.* **2018**, *8*, 1–7. [CrossRef]
50. Ida, T.; Iwazaki, H.; Kawaguchi, Y.; Kawauchi, S.; Ohkura, T.; Iwaya, K.; Tsuda, H.; Saitoh, D.; Sato, S.; Iwai, T. Burn depth assessments by photoacoustic imaging and laser Doppler imaging. *Wound Repair Regen.* **2016**, *24*, 349–355. [CrossRef] [PubMed]
51. Wei, C.W.; Nguyen, T.M.; Xia, J.; Arnal, B.; Wong, E.Y.; Pelivanov, I.M.; O'Donnell, M. Real-time integrated photoacoustic and ultrasound (PAUS) imaging system to guide interventional procedures: Ex vivo study. *IEEE Trans. Ultrason. Ferroelectr. Freq. Control* **2015**, *62*, 319–328. [CrossRef] [PubMed]
52. Fang, Q.; Boas, D.A. Monte Carlo Simulation of Photon Migration in 3D Turbid Media Accelerated by Graphics Processing Units. *Opt. Express* **2009**, *17*, 20178. [CrossRef] [PubMed]
53. Rich, L.J.; Chamberlain, S.R.; Falcone, D.R.; Bruce, R.; Heinmiller, A.; Xia, J.; Seshadri, M. Performance Characteristics of Photoacoustic Imaging Probes with Varying Frequencies and Light-delivery Schemes. *Ultrason. Imaging* **2019**, *41*, 319–335. [CrossRef] [PubMed]
54. Jacques, S.L. Optical properties of biological tissues: A review. *Phys. Med. Biol.* **2013**, *58*, 5007–5008. [CrossRef]
55. Pavan, T.Z.; Madsen, E.L.; Frank, G.R.; Carneiro, A.A.O.; Hall, T.J. Nonlinear elastic behavior of phantom materials for elastography. *Phys. Med. Biol.* **2010**, *55*, 2679. [CrossRef]
56. Uliana, J.H.; Sampaio, D.R.T.; Carneiro, A.A.O.; Pavan, T.Z. Photoacoustic-based thermal image formation and optimization using an evolutionary genetic algorithm. *Res. Biomed. Eng.* **2018**, *34*, 147–156. [CrossRef]
57. Naser, M.A.; Sampaio, D.R.; Muñoz, N.M.; Wood, C.A.; Mitcham, T.M.; Stefan, W.; Sokolov, K.V.; Pavan, T.Z.; Avritscher, R.; Bouchard, R.R. Improved Photoacoustic-Based Oxygen Saturation Estimation With SNR-Regularized Local Fluence Correction. *IEEE Trans. Med. Imaging* **2019**, *38*, 561–571. [CrossRef] [PubMed]
58. Liu, S.; Feng, X.; Jin, H.; Zhang, R.; Luo, Y.; Zheng, Z.; Gao, F.; Zheng, Y. Handheld Photoacoustic Imager for Theranostics in 3D. *IEEE Trans. Med. Imaging* **2019**, *38*, 2037–2046. [CrossRef]
59. Singh, C.P.; Bindra, K.S.; Bhalerao, G.M.; Oak, S.M. Investigation of optical limiting in iron oxide nanoparticles. *Opt. Express* **2008**, *16*, 8440. [CrossRef]
60. Jacques, S.L.; Prahl, S. Tabulated Molar Extinction Coefficient for Hemoglobin in Water. Available online: https://omlc.org/spectra/hemoglobin/index.html (accessed on 16 July 2020).
61. Bushberg, J.T.; Seibert, J.A.; Leidholdt, E.M.; Boone, J.M. *The Essential Physics of Medical Imaging*, 3rd ed.; Lippincott Williams & Wilkins: Philadelphia, PA, USA, 2011.
62. Alles, E.J.; Jaeger, M.; Bamber, J.C. Photoacoustic clutter reduction using short-lag spatial coherence weighted imaging. *IEEE Int. Ultrason. Symp. IUS* **2014**, 41–44. [CrossRef]
63. Netter, F.H. *Atlas of Human Anatomy*, 6th ed.; Sauders Elsevier: Philadelphia, PA, USA, 2014; Volume 1.
64. Lee, H.D.; Shin, J.G.; Hyun, H.; Yu, B.A.; Eom, T.J. Label-free photoacoustic microscopy for in-vivo tendon imaging using a fiber-based pulse laser. *Sci. Rep.* **2018**, *8*, 1–9. [CrossRef] [PubMed]
65. Sabino, C.P.; Deana, A.M.; Yoshimura, T.M.; da Silva, D.F.; França, C.M.; Hamblin, M.R.; Ribeiro, M.S. The optical properties of mouse skin in the visible and near infrared spectral regions. *J. Photochem. Photobiol.*

B Biol. **2016**, *160*, 72–78. [CrossRef] [PubMed]

66. Cook, M.J. *The Anatomy of the Laboratory Mouse*; Academic Press: London, UK; New York, NY, USA, 1965.
67. Choi, W.; Park, E.Y.; Jeon, S.; Kim, C. Clinical photoacoustic imaging platforms. *Biomed. Eng. Lett.* **2018**, *8*, 139–155. [CrossRef] [PubMed]

14

Tomographic Ultrasound and LED-Based Photoacoustic System for Preclinical Imaging

Kalloor Joseph Francis [1,*], Richell Booijink [2], Ruchi Bansal [2] and Wiendelt Steenbergen [1,*]

[1] Biomedical Photonics Imaging (BMPI), Technical Medical Center, University of Twente, 7522 NH Enschede, The Netherlands

[2] Translational Liver Research, Medical Cell BioPhysics (MCBP), Technical Medical Center, University of Twente, 7522 NH Enschede, The Netherlands; r.bansal@utwente.nl (R.B.); r.s.booijink@utwente.nl (R.B.)

* Correspondence: f.kalloorjoseph@utwente.nl (K.J.F.); w.steenbergen@utwente.nl (W.S.)

Abstract: Small animals are widely used as disease models in medical research. Noninvasive imaging modalities with functional capability play an important role in studying the disease state and treatment progress. Photoacoustics, being a noninvasive and functional modality, has the potential for small-animal imaging. However, the conventional photoacoustic tomographic systems use pulsed lasers, making it expensive, bulky, and require long acquisition time. In this work, we propose the use of photoacoustic and ultrasound tomographic imaging with LEDs as the light source and acoustic detection using a linear transducer array. We have demonstrated full-view tomographic imaging of a euthanized mouse and a potential application in liver fibrosis research.

Keywords: tomography; photoacoustic; ultrasound; small animal; liver; fibrosis

---

1. Introduction

Studying different diseases and developing new drugs in a controlled environment is vital in biomedical research. Small animals are widely used for this purpose, as they allow for controlled disease staging and evaluating the performance of drugs through histopathological validation [1]. Longitudinal monitoring of disease progression and treatment response to drugs can improve the outcome of preclinical studies and can reduce the number of laboratory animal deaths. Imaging modalities can be used for longitudinal monitoring of small animal models. However, there are limitations in using conventional imaging modalities such as MRI, CT, and ultrasound for small animal imaging [2]. Micro MRI is costly and has a slow data acquisition. Micro CT and PET, on the other hand, use ionizing radiation, which hinders longitudinal observations [2]. Ultrasound (US) is a noninvasive and real-time imaging modality but, being a structural imaging modality, in most cases it cannot quantify disease state. Photoacoustic (PA) imaging is a new modality that has functional and molecular capability while being noninvasive and real-time. Thus, PA is considered to be ideal for small animal imaging [3].

PA imaging utilizes pulsed light excitation to induce a temperature rise in optical absorbing structures inside the tissue resulting in thermoelastic expansion and acoustic wave generation. These acoustic waves are detected for imaging [4]. The advantage of PA imaging is that with optical excitation and acoustic detection it combines optical contrast at ultrasound resolution. Additionally, the use of ultrasound transducers enables us to combine PA imaging with conventional US imaging providing co-registered structural and functional imaging of the tissue. Several PA and US imaging systems were successfully demonstrated for small-animal whole-body imaging [3,5,6]. However, the use of a pulsed laser source in these systems not only makes them expensive but demands laser safe small animal labs, eye safety goggles, and additional manpower to operate the system. Therefore, for the wide use of PA imaging in small animal labs, there is a requirement for low cost, compact, safe to use tomographic systems which can be operated by a non-expert. Recent developments in LED-based PA imaging, being compact, low-cost, and safe to use, offer promising avenues to fill this gap [7]. LED-based handheld PA systems were used previously for small animal studies for imaging superficial structures such as tumors [8], wounds [9], and knee joints [7,10]. A limitation of the hand-held PA system using a linear transducer array is the limited view of the target tissue due to the directional sensitivity of the transducer. Additionally, with a small number of LED elements arranged on either side of the transducer, the imaging depth is shallow. We have recently developed a tomographic imaging configuration using a linear transducer array and four LED arrays, to overcome the limited view and to improve the imaging depth [11,12]. The system was originally developed for imaging finger joints for diagnosis and monitoring of rheumatoid arthritis [11].

In this study, we propose the application of our tomographic US and LED-based PA system for preclinical research. First, we demonstrate full-view tomographic imaging of the abdominal region of a mouse. We also compare the results with B-scan images obtained using a handheld probe. Further, we present a potential application of the system in liver fibrosis research. A large number of preclinical studies are currently being performed in small animals to develop antifibrotic therapies. However, the outcome of the preclinical study relies on endpoint histopathological analysis. A noninvasive imaging technique can provide longitudinal monitoring of animals and can improve the study outcome. We present the use of noninvasive and low-cost US and PA tomographic imaging system for liver imaging and compared the outcome with histology images.

2. Materials and Methods

An LED-based photoacoustic and ultrasound imaging system, AcousticX (Cyberdyne Inc., Japan), was used in this work. Four LED arrays having 576 elements (36 × 4 array) were used as the light source. We used LEDs having a wavelength of 850 nm, and each array has a pulse energy of 200 μJ with a pulse duration of 70 ns. We used a linear transducer array (128 elements) with a center frequency 7 MHz with 80% bandwidth for acoustic detection. A tomographic imaging configuration with four LED arrays and transducer scanning around the sample was used in this study.

PA imaging using a linear transducer array suffers from low image quality due to incomplete acoustic detection. To overcome the limited view problem in linear array-based imaging, we recently developed a tomographic imaging configuration [11]. The system consists of an imaging probe with a linear transducer array and four LED arrays as shown in Figure 1a. Two LED arrays were placed parallel to the long axis of the transducer, geometrically pointing towards the focus of the transducer (20 mm depth). The other two LED arrays were placed on either side of the transducer along its short axis at an angle of 105° with the transducer surface. These two LED arrays were also placed at an angle of 5° with the imaging plane to minimize the acoustic reflections being detected. In this way, the object to be imaged is illuminated from three sides. The probe is then scanned around the object for tomographic imaging. Based on a simulation study, we have estimated that 16 angular views with an angular step of 22.5° is sufficient to form a full-view tomographic image [11]. The illumination configuration was also developed to provide a significant overlapping region between two angular scans. Interested readers can refer to the work in [11,12] for more details. A 3D printed holder encompassing the transducer and LED arrays to form the imaging probe is shown in Figure 1b. For small animal imaging, the probe was mounted on a motorized linear and circular scanning system, installed on top of a water tank as shown in Figure 1c. A 3D printed small animal holder was used to keep the mouse in place for imaging (Figure 1c).

Male Balb/c mice (8 weeks old) were used in this study. All the animals used in the study received ad libitum normal chow diet and normal water, and were housed with 12h-light/12h-dark cycle. All the animal experiments were carried out strictly according to the ethical guidelines for the Care and Use of Laboratory Animals (Utrecht University, The Netherlands). A proof-of-concept study was performed whereby liver fibrosis was induced in one mouse by a single injection of 1ml/kg of carbon tetrachloride (CCl_4), and the control animal received olive oil. Mice were euthanized and imaged immediately using the PA and US tomographic system. The hair with the outer skin layer of the animals was removed around the abdominal region before imaging. After the imaging experiments, the livers of the animals were collected and fixed with cryomatrix in isopentane. Fixed livers were sectioned into 5 μm sections and immunohistological analysis using collagen I (fibrosis marker) antibody was performed.

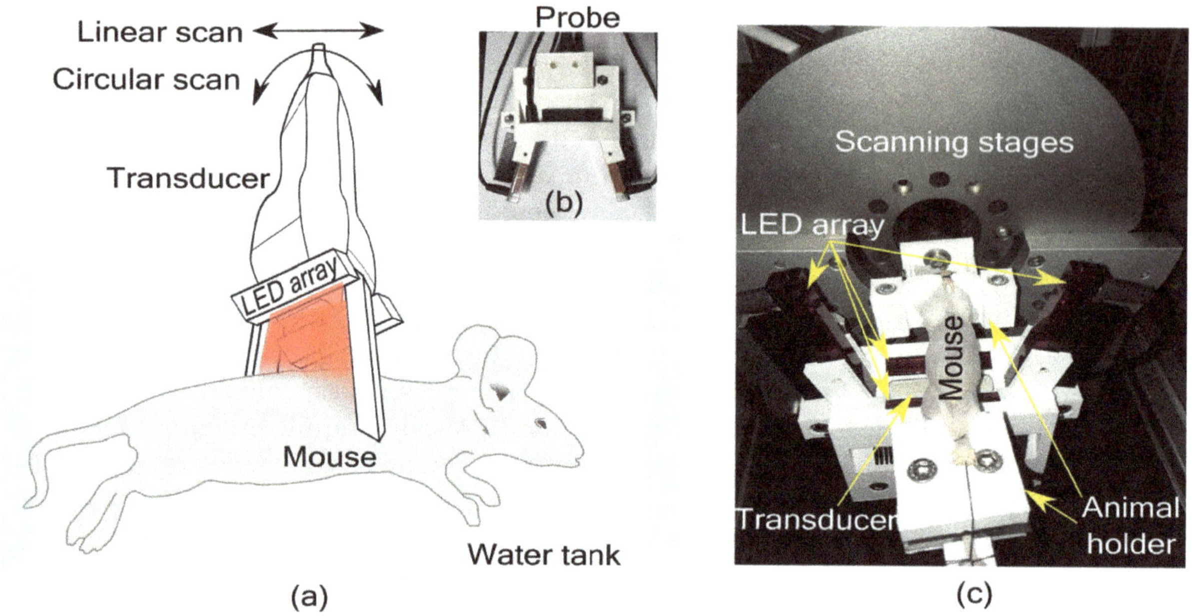

Figure 1. Small animal tomographic imaging system. (**a**) Schematic of the set-up with the imaging probe scanning around the mouse in a water tank. (**b**) Imaging probe with linear transducer array and four LED arrays in a 3D printed holder. (**c**) Photograph of the imaging set-up showing mouse holder, imaging probe and the scanning stages.

Two scanning techniques were used in this study, involving a combination of circular and linear scans. To obtain a complete tomographic image, a circular scanning of the entire 360° was performed. Combined PA and US imaging were performed at each angular step. Typically, a circular scan takes 42.5 secs. However, due to memory limitations of the system, the RF data was saved after each 180° scan and combined in the postprocessing stage. Multiple tomographic images of the abdominal area were obtained by translating the probe to a different location and repeating the circular scan. In the second experiment, the liver region was considered as the region of interest. Here, a limited view tomographic imaging was performed by spatial compounding of B-scan images from three angles (20° steps). In this case, linear scans were performed for the entire length (15 mm length) of the liver at each angular step. Each linear scan took 8.5 secs and the 20° circular scan took 2.5 secs. The US and PA B-scan images were formed by delay and sum algorithm. For speckle reduction and to improve the contrast of the US image, Bayesian mean filtering using an open source software was used [13]. To form tomographic images, the B-scan images from both US and PA imaging were rotated to the acquired angle and spatially compounded using a custom developed MATLAB program [14].

3. Results and Discussion

In Figure 2a–c, co-registered ultrasound and photoacoustic B-scan images of a mouse abdomen, obtained from three different angles, have been presented. The images demonstrate the limited view problem in small animal imaging using a linear transducer array. The limited view arises from the directional sensitivity of the transducer resulting in structures oriented away from the transducer being undetected. The tomographic images obtained from spatial compounding of the B-scan images are shown in Figure 2d–f. The ultrasound image shows the capability of the tomographic system to image major abdominal organs such as the liver, kidney, spleen, stomach, and intestines. Additionally, anatomical structures such as skin and spinal cord are also imaged in this mode. Kidney and lobes of the liver can be seen as hypoechogenic regions, while the stomach, spleen, and intestine are visible as hyperechogenic regions. In PA images major blood vessels are visible beneath the skin and around the spinal cord. In addition to that, high PA signals were also observed from the liver, kidney, and spleen. For the imaging configuration used in this work, it was estimated that PA signal strength drops to 30% at a depth of 9.7 mm in soft tissue [11]. This finding also holds in this study, as most of the structures visible in PA images are within the 10 mm depth from the skin surface. Illumination from three sides and spatial compounding from several angles enable PA tomographic imaging to visualize most of the absorbing structures in the small animal. The abdominal diameter of Balb/c mice is mostly less than 30 mm and most of the organs of interest are within the 10 mm depth from the skin surface, making the system useful for small animal studies. However, there is indeed a region at the center where the signal to noise ratio is low, which can only be improved with better illumination methods. Another challenge in PA imaging is reflection artifacts from multiple structures inside the small animal body. There are several methods proposed to solve reflection artifacts in PA images [15]. Methods for improving the imaging depth and removing artifacts will be considered in the future. In this study, we have imaged a euthanized animal; however, imaging a live animal in this set-up is also possible by positioning the scanning stages such that the snout of the animal is above the water while the rest of the body immersed and/or using a breathing mask. Imaging speed is another factor that needs to be considered while imaging a live animal. The current scanning time is 42.5 secs, which is longer when compared with the state-of-the-art system using a full ring transducer [3]. However, it is possible to synchronize the breathing cycle of the animal with the acquisition and by using postprocessing to reduce image distortion due to motion while acquisition [16].

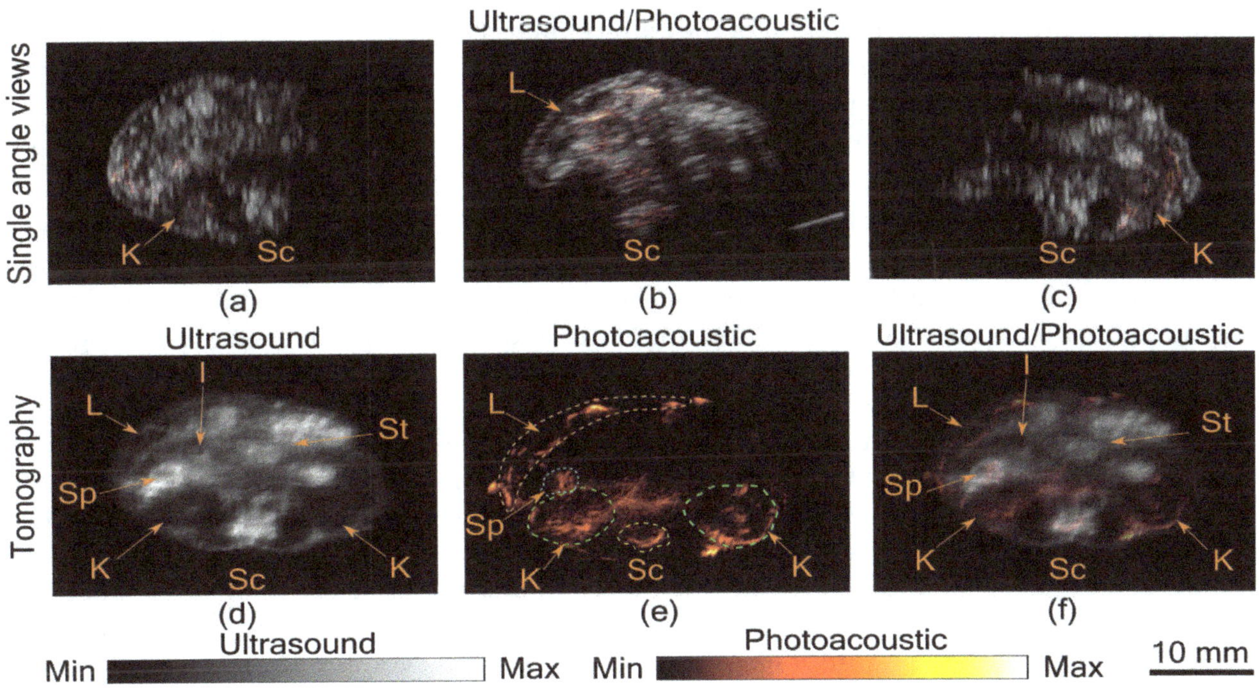

Figure 2. Tomographic photoacoustic and ultrasound imaging. (**a–c**) Co-registered ultrasound and photoacoustic B-Scan images of mouse abdomen, acquired from three different angles. Tomographic (**d**) ultrasound, (**e**) photoacoustic, and (**f**) co-registered ultrasound and photoacoustic image. Several organs in the abdominal region indicated by Sc-spinal cord, K-kidney, L-liver, Sp -spleen, St-stomach, and I-intestine. Dashed lines are used to mark the organs in the photoacoustic image.

In Figure 2, the liver is visible in both US and PA. Being a superficial organ, small animal liver imaging is one of the potential applications where the proposed system can be used. To demonstrate this aspect, tomographic imaging of a control and a fibrotic mouse was performed. Figure 3a,h shows five tomographic slices of control and fibrotic mouse, respectively, with the liver in the top region of the image. Remarkable differences can be observed between control and fibrotic liver in both US and PA images. To analyze this difference, let us consider a pair of US and PA images of the liver from both control and fibrotic mouse shown in Figure 3b,c,e,f. The liver is marked with a green boundary. Two lobes of the liver are visible in the US images. In the US image, the difference in control and fibrotic liver is evident with the difference in echogenicity. Echogenicity can be characterized by the brightness level or the mean value of the region of interest. The mean pixel value was calculated with the liver as the region of interest. For the control animal, the calculated mean value was 0.13 ± 0.02, while it was 0.25 ± 0.03 for the fibrotic case. Additionally, heterogeneity computed using the variance was found to be 0.52 ± 0.11 for the control liver and 0.85 ± 0.10 for the fibrotic liver. These metrics were computed over the liver region with multiple tomographic slices stacked and normalized with the maximum value. The difference in structure evidenced in the US image is due to the hepatic nodularity developed due to scar formation in fibrotic liver [17]. In addition to the differences in US images, the PA images in Figure 3c,f show a difference in contrast between control and fibrotic liver. The contrast value computed for the liver region for the control animal was 0.48 ± 0.08 and 0.69 ± 0.08 for the fibrotic case. The primary reason for the high PA contrast in the fibrotic liver is due to the neovasculature in hypoxic liver cells [18]. Angiogenesis or neovascularization plays a crucial role in the progression of liver fibrosis and is also considered as an early indicator of fibrosis thus PA imaging can be used for monitoring the disease progression, while heterogeneity observed with US imaging reflects scar formation at a later stage of the disease [18]. The liver fibrosis was further confirmed using histopathological analysis. Figure 3d,g show histology images of control and fibrotic liver respectively with Collagen I immunostainings. The fibrotic liver (Figure 3g) shows an increased level of collagen bridges resulting from an accumulation of the extracellular matrix protein. These results are also in line with our previous small animal liver fibrosis study [19]. The main improvement we achieved in this work is the superior image quality from the tomographic system and the use of LED-based PA and US imaging. Further works will focus on including more animals in the study and developing a facility to image live animals.

The advantage of using an LED-based PA system is primarily the cost-effectiveness of the system. Nanosecond pulsed lasers and laser diodes are commonly used for tomographic imaging. The cost for a pulsed laser is approximately 70–200k$, and for laser diodes, with drivers, the cost ranges from 10–25k$. For LEDs with driving electronics, the cost is as lower as 10–15k$ [20]. Another benefit is that LED arrays can be integrated within the imaging probe, hence the system can be compact and suitable for small animal labs. Additionally, there is no requirement for a laser-safe imaging facility. However, the limitations are the low pulse energy resulting in low imaging depth, to an extent, this can be addressed using LED arrays with a large number of elements and frame averaging. The longer pulse duration (30–100 ns) achieved with driving circuits for LEDs is sufficient for stress confinement in tomographic imaging applications where the expected resolution is 1mm. However, unlike lasers, wavelength tuning is not possible with LED-based illumination. LED arrays with elements having multiple wavelengths were tested for oxygen saturation imaging compromising pulse energy and imaging depth. Importantly, for different imaging applications, a wide choice of LEDs is available ranging from visible to near-infrared wavelengths (470–980nm). Custom-developed power LED arrays arranged around the small animal along with ring US transducer can be an ideal configuration for small animal imagers in the future.

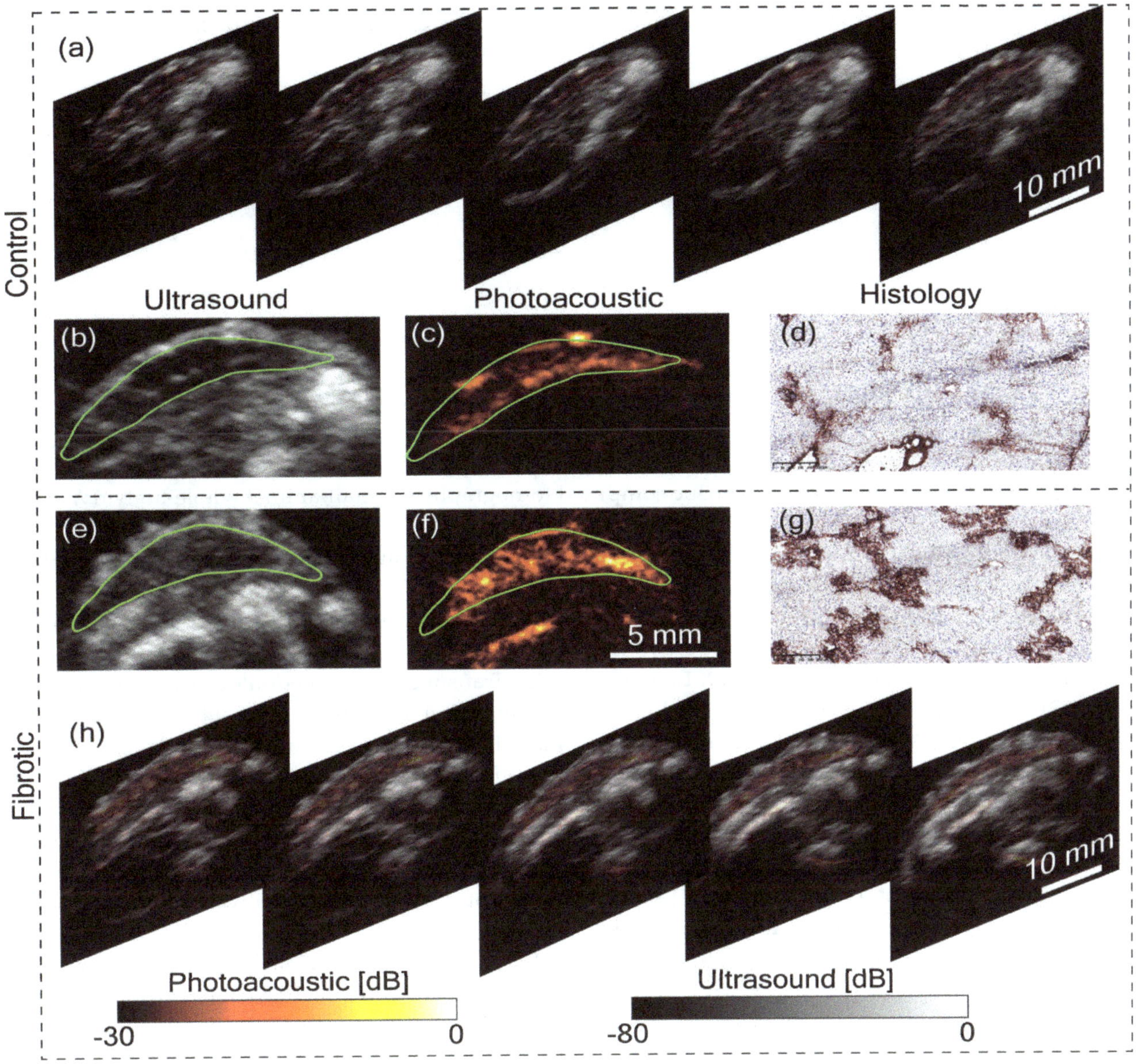

Figure 3. Tomographic imaging of the liver. (**a**) Tomographic photoacoustic and ultrasound images of a control mouse showing the liver at a scanning step of 2 mm. (**b**) Ultrasound image of the liver and (**c**) corresponding photoacoustic image. The green line markers the liver region. (**d**) Histology image of the control liver stained with Collagen I (fibrosis marker). (**e**) Ultrasound image of a mouse liver with fibrosis (CCl_4-treated) and (**f**) corresponding photoacoustic image. (**g**) Histology image of the fibrotic liver stained with collagen I (fibrosis marker). (**h**) Tomographic photoacoustic and ultrasound images of the fibrotic mouse showing liver at a scanning step of 2 mm.

4. Conclusions

In this work, a tomographic ultrasound and LED-based photoacoustic system was demonstrated for small animal imaging. Results show that the tomographic ultrasound imaging can be used to distinguish major organs in the abdominal region of a small animal. The tomographic photoacoustic imaging is capable of imaging an approximate depth of 10 mm from the surface of the skin, allowing imaging of blood vessels and major organs. Limited imaging depth and artifacts are some of the hurdles for photoacoustic imaging in this proposed configuration. The applicability of the proposed imaging system is demonstrated in small animal liver imaging in a fibrotic mouse model. An increase in photoacoustic contrast and ultrasound echogenicity was observed in the fibrotic liver compared to that of the control mouse. The proposed tomographic ultrasound and photoacoustic imaging system offer a cost-effective, compact, and eye-safe alternative for the expensive laser-based system for small animal research.

Author Contributions: K.J.F.- conceptualization, methodology, imaging experiments, data processing, analysis, draft preparation; R.B. (Richell Booijink) - histopathological analysis; R.B. (Ruchi Bansal) - conceptualization, small animal handling, review and editing, W.S. - supervision, project administration, funding acquisition, review and editing. All authors have read and agreed to the published version of the manuscript.

References

1. Andersen, M.L.; Winter, L.M. Animal models in biological and biomedical research-experimental and ethical concerns. *An. Acad. Bras. CiÊNcias* **2019**, *91*, e20170238.
2. Xia, J.; Wang, L.V. Small-animal whole-body photoacoustic tomography: A review. *IEEE Trans. Biomed. Eng.* **2013**, *61*, 1380–1389.
3. Li, L.; Zhu, L.; Ma, C.; Lin, L.; Yao, J.; Wang, L.; Maslov, K.; Zhang, R.; Chen, W.; Shi, J.; others. Single-impulse panoramic photoacoustic computed tomography of small-animal whole-body dynamics at high spatiotemporal resolution. *Nat. Biomed. Eng.* **2017**, *1*, 1–11.
4. Ntziachristos, V.; Ripoll, J.; Wang, L.V.; Weissleder, R. Looking and listening to light: The evolution of whole-body photonic imaging. *Nat. Biotechnol.* **2005**, *23*, 313–320.
5. Jeon, M.; Kim, J.; Kim, C. Multiplane spectroscopic whole-body photoacoustic imaging of small animals in vivo. *Med Biol. Eng. Comput.* **2016**, *54*, 283–294.
6. Merčep, E.; Herraiz, J.L.; Deán-Ben, X.L.; Razansky, D. Transmission–reflection optoacoustic ultrasound (TROPUS) computed tomography of small animals. *Light. Sci. Appl.* **2019**, *8*, 1–12.
7. Zhu, Y.; Xu, G.; Yuan, J.; Jo, J.; Gandikota, G.; Demirci, H.; Agano, T.; Sato, N.; Shigeta, Y.; Wang, X. Light emitting diodes based photoacoustic imaging and potential clinical applications. *Sci. Rep.* **2018**, *8*, 1–12.
8. Xavierselvan, M.; Mallidi, S. LED-Based Functional Photoacoustics—Portable and Affordable Solution for Preclinical Cancer Imaging. In *LED-Based Photoacoustic Imaging*; Springer: Singapore, 2020; pp. 303–319.
9. Hariri, A.; Chen, F.; Moore, C.; Jokerst, J.V. Noninvasive staging of pressure ulcers using photoacoustic imaging. *Wound Repair Regen.* **2019**, *27*, 488–496.
10. Francis, K.J.; Xavierselvan, M.; Singh, M.K.A.; Mallidi, S.; Van Der Laken, C.; Van De Loo, F.; Steenbergen, W. LED-based photoacoustic imaging for early detection of joint inflammation in rodents: towards achieving 3Rs in rheumatoid arthritis research. In *Photons Plus Ultrasound: Imaging and Sensing 2020. International Society for Optics and Photonics*; SPIE: San Francisco, CA, USA, 2020; Vol. 11240, p. 112400M.
11. Francis, K.J.; Boink, Y.E.; Dantuma, M.; Singh, M.K.A.; Manohar, S.; Steenbergen, W. Tomographic imaging with an ultrasound and LED-based photoacoustic system. *Biomed. Opt. Express* **2020**, *11*, 2152–2165.
12. Francis, K.J.; Boink, Y.E.; Dantuma, M.; Singh, M.K.A.; Manohar, S.; Steenbergen, W. Light Emitting Diodes Based Photoacoustic and Ultrasound Tomography: Imaging Aspects and Applications. In *LED-Based Photoacoustic Imaging*; Springer: Berlin/Heidelberg, Germany, 2020; pp. 245–266.
13. Coupé, P.; Hellier, P.; Kervrann, C.; Barillot, C. Nonlocal means-based speckle filtering for ultrasound images. *IEEE Trans. Image Process.* **2009**, *18*, 2221–2229.
14. Francis, K.J.; Chinni, B.; Channappayya, S.S.; Pachamuthu, R.; Dogra, V.S.; Rao, N. Multiview spatial compounding using lens-based photoacoustic imaging system. *Photoacoustics* **2019**, *13*, 85–94.
15. Nguyen, H.N.Y.; Steenbergen, W. Reducing artifacts in photoacoustic imaging by using multi-wavelength excitation and transducer displacement. *Biomed. Opt. Express* **2019**, *10*, 3124–3138.
16. Ron, A.; Davoudi, N.; Deán-Ben, X.L.; Razansky, D. Self-gated respiratory motion rejection for optoacoustic tomography. *Appl. Sci.* **2019**, *9*, 2737.
17. Viganò, M.; Visentin, S.; Aghemo, A.; Rumi, M.G.; Ronchi, G.; Colli, A.; Colucci, A.; Paggi, S.; Fraquelli, M.; Conte, D. US features of liver surface nodularity as a predictor of severe fibrosis in chronic hepatitis C. *Radiology* **2005**, *234*, 641.

18. Bocca, C.; Novo, E.; Miglietta, A.; Parola, M. Angiogenesis and fibrogenesis in chronic liver diseases. *Cell. Mol. Gastroenterol. Hepatol.* **2015**, *1*, 477–488.
19. van den Berg, P.J.; Bansal, R.; Daoudi, K.; Steenbergen, W.; Prakash, J. Preclinical detection of liver fibrosis using dual-modality photoacoustic/ultrasound system. *Biomed. Opt. Express* **2016**, *7*, 5081–5091.
20. Zhu, Y.; Feng, T.; Cheng, Q.; Wang, X.; Du, S.; Sato, N.; Kuniyil Ajith Singh, M.; Yuan, J. Towards Clinical Translation of LED-Based Photoacoustic Imaging: A Review. *Sensors* **2020**, *20*, 2484.

Permissions

All chapters in this book were first published by MDPI; hereby published with permission under the Creative Commons Attribution License or equivalent. Every chapter published in this book has been scrutinized by our experts. Their significance has been extensively debated. The topics covered herein carry significant findings which will fuel the growth of the discipline. They may even be implemented as practical applications or may be referred to as a beginning point for another development.

The contributors of this book come from diverse backgrounds, making this book a truly international effort. This book will bring forth new frontiers with its revolutionizing research information and detailed analysis of the nascent developments around the world.

We would like to thank all the contributing authors for lending their expertise to make the book truly unique. They have played a crucial role in the development of this book. Without their invaluable contributions this book wouldn't have been possible. They have made vital efforts to compile up to date information on the varied aspects of this subject to make this book a valuable addition to the collection of many professionals and students.

This book was conceptualized with the vision of imparting up-to-date information and advanced data in this field. To ensure the same, a matchless editorial board was set up. Every individual on the board went through rigorous rounds of assessment to prove their worth. After which they invested a large part of their time researching and compiling the most relevant data for our readers.

The editorial board has been involved in producing this book since its inception. They have spent rigorous hours researching and exploring the diverse topics which have resulted in the successful publishing of this book. They have passed on their knowledge of decades through this book. To expedite this challenging task, the publisher supported the team at every step. A small team of assistant editors was also appointed to further simplify the editing procedure and attain best results for the readers.

Apart from the editorial board, the designing team has also invested a significant amount of their time in understanding the subject and creating the most relevant covers. They scrutinized every image to scout for the most suitable representation of the subject and create an appropriate cover for the book.

The publishing team has been an ardent support to the editorial, designing and production team. Their endless efforts to recruit the best for this project, has resulted in the accomplishment of this book. They are a veteran in the field of academics and their pool of knowledge is as vast as their experience in printing. Their expertise and guidance has proved useful at every step. Their uncompromising quality standards have made this book an exceptional effort. Their encouragement from time to time has been an inspiration for everyone.

The publisher and the editorial board hope that this book will prove to be a valuable piece of knowledge for researchers, students, practitioners and scholars across the globe.

List of Contributors

John Mello Camille C. Guzman
Department of Biomedical Engineering, National Cheng Kung University, Tainan 701, Taiwan

Sheng-Min Hsu
Department of Ophthalmology, National Cheng Kung University Hospital, Tainan 701, Taiwan

Han-Sheng Chuang
Department of Biomedical Engineering, National Cheng Kung University, Tainan 701, Taiwan
Center for Micro/Nano Science and Technology, National Cheng Kung University, Tainan 701, Taiwan

Wei-Hsuan Sung
College of Medicine, Chang Gung University, Taoyuan 33302, Taiwan
Chang Gung Memorial Hospital Linkou Medical Center, Taoyuan 33305, Taiwan

Chung-Yao Yang
Chang Gung Memorial Hospital Linkou Medical Center, Taoyuan 33305, Taiwan
Hygeia Touch Inc., Taipei 10441, Taiwan

Ching-Yi Liu
Hygeia Touch Inc., Taipei 10441, Taiwan

Cheng-Han Chen
Department of Emergency Medicine, Taipei Veterans General Hospital, Taipei 11217, Taiwan
School of Medicine, National Yang-Ming University, Taipei 11221, Taiwan
Institute of Biomedical Engineering, National Tsing Hua University, Hsinchu 30013, Taiwan

Chao-Min Cheng and Yu-Ting Tsao
Institute of Biomedical Engineering, National Tsing Hua University, Hsinchu 30013, Taiwan

Ching-Fen Shen
Department of Pediatrics, National Cheng Kung University Hospital, College of Medicine, National Cheng Kung University, Tainan 70403, Taiwan

Mitrayana and Mirza Satriawan
Department of Physics, Universitas Gadjah Mada, Yogyakarta 55281, Indonesia

Donni Kis Apriyanto
Department of Physics, University of Lampung, Bandar Lampung 35141, Indonesia

Seema Rani, Sanchita Bandyopadhyay-Ghosh and Subrata Bandhu Ghosh
Engineered Biomedical Materials Research and Innovation Centre (EnBioMatRIC), School of Automobile, Mechanical and Mechatronics Engineering (SAMM), Manipal University Jaipur, Rajasthan 303007, India

Guozhen Liu
Graduate School of Biomedical Engineering, Faculty of Engineering, The University of New South Wales, Sydney NSW 2052, Australia

Maju Kuriakose and Christopher D. Nguyen
Department of Biomedical Engineering, Tufts University, Medford, MA 02155, USA

Mithun Kuniyil Ajith Singh
Research and Business Development Division, CYBERDYNE INC., Stationsplein 45, A4.004, 3013 AK Rotterdam, The Netherlands
Research & Business Development Division, Cyberdyne INC, Cambridge Innovation Center, 3013 Rotterdam, The Netherlands

Joost Holthof and Jithin Jose
FUJIFILM VisualSonics, 1114 AB Amsterdam, The Netherlands

Valeria Grasso
FUJIFILM VisualSonics, 1114 AB Amsterdam, The Netherlands
Institute for Animal Science, Hannover Medical School, 30625 Hannover, Germany

Jiawei Tang, Mingyang Lu and Wuliang Yin
School of Electrical and Electronics Engineering, The University of Manchester, Manchester M13 9PL, UK

Yuedong Xie
School of Instrumentation and Optoelectronic Engineering, Beihang University, Beijing 100036, China
Beijing Advanced Innovation Center for Big Data-based Precision Medicine, Beihang University, Beijing 100036, China

Marvin Xavierselvan
Department of Biomedical Engineering, Tufts University, Medford, MA 02155, USA

Srivalleesha Mallidi
Department of Biomedical Engineering, Tufts University, Medford, MA 02155, USA
Wellman Center for Photomedicine, Massachusetts General Hospital, Harvard Medical School, Boston, MA 02114, USA

Wenfeng Xia
School of Biomedical Engineering & Imaging Sciences, King's College London, King's Health Partners, St Thomas' Hospital, London SE1 7EH, UK

Chaoming Fang and Yixuan Wang
School of Instrumentation and Optoelectronic Engineering, Beihang University, Beijing 100083, China

Bowei He
School of Automation Science and Electrical Engineering, Beihang University, Beijing 100083, China

Jin Cao
Department of Psychiatry, Massachusetts General Hospital, Harvard Medical School, Boston, MA 02138, USA

Shuo Gao
School of Instrumentation and Optoelectronic Engineering, Beihang University, Beijing 100083, China
Beijing Advanced Innovation Center for Big Data-Based Precision Medicine, Beihang University, Beijing 100083, China

Haoyang Chen, Sumit Agrawal, Ajay Dangi, Christopher Wible, Mohamed Osman, Lidya Abune, Huizhen Jia and Yong Wang
Department of Biomedical Engineering, The Pennsylvania State University, State College, PA 16802, USA

Randall Rossi
Huck Institutes of the Life Sciences, The Pennsylvania State University, State College, PA 16802, USA

Sri-Rajasekhar Kothapalli
Department of Biomedical Engineering, The Pennsylvania State University, State College, PA 16802, USA
Penn State Cancer Institute, The Pennsylvania State University, Hershey, PA 17033, USA
Graduate Program in Acoustics, The Pennsylvania State University, State College, PA 16802, USA

Sidan Du
Department of Electronic Science and Engineering, Nanjing University, Nanjing 210023, China

Yunhao Zhu and Jie Yuan
Department of Electronic Science and Engineering, Nanjing University, Nanjing 210023, China
Department of Biomedical Engineering, University of Michigan, Ann Arbor, MI 48109, USA

Xueding Wang
Department of Biomedical Engineering, University of Michigan, Ann Arbor, MI 48109, USA

Ting Feng
Department of Electronic and Optical Engineering, Nanjing University of Science and Technology, Nanjing 210094, China
Institution of Acoustics, Tongji University, Shanghai 200092, China

Qian Cheng
Institution of Acoustics, Tongji University, Shanghai 200092, China

Naoto Sato
Research and Development Division, CYBERDYNE INC, Tsukuba 3050818, Japan

João H. Uliana, Diego R. T. Sampaio, Guilherme S. P. Fernandes, Antonio A. O. Carneiro and Theo Z. Pavan
Department of Physics, FFCLRP, University of São Paulo, Ribeirão Preto 14040-901, SP, Brazil

María S. Brassesco
Department of Biology, FFCLRP, University of São Paulo, Ribeirão Preto 14040-901, SP, Brazil

Marcello H. Nogueira-Barbosa
Department of Medical Images, Hematology and Clinical Oncology, Ribeirão Preto Medical School, University of São Paulo, Ribeirão Preto 14040-901, SP, Brazil

Kalloor Joseph Francis and Wiendelt Steenbergen
Biomedical Photonics Imaging (BMPI), Technical Medical Center, University of Twente, 7522 NH Enschede, The Netherlands

Index

www.ingramcontent.com/pod-product-compliance
Lightning Source LLC
LaVergne TN
LVHW060516210926
848485LV00005B/1091
* 9 7 8 1 6 3 9 2 7 6 0 2 8 *